# Current Clinical Urology

Eric A. Klein, MD, Series Editor

AF712806

For further volumes:
http://www.springer.com/series/7635

# Urological Men's Health

## A Guide for Urologists and Primary Care Physicians

*Editor*

Daniel A. Shoskes, MD, MSc, FRCS(C)

*Department of Urology, The Glickman Urologic and Kidney Institute, Cleveland Clinic, Cleveland, OH, USA*

Humana Press

*Editor*
Daniel A. Shoskes, MD, MSc, FRCS(C)
Department of Urology
The Glickman Urologic and Kidney Institute
Cleveland Clinic
Cleveland, OH, USA

ISBN 978-1-4939-6003-3    ISBN 978-1-61779-900-6 (eBook)
DOI 10.1007/978-1-61779-900-6
Springer NewYork Heidelberg Dordrecht London

© Springer Science+Business Media New York 2012
Softcover re-print of the Hardcover 1st edition 2012
This work is subject to copyright. All rights are reserved by the Publisher, whether the whole or part of the material is concerned, specifically the rights of translation, reprinting, reuse of illustrations, recitation, broadcasting, reproduction on microfilms or in any other physical way, and transmission or information storage and retrieval, electronic adaptation, computer software, or by similar or dissimilar methodology now known or hereafter developed. Exempted from this legal reservation are brief excerpts in connection with reviews or scholarly analysis or material supplied specifically for the purpose of being entered and executed on a computer system, for exclusive use by the purchaser of the work. Duplication of this publication or parts thereof is permitted only under the provisions of the Copyright Law of the Publisher's location, in its current version, and permission for use must always be obtained from Springer. Permissions for use may be obtained through RightsLink at the Copyright Clearance Center. Violations are liable to prosecution under the respective Copyright Law.
The use of general descriptive names, registered names, trademarks, service marks, etc. in this publication does not imply, even in the absence of a specific statement, that such names are exempt from the relevant protective laws and regulations and therefore free for general use.
While the advice and information in this book are believed to be true and accurate at the date of publication, neither the authors nor the editors nor the publisher can accept any legal responsibility for any errors or omissions that may be made. The publisher makes no warranty, express or implied, with respect to the material contained herein.

Humana Press is a brand of Springer
Springer is part of Springer Science+Business Media (www.springer.com)

# Preface

Men's Health is a rapidly growing, controversial, and shifting topic. The stereotypical dislike of men going to the doctor is often based in fact, especially for preventative visits. Indeed, it is often with the onset of voiding or erectile problems that men make the plunge to seek medical help. As a result, the Urologist is often the initial gatekeeper for male patients, whose mild erection problems may mask serious cardiovascular disease, diabetes, lipid disorders, or hypogonadism. There has been an increasing trend to make Urology the male "home" for healthcare, analogous to the role of Gynecology for women. While a Urologist may not want to take on this role, it is incumbent on us to identify these contributing systemic problems and refer when appropriate.

This book will cover the major urologic conditions that impact the health and well-being of the adult male. It will begin with an overview of men's preventative health in general, as practiced by a world leading Executive Health center. It will then cover the major genitourinary malignancies and address the latest controversies in screening and treatment selection. The conditions that don't shorten life but have a major impact on the quality of life and health care expenditure—BPH, urinary incontinence, infertility, urethral strictures, erectile dysfunction, urinary tract infections, and chronic pelvic pain—will be addressed next. Also included will be chapters on herbal and complementary therapy, psychological and spousal support in urologic illness, and the links between genitourinary disease and general vascular endothelial dysfunction.

I would like to thank the series editor Eric Klein MD for his support of this volume and the staff at Springer, especially Kevin Wright, for their hard work in making this possible.

Cleveland, OH, USA Daniel A. Shoskes

# Contents


1 **Evidence-Based and Age-Appropriate Preventive Health Evaluations in Men** ........ 1
Raul J. Seballos

2 **Clinical Testing of Endothelial Function in Erectile Dysfunction** ........ 13
Titte R. Srinivas and Mark S. Segal

3 **Controversies and Opportunities for PSA Screening** ........ 23
Benjamin Cohen and Eric A. Klein

4 **A Phenotypic Approach to the Evaluation and Treatment of Men with Chronic Pelvic Pain Syndrome** ........ 29
Kiranpreet Khurana and Daniel A. Shoskes

5 **Recurrent Urinary Tract Infections in Men** ........ 39
Stacey C. Carter, Mya E. Levy, and Scott I. Zeitlin

6 **Evaluation and Medical Management of BPH and LUTS in Men** ........ 55
Bilal Chughtai, Richard Lee, Matthew Hall, and Alexis E. Te

7 **The Surgical Treatment of Benign Prostatic Hyperplasia** ........ 67
James C. Ulchaker

8 **Rational Herbal and Complementary Interventions for Prevention and Treatment of Urological Disorders in Men** ........ 77
Mark A. Moyad

9 **Androgen Decline in the Aging Male: Making Sense of the "Male Menopause"** ........ 89
Daniel A. Shoskes

10 **Evaluation and Treatment of Peyronie's Disease** ........ 97
Lawrence S. Hakim

**11 Primary Care Evaluation and Treatment of Erectile Dysfunction** ... 105
Martin Miner and Jacob Rajfer

**12 Surgical Treatment for Erectile Dysfunction** ... 121
Drogo K. Montague

**13 Managing Overactive Bladder and Urinary Incontinence in the Male** ... 129
Humphrey Atiemo and J. Quentin Clemens

**14 Treatment of Localized Prostate Cancer** ... 141
Andrew J. Stephenson

**15 Management of Urethral Strictures in Men** ... 155
Richard A. Santucci and Mang L. Chen

**16 Medical and Surgical Interventions in Male Fertility** ... 169
Kevin Chandler and Edmund Sabanegh Jr.

**17 Evaluation and Therapy of Chronic Scrotal Content Pain and Epididymitis** ... 181
Jonas S. Benson and Laurence A. Levine

**18 Psychosocial Factors in Painful Urogenital Conditions in Men** ... 189
Dean A. Tripp and Jessica Ginting

**Index** ... 209

# Contributors

**Humphrey Atiemo, MD** Department of Urology, University of Michigan Medical Center, Ann Arbor, MI, USA

**Jonas S. Benson, MD** Department of Urology, Rush University Medical Center, Chicago, IL, USA

**Stacey C. Carter, MD** Department of Urology, David Geffen School of Medicine at UCLA, Los Angeles, CA, USA

**Kevin Chandler, MD** Department of Urology, Cleveland Clinic, Cleveland, OH, USA

**Mang L. Chen, MD** Department of Urology, Detroit Receiving Hospital, Detroit, MI, USA

**Bilal Chughtai, MD** Department of Urology, Weill Cornell Medical Center, New York, NY, USA

**J. Quentin Clemens, MD, FACS, MSCI** Department of Urology, University of Michigan Medical Center, Ann Arbor, MI, USA

**Benjamin Cohen, MD** Glickman Urological and Kidney Institute, Cleveland Clinic, Cleveland, OH, USA

**Jessica Ginting, MSc** Department of Psychology, Queen's University, Kingston, ON, Canada

**Lawrence S. Hakim, MD, FACS** Department of Urology, Cleveland Clinic Florida, Weston, FL, USA

**Matthew Hall, MD, BS** Department of Urology, Mount Sinai School of Medicine, New York, NY, USA

**Kiranpreet Khurana, MD** Department of Urology, The Glickman Urologic and Kidney Institute, Cleveland Clinic, Cleveland, OH, USA

**Eric A. Klein, MD** Glickman Urological and Kidney Institute, Cleveland Clinic, Cleveland, OH, USA

**Richard Lee, MD** Department of Urology, Weill-Cornell Medical College of Cornell University, New York, NY, USA

**Laurence A. Levine, MD** Department of Urology, Ruch University Medical Center, Chicago, IL, USA

**Mya E. Levy, MD** Department of Urology, David Geffen School of Medicine at UCLA, Los Angeles, CA, USA

**Martin Miner, MD** Department of Family Medicine and Urology, Warren Albert School of Medicine, Brown University, Men's Health Center, The Miriam Hospital, Providence, RI, USA

**Drogo K. Montague, MD** Center for Genitourinary Reconstruction, Glickman Urologic and Kidney Institute, Cleveland Clinic, Cleveland, OH, USA

**Mark A. Moyad, MD, MPH** Jenkins/Pokempner Director of Preventative and Alternative Medicine, Department of Urology, University of Michigan Medical Center, Ann Arbor, MI, USA

**Jacob Rajfer, MD** Department of Urology, UCLA School of Medicine, Los Angeles, CA, USA

Harbor-UCLA Medical Center, Torrance, CA, USA

**Edmund Sabanegh Jr., MD** Department of Urology, Cleveland Clinic, Cleveland, OH, USA

**Richard A. Santucci, MD, FACS** Department of Urology, The Detroit Medical Center, Detroit, MI, USA

**Raul J. Seballos, MD, FACP** Department of Preventive Medicine, Wellness Institute, Cleveland Clinic, Cleveland, OH, USA

**Mark S. Segal, MD, PhD** Division of Nephrology, Hypertension and Transplantation, University of Florida, Gainsville, FL, USA

**Daniel A. Shoskes, MD, MSc, FRCS(C)** Department of Urology, The Glickman Urologic and Kidney Institute, Cleveland Clinic, Cleveland, OH, USA

**Titte R. Srinivas, MD** Department of Nephrology and Hypertension, Glickman Urologic and Kidney Institute, Cleveland Clinic, Cleveland, OH, USA

**Andrew J. Stephenson, MD, FACS, FRCS(C)** Glickman Urological and Kidney Institute, Cleveland Clinic, Cleveland, OH, USA

Cleveland Clinic Lerner College of Medicine, Case Western Reserve University, Cleveland, OH, USA

**Alexis E. Te, MD** Department of Urology, Weill Cornell Medical Center, Brady Prostate Center and Urodynamic Laboratory, New York Presbyterian-Cornell, New York, NY, USA

**Dean A. Tripp, PhD** Departments of Psychology, Anesthesiology & Urology, Queen's University, Kingston, ON, Canada

**James C. Ulchaker, MD, FACS** Glickman Urologic and Kidney Institute, Cleveland Clinic, Cleveland, OH, USA

**Scott I. Zeitlin, MD** Department of Urology and OB/GYN, David Geffen School of Medicine at UCLA, VA Greater Los Angeles Healthcare System, Los Angeles, CA, USA

# Evidence-Based and Age-Appropriate Preventive Health Evaluations in Men

1

Raul J. Seballos

## Introduction

The annual physical examination or preventive health evaluation (PHE) usually consists of a focused history, physical examination, laboratory testing, and immunizations. Counseling and risk assessment for potential health problems are also part of the evaluation. More invasive diagnostic procedures, such as a colonoscopy, may be ordered. Three driving factors for the PHE is the belief that the exam detects subclinical illness, the belief that the annual exam is of proven value, and the fear of negative outcomes. The purpose of the PHE, for health promotion and screening of disease risk factors and subclinical illness, remains controversial. Over the past two decades, the American College of Physicians, the American Medical Association, the U.S. Preventive Services Task Force (USPSTF), and the U.S. Public Health Service have all agreed that routine annual checkups for healthy adults should be abandoned in favor of a more selective approach to preventing and detecting health problems. Nevertheless, the public has a high expectation for a comprehensive annual physical examination and extensive routine testing [1]. Nearly two thirds of physicians and patients surveyed believe that it is important to undergo an annual physical evaluation and is important to strengthen the physician–patient relationship [2]. Mehrotra et al. reported that between 2002 and 2004, an estimated 44.4 million adults per year received a PHE. Together with a preventive gynecological examinations (19.4 million women per year), these were one of the most common reasons adults saw their physicians [3].

According the U.S. Agency for Healthcare Research and Quality (AHRQ), men generally die younger than women and have higher death rates from heart disease, cancer, stroke, and AIDS [4]. A U.S. survey found that women are three times more likely than men to see a doctor on a regular basis. Men are 24% less likely than women to have visited a doctor within the past year and are 22% more likely to have neglected their cholesterol tests. Men are 28% more likely than women to be hospitalized for congestive heart failure. Men are 32% more likely than women to be hospitalized for long-term complications of diabetes and are more than twice as likely as women to have a leg or foot amputated due to complications from diabetes. Lastly, men are 24% more likely than women to be hospitalized for pneumonia that could have been prevented by getting an immunization [4].

This chapter serves as a resource for healthcare providers by reviewing the evidence-based and age-appropriate strategies to the care of men. The USPSTF was convened by the Public Health Service to rigorously evaluate clinical research in order to assess the merits of preventive measures,

R.J. Seballos, MD, FACP (✉)
Department of Preventive Medicine, Wellness Institute, Cleveland Clinic, 9500 Euclid Avenue, Desk A-11, Cleveland, OH 44195, USA
e-mail: seballr@ccf.org

D.A. Shoskes (ed.), *Urological Men's Health: A Guide for Urologists and Primary Care Physicians*, Current Clinical Urology, DOI 10.1007/978-1-61779-900-6_1,
© Springer Science+Business Media New York 2012

including screening tests, counseling, immunizations, and preventive medications. Their most up-to-date USPSTF recommendations for adults are available in their web site [5]. In keeping with the spirit of "selective approach to preventing and detecting health problems" and to "individualize the visit to meet the specific needs of the patient," only those recommendations that are strongly recommended (grade "A") and recommended (grade "B") are discussed. Table 1.1, which has been modified for men only, is the USPSTF recommendation of services that have received an "A" or a "B" grade from the Task Force [7]. Lastly, services that the USPSTF recommends against routinely providing (grade "D") to asymptomatic male patients, where they found at least fair evidence that the service is ineffective or that harms outweighs benefits, will be discussed.

Starting at age 18, the USPSTF recommends all adults be screened for blood pressure. Blood pressures should be monitored every 1–2 years or more frequently if borderline high. Persons should be seated quietly for at least 5 min in a chair (rather than on an exam table), with feet on the floor, and arm supported at heart level. Appropriate-sized cuff bladder, encircling at least 80% of the arm, should be used to ensure accuracy. At least two measurements should be made. The USPSTF found good evidence that screening and treatment for high blood pressure cause little major harm, and that treatment of high blood pressure in adults substantially decreases the incidence of cardiovascular events. The USPSTF concluded that there was high certainty that the net benefit of screening for high blood pressure in adults was substantial.

## Blood Pressure

The lifetime risk for cardiovascular disease (CVD) is 2 in 3 for men and 1 in 2 for women at 40 years of age [8]. According to JNC 7, normal blood pressure is <120/80 mm Hg. A blood pressure of 120–129/80–89 mm Hg is in the "pre-hypertension category." The primary goal of hypertensive therapy is to control blood pressure at a level of <140/90 mm Hg. For patients with diabetes or renal disease, the goal blood pressure is <130/80 mm Hg [9]. Hypertension remains to be a significant risk factor for CVD. Twenty-nine percent of U.S. adults ≥ 18 years of age were hypertensive. An additional 37% of U.S. adults had pre-hypertension, and 7% of adults with hypertension had never been told that they had hypertension. The prevalence of hypertension was nearly equal between men and women. Among hypertensive adults, 78% were aware of their condition, 68% were using antihypertensive medication, and >64% of those treated were controlled [8]. In the USA, hypertension is responsible for 35% of myocardial infarctions (MIs) and strokes, 49% of episodes of heart failure, and 24% of premature deaths. Additional complications of hypertension include end-stage renal disease, retinopathy, and aortic aneurysm.

## Cholesterol

Data from NHANES 1999–2002 (NCHS) showed that nearly two thirds of participants whose test results indicated high blood cholesterol (or who were taking a cholesterol lowering medication) had been told by a provider that they had high cholesterol. Women were less likely than men, and blacks and Mexican Americans were less likely than were whites, to be aware of their condition. Fewer than half of Mexican Americans with high cholesterol were aware of their condition [10, 11]. Good-quality evidence shows that total cholesterol, low density lipoprotein-cholesterol (LDL-C), and high density lipoprotein-cholesterol (HDL-C) are independent predictors of coronary heart disease (CHD) risk, and ratios of total cholesterol to HDL-C (total cholesterol/HDL-C) or LDL-C to HDL-C (LDL-C/HDL-C) classify risk better than total cholesterol alone. The risk for CHD is highest in those with a combination of risk factors.

The USPSTF strongly recommends screening for cholesterol abnormalities starting at age 35. However, if the patient is at an increased risk for CVD, cholesterol screening should begin at age 20. A fasting (at least 8 h) lipid profile should be tested every 5 years, or more frequently based on

**Table 1.1** USPSTF A and B recommendations [6]. The U.S. Preventive Services Task Force (USPSTF) recommends that clinicians discuss these preventive services with eligible patients and offer them as a priority. All these services have received an "A" (strongly recommended) or a "B" (recommended) grade from the Task Force. Adapted for men [6]

| Recommendation for men | Comments | Age specified | Grade | Date in effect |
|---|---|---|---|---|
| Abdominal aortic aneurysm screening | Recommends one-time screening for abdominal aortic aneurysm by ultrasonography in men who have ever smoked | 65–75 | B | February 2005 |
| Alcohol misuse counseling | Recommends screening and behavioral counseling interventions to reduce alcohol misuse by adults in primary care settings | All adults | B | April 2004 |
| Aspirin to prevent cardiovascular disease (CVD) | Recommends the use of aspirin for men when the potential benefit due to a reduction in myocardial infarctions outweighs the potential harm due to an increase in gastrointestinal hemorrhage | 45–79 | A | March 2009 |
| Blood pressure screening in adults | Strongly recommends screening for high blood pressure in all adults | ≥18 | A | December 2007 |
| Cholesterol abnormalities screening: men 35 and older | Strongly recommends screening men for lipid disorders | ≥35 | A | June 2008 |
| Cholesterol abnormalities screening: men younger than 35 | Recommends screening men aged 20–35 for lipid disorders if they are at increased risk for coronary heart disease | 20–35 | B | June 2008 |
| Colorectal cancer screening | Strongly recommends screening for colorectal cancer using fecal occult blood testing, sigmoidoscopy, or colonoscopy, in adults, beginning at age 50 years and continuing until age 75 years. The risks and benefits of these screening methods vary | ≥50 | A | October 2008 |
| Depression screening: adults | Recommends screening adults for depression when staff-assisted depression care supports are in place to assure accurate diagnosis, effective treatment, and follow-up | All adults | B | December 2009 |
| Diabetes screening | The USPSTF recommends screening for type 2 diabetes in asymptomatic adults with sustained blood pressure (either treated or untreated) >135/80 mm Hg | All adults | B | June 2008 |
| Healthy diet counseling | The USPSTF recommends intensive behavioral dietary counseling for adult patients with hyperlipidemia and other known risk factors for cardiovascular and diet-related chronic disease. Intensive counseling can be delivered by primary care clinicians or by referral to other specialists, such as nutritionists or dietitians | All adults | B | January 2003 |
| HIV screening | Strongly recommends that clinicians screen for human immunodeficiency virus (HIV) all adolescents and adults at increased risk for HIV infection | 13–64 | A | July 2005 |
| Obesity screening and counseling: adults | Recommends that clinicians screen all adult patients for obesity and offer intensive counseling and behavioral interventions to promote sustained weight loss for obese adults | All adults | B | December 2003 |

(continued)

**Table 1.1** (continued)

| Recommendation for men | Comments | Age specified | Grade | Date in effect |
|---|---|---|---|---|
| STIs counseling | Recommends high-intensity behavioral counseling to prevent sexually transmitted infections (STIs) for all sexually active adolescents and for adults at increased risk for STIs | All adults | B | October 2008 |
| Tobacco use counseling and interventions | Strongly recommends that clinicians ask all adults about tobacco use and provide tobacco cessation interventions for those who use tobacco products | All adults | A | April 2009 |
| Syphilis screening | Strongly recommends that clinicians screen persons at increased risk for syphilis infection | All adults | A | July 2004 |

results and risk profile. The profile should include fasting measurement of total cholesterol and HDL-C. At least two serum lipid measurements are necessary to ensure that true values are within 10% of the mean of the measurements.

## Diabetes

According to the latest statistics from the American Diabetes Association (ADA), 25.8 million children and adults in the USA (8.3% of the population) have diabetes. Of these, 7 million do not know they have diabetes [12]. There are 79 million people who have pre-diabetes [a fasting plasma glucose (FPG) of 100–125 mg/dl and/or a hemoglobin A1c of 5.7–6.4%].

In 2008, the USPSTF recommended that all asymptomatic adults, with sustained blood pressure (treated or untreated) >135/80 mm Hg, be screened for diabetes. Three tests can be used: FPG, hemoglobin A1c (A1c), or 2-hour oral glucose tolerance test. In contrast, the ADA recommends all adults of any age be screened for diabetes if they are overweight [body mass index (BMI)$\geq$25 kg/m$^2$] and have one or more additional risk factors: physical inactivity, first-degree relative with diabetes members of a high-risk ethnic population (e.g., African American, Latino, Native American, Asian American, Pacific Islander), women who delivered a baby weighing >9 lb or were diagnosed with gestational diabetes, hypertension ($\geq$140/90 mm Hg or on therapy for hypertension), HDL-C level <35 mg/dl and/or a triglyceride level >250 mg/dl, women with polycystic ovary syndrome, A1c$\geq$5.7%, impaired glucose tolerance, or previously impaired fasting glucose, other clinical conditions associated with insulin resistance (e.g., severe obesity, acanthosis nigricans), and history of CVD [12]. In the absence of above criteria, testing for diabetes should start at age 45. If results are normal, testing should be repeated at least at 3-year intervals, with consideration of more frequent testing depending on initial results and risk status.

## Obesity and Health Diet Counseling

The USPSTF found good evidence that BMI, calculated as weight in kilograms divided by height in meters squared, is reliable and valid for identifying adults at increased risk for mortality and morbidity due to overweight and obesity. About one third of the U.S. population is obese (BMI$\geq$30 kg/m$^2$) [13, 14]. Obesity is a risk factor for a variety of chronic conditions including diabetes, hypertension, high cholesterol, stroke, coronary heart disease, certain cancers (colon, kidney, gallbladder, breast, and endometrium), sleep apnea, gallbladder disease, and certain musculoskeletal disorders, such as osteoarthritis of the knee. It is also associated with decreased life expectancy. The cost of care for obesity is increasing, and now estimated to be $147 billion dollars (in 2008 dollars) [15].

The USPSTF recommends that clinicians screen all adult patients for obesity and offer *intensive* counseling and behavioral interventions to promote sustained weight loss for *obese* adults.

A high-intensity intervention is more than one person-to-person (individual or group) session per month for at least the first 3 months of the intervention. However, the effectiveness of interventions with obese people may not be generalizable to adults who are overweight [16]. Successful interventions typically included two to three components (diet, exercise, and behavioral therapy). The effectiveness of interventions to promote weight loss is derived mostly from women (especially white women). While the data may be limited, the USPSTF felt that these interventions may be used with obese men and other population groups, taking into account cultural and other individual factors. In addition, the USPSTF recommends intensive behavioral dietary counseling for adult patients with hyperlipidemia and other known risk factors for cardiovascular and diet-related chronic disease. Intensive counseling can be delivered by primary care clinicians or by nutritionists or dietitians.

## Aspirin to Prevent CVD

Heart disease is the number one and cerebrovascular disease is the number four cause of death in the USA [17]. Aspirin has been recommended to reduce the risk of MI and stroke. However, aspirin use has been associated with gastrointestinal (GI) bleeding and hemorrhagic stroke. The net benefit of aspirin depends on the initial risk and overall risks for CVD events and GI bleeding. The Framingham Risk calculator is available in the Internet and can be used to predict a person's 10-year risk for "hard" CHD outcomes (MI and coronary death) [18].

In March 2009, the USPSTF found good evidence that aspirin decreases the incidence of MI in men and ischemic strokes in women. They recommended the use of aspirin for men ages 45–79 when the potential benefit due to a reduction in MI outweighs the potential harm due to an increase in GI bleeding [19]. In contrast, the USPSTF recommended the use of aspirin for women ages 45–79 when the potential benefit due to a reduction in ischemic stroke outweighs the aforementioned risk of aspirin use. There was

**Table 1.2** Ten-year coronary heart disease (CHD) risk levels at which the number of cardiovascular disease events prevented is closely balanced to the number of serious bleeding events. Shared decision making is strongly encouraged with persons whose risk is close to (either above or below) these estimates of 10-year risk levels. As the potential cardiovascular disease reduction benefit increases above harms, the recommendation to take aspirin should become stronger

| Age (years) | Men 10-Year CHD risk (%) | Women 10-Year stroke risk (%) |
|---|---|---|
| 45–59 | ≥4 | ≥3 |
| 60–69 | ≥9 | ≥8 |
| 70–79 | ≥12 | ≥11 |

insufficient evidence to recommend for or against taking aspirin for men and women older than age 80 to reduce the risk of CVD. The optimum dose of aspirin for preventing CVD events is not known. However, 75 mg/day seems as effective as higher dosages. The risk for gastrointestinal bleeding may increase with dose.

Table 1.2 shows the 10-year CHD risk levels at which the number of CVD events prevented is closely balanced to the number of serious bleeding events. For example, a man age 55 who has a calculated 10-year risk for CHD of 10% should be encouraged to take aspirin as the potential benefit is greater than the risk for serious bleeding of about 4% for men age 45–59. In contrast, a man age 55 with a calculated 10-year risk for CHD of 3% should not be recommended aspirin as the risk for complications outweighs its benefit. As the potential benefit increases above potential harms, the recommendation to take aspirin should become stronger.

In 2010, the ADA recommended low-dose aspirin (75–162 mg/day) for men of age > 50 and women of age > 60 with type 1 or 2 diabetes at increased cardiovascular risk (10-year risk > 10%). These include most diabetic men of age > 50 who have at least one additional major risk factor (family history of CVD, hypertension, smoking, dyslipidemia, or albuminuria) [12]. Aspirin use was not recommended in men under 50 who have diabetes but no other major risk factors for heart disease.

## Abdominal Aortic Aneurysm

An abdominal aortic aneurysm (AAA) is present when the infrarenal aortic diameter exceeds 3.0 cm. The prevalence of AAAs 2.9–4.9 cm in diameter ranges from 1.3% in men age 45–54 to 12.5% in men age 75–84 [8]. Large AAAs tend to expand more rapidly than small AAAs and are higher risk for rupture, and accounted for about 13,800 deaths in the USA in 2009 [8]. The major risk factors for AAA include male sex, a history of ever smoking (>100 cigarettes in a person's lifetime in most surveys), and age≥65. Other lesser risk factors include family history, CHD, claudication, hypercholesterolemia, hypertension, cerebrovascular disease, and increased height. Factors associated with decreased risk include female sex, diabetes mellitus, and black race.

In 2005, the USPSTF recommended a one-time screening for AAA by ultrasonography in men ages 65–75 who have ever smoked [20]. There was good evidence that screening for AAA and surgical repair of large AAAs (5.5 cm or more) in men ages 65–75 who have ever smoked (current and former smokers) leads to decreased AAA-specific mortality. The USPSTF made no recommendation for or against screening non-smoking men ages 65–75 who were lifetime non-smokers. The USPSTF recommended against routine screening for AAA in women.

## Colorectal Cancer

Colorectal cancer is the third most common type of cancer and the second leading cause of cancer death in the USA. As many as 18,000 lives could be saved yearly if colorectal cancer screening was appropriately done [21]. In 2008, the USPSTF strongly recommended screening for colorectal cancer beginning at age 50 using fecal occult blood testing, sigmoidoscopy, or colonoscopy and continuing until age 75 [21]. More specifically, the American Gastroenterological Society recommended flexible sigmoidoscopy every 5 years, or colonoscopy every 10 years, or double contrast barium enema every 5 years, or computed tomographic colonography every 5 years to detect adenomatous polyps and cancer [22].

## Human Immunodeficiency Virus Screening

In 2006, just over one million persons living in the USA have human immunodeficiency virus (HIV). Unfortunately, about 21% (approximately 232,700 persons) did not know they were infected with HIV [23]. The Centers for Disease Control and Prevention (CDC) estimates that 56,300 new HIV infections occurred in the USA in 2006. Of these new infections, 54% are estimated to be acquired from the 25% of infected people who are unaware of their serostatus [24]. The rational for screening is that persons not aware of being infected by HIV will not undergo early treatment that can reduce the morbidity and mortality associated with HIV. In addition, they may not have the knowledge to protect their sex or drug-use partners from becoming infected. Knowing whether one is positive or negative for HIV confers clinical benefits in healthy decision making.

In July 2005, the USPSTF strongly recommended that clinicians screen for HIV in all adolescents and adults at increased risk for HIV infection in all health-care settings, including hospital emergency departments, urgent care clinics, inpatient services, sexually transmitted disease (STD) clinics, tuberculosis clinics, and primary care offices [25]. High-risk persons include: men who have had sex with men after 1975; men and women having unprotected sex with multiple partners; past or present injection drug users; men and women who exchange sex for money or drugs or have sex partners who do; individuals whose past or present sex partners were HIV-infected, bisexual, or injection drug users; persons being treated for STDs; and persons with a history of blood transfusion between 1978 and 1985. People at high risk for HIV infection should be screened annually. There is no recommendation for or against screening for HIV in low-risk patients.

In September 2006, the CDC recommended all individuals between 13 and 64 years of age be screened for HIV regardless of recognized risk factors [26]. Subsequently, in November 2006, the USPSTF confirmed its "C" recommendation (no recommendation for or against screening) for screening nonpregnant adolescents and adults who are not at increased risk for HIV infection. In conclusion, health-care providers should assess risk factors for HIV infection by obtaining a careful sexual history and inquiring about injection drug use in all patients. Periodic screening for infection with HIV is recommended for all persons at increased risk of infection.

## Other Grade A Recommendations

During the PHE, health-care providers are strongly recommended to ask all adults about tobacco use and provide tobacco cessation interventions for users. Tobacco use, particularly cigarette smoking, is the leading cause of death in the USA. Smoking is associated with a two- to threefold increased risk of dying from CHD. On average, active or former smokers die 14 years earlier than nonsmoker. Approximately 260,000 men die yearly directly from smoking [27]. In addition, secondhand smoke contributes to about 38,000 deaths annually.

In 2004, the USPSTF found adequate evidence that screening tests can accurately detect syphilis infection and that antibiotics can cure syphilis. Clinicians are strongly recommended to screen persons at increased risk for syphilis infection. Populations at increased risk for syphilis infection include men who have sex with men and engage in high-risk sexual behavior, commercial sex workers, persons who exchange sex for drugs, and those in adult correctional facilities [28].

## Other Grade B Recommendations

Other Grade B recommendations by the USPSTF that should be part of the PHE in a primary care setting include: screening and behavioral counseling interventions to reduce alcohol misuse by adults (including pregnant women) [29] and screening adults for depression when staff-assisted depression care supports are in place to assure accurate diagnosis, effective treatment, and follow-up [30]. Lastly, the USPSTF recommended high-intensity behavioral counseling to prevent sexually transmitted infections (STIs) for all sexually active adolescents and for adults at increased risk for STIs. These include adults with current STIs or infections within the past year are at increased risk for future STIs. In addition, adults who have multiple current sexual partners [31].

## Grade D Recommendations

In 2007, the USPSTF recommended against routine use of *aspirin and nonsteroidal anti-inflammatory drugs (NSAIDs) to prevent colorectal cancer* in individuals at average risk for colorectal cancer [32]. This recommendation applies to asymptomatic adults at average risk for colorectal cancer, including those with a family history of colorectal cancer. This recommendation does not apply to individuals with familial adenomatous polyposis, hereditary nonpolyposis colon cancer syndromes (Lynch I or II), or a history of colorectal cancer or adenomas. In addition, the USPSTF has recommended against routine screening for pancreatic cancer in asymptomatic adults using abdominal palpation, ultrasonography, or serologic markers.

The USPSTF recently recommended against *screening for testicular cancer* in adolescent or adult males. Testicular cancer (a primary germ-cell tumor of the testis) is the most common cancer among males ages 15–34 [33]. However, it is a relatively rare compared with other types of cancer with an annual incidence rate of 5.4 cases per 100,000 males. Most cases are discovered accidentally by patients or their partners. There is inadequate evidence that screening by a health-care provider or patient self-examination has a higher yield or greater accuracy for detecting testicular cancer at earlier (and more curable) stages. The American Cancer Society (ACS) recommends a testicular exam as part of a routine cancer-related checkup, and most doctors agree that examining a man's testicles be part of a general physical exam. The ACS advises men to be aware of testicular cancer and to see a doctor right away if they find a lump in a testicle. Because regular testicular self-exams have not been studied enough to show they reduce the death rate from this cancer, the ACS does not have a recommendation on regular testicular self-exams for all men. However, some doctors recommend that all men do monthly testicular self-exams after puberty [34].

The USPSTF also recommended against the *use of beta-carotene supplements*, either alone or in combination, for the prevention of cancer or CVD. However, there was insufficient evidence (grade "I") to recommend for or against the use of supplements of vitamins A, C, or E; multivitamins with folic acid; or antioxidant combinations for the prevention of cancer or CVD [35].

In 2007, the USPSTF recommended against *screening for asymptomatic carotid artery stenosis* (CAS) in the general adult population [36]. This recommendation applies to adults *without* neurologic signs or symptoms, including a history of transient ischemic attacks or stroke. Stroke is a leading cause of death and disability in the USA, but only a small proportion of all disabling strokes are due to CAS. The most feasible screening test for severe CAS (60%–99% stenosis) is duplex ultrasonography, which has moderate sensitivity and specificity but has many false-positive results. Similarly, the USPSTF found only fair evidence that screening with ankle brachial index (ABI) can detect adults with asymptomatic peripheral arterial disease (PAD) and recommended against *screening for PAD* as harms of routine screening exceeded benefits [37].

The American Society of Neuroimaging in 2007 recommended against screening for CAS in unselected populations, but advised that screening of adults age 65 years or older with 3 or more cardiovascular risk factors should be considered [38]. More recently, the Society for Vascular Surgery recommended ultrasound scan of the carotid arteries to assess stroke risk and ABI to identify PAD and risk of heart disease for individuals age 55 years or older with cardiovascular risk factors, such as a history of hypertension, diabetes mellitus, smoking, hypercholesterolemia, or known CVD [39].

In adults at low risk for CHD, the USPSTF recommended against routine screening with resting electrocardiography, exercise treadmill test, or electron-beam computerized tomography scanning for coronary calcium for either the presence of severe coronary artery stenosis or the prediction of CHD events in adults at low risk for CHD events. However, in those patients with intermediate risk for CHD events, there was insufficient evidence (grade "I") to screen for or against for either the presence of severe coronary artery stenosis or the prediction of CHD events [40].

Other grade "D" recommendations that the USPSTF recommended screening against included routine screening for chronic hepatitis B virus infection and hepatitis C virus infection in asymptomatic adults who are *not* at increased risk (general population) for infection. In addition, they recommended against routine serological screening for herpes simplex virus in asymptomatic adolescents and adults [5]. The USPSTF also recommended against routine genetic screening for hereditary hemochromatosis in the asymptomatic general population and screening adults for chronic obstructive pulmonary disease using spirometry [5].

## Immunizations (See Table 1.3)

**Table 1.3** Some of the recommended adult immunizations

| Vaccination | Who | Frequency |
|---|---|---|
| Influenza vaccine | All adults | Annually |
| Human papilloma vaccine | Males ages 9–26 | One series of three vaccines |
| Diphtheria/tetanus/ pertussis vaccine (Tdap) | All adults ages 19–64 | One time in place of the diphtheria/tetanus booster |
| Diphtheria/tetanus vaccine (Td) | All adults up to age 65<br>Adults ≥ 65 | Every 10 years<br>Single vaccination only |
| Varicella zoster | Adults ≥ 60 | Single vaccination only; no revaccination required |
| Pneumococcal vaccine | All adults ≥ 65 or any age at high risk (all adult smokers, diabetics, cancer) | Initial vaccination |

## Influenza Vaccine

Nearly 50,000 adults die each year in the USA from vaccine-preventable diseases with influenza being the most common. The most recent adult immunization was released in January 2011 [41]. Over the past 30 years (between 1976 and 2006), estimates of deaths due to the flu range from 3,000 to 49,000 seasonally. Certain groups are at higher risk for complications. These include older people, young children, pregnant women and people with certain health conditions (such as asthma, diabetes, or heart disease), and persons who live in facilities like nursing homes. The influenza vaccine is recommended for everyone over 6 months old, even healthy adults ages 19–49 without risk factors [41].

## Human Papilloma Virus Vaccine

The human papilloma virus (HPV) is the most common STI in the USA. More than 40 types of HPV are passed on through sexual contact. Most men who get HPV never develop any symptoms. In men, HPV can infect the genital areas, including the skin on and around the penis or anus. They can also infect the mouth and throat. Each year, there are about 400 men get HPV-associated penile cancer, 1,500 men get HPV-associated anal cancer, and 5,600 men get HPV-associated oropharyngeal cancers. Although anal cancer is uncommon in the general population, the incidence is increasing. HPV is associated with approximately 90% of anal cancer [42]. In October 2009, the FDA approved use of the quadrivalent HPV4 vaccine (Gardasil) for the prevention of genital warts (condyloma acuminata) due to HPV types 6 and 11 in boys and men, ages 9–26. In December 2010, the FDA approved Gardasil for the prevention of anal cancer and associated precancerous lesions due to HPV types 6, 11, 16, and 18 in both females and males ages 9–26. The CDC has not yet recommended the use of Gardasil for males in these age groups because studies suggest that the best way to prevent the most disease due to HPV is to vaccinate as many girls and women as possible. Parents of boys and young men can decide if Gardasil is right for them after discussing the risks and benefits of the vaccine with their health-care providers [41].

## Td (Tetanus, Diphtheria) and Tdap (Tetanus, Diphtheria, Pertussis) Vaccines

Pertussis (whooping cough) is caused by the bacterium *Bordetella pertussis* and is a highly contagious respiratory disease. Over the past 5 years, between 10,000 and 27,000 whooping cough cases have been reported each year. Household members are the main source of infection but outbreaks in daycare centers, schools and hospitals have increased. The major reason for the resurgence of whooping cough is due to waning protection from childhood vaccination. All adults should get a booster dose of Td (Tetanus, Diphtheria) every 10 years. Adults under 65 who have never gotten Tdap (Tetanus, Diphtheria, Pertussis) should substitute it for the next booster dose. Adults under age 65 who expect to have close contact with an infant younger than age 12 months (including women who may become pregnant) should get a dose of Tdap. Waiting at least 2 years since the last dose of Td is suggested, but not required. In addition, health-care workers under 65 who have direct patient contact in hospitals or clinics should get a dose of Tdap [41].

## Varicella Zoster Virus Vaccine

Varicella zoster virus (VZV) can reactivate clinically decades after initial infection to cause herpes zoster (shingles). One in three persons will develop shingles in their lifetime, and approximately one million cases per year are reported in the USA [43]. Postherpetic neuralgia, a chronic pain condition that can last months or even years, is a common complication of the VZV infection. In 2008, the Advisory Committee on Immunization Practices (ACIP) recommended a one-time Shingles vaccination for all adults age $\geq 60$ regardless of whether they recall having had chickenpox or not. There is no maximum age for getting the shingles vaccine. Although approved by the FDA for adults 50 and older, the CDC has yet to recommend starting the shingles vaccine starting at age 50 [41].

## Pneumococcal Vaccine

Pneumococcal disease is caused by *Streptococcus pneumonia* transmitted through respiratory droplets. The most serious complications include bacteremia, meningitis, and pneumonia. Annually, there are about 900,000 cases of community-acquired pneumonia with 175,000 Americans being hospitalized. The pneumococcal vaccine is recommended for all adults age ≥ 65. It is also recommended for adults age 19–64 with chronic medical conditions (lung, heart, liver, kidney or sickle cell disease, diabetes, alcoholism, asthma), immunocompromising conditions (HIV/AIDS, lymphoma or leukemia, damaged or no spleen) or those receiving treatment (steroids, radiation therapy, etc.), cochlear implants or cerebrospinal fluid leaks, cigarette smokers, nursing home residents, and Alaska Native and American Indian adults age 50–64 if recommended by local public health authorities in areas where risk of invasive disease is increased. A one-time booster is recommended ≥ 5 years after the first dose for the following adults: age ≥ 65 if the first dose was given prior to age 65; age 19–64 with chronic renal failure or nephrotic syndrome; functional or anatomic asplenia; immunocompromising conditions. The pneumococcal vaccine can be given at any time and can be given concurrently with the influenza vaccine [41].

Other immunizations recommended by the CDC include MMR (measles, mumps, rubella), hepatitis A, hepatitis B, meningococcal, and polio. These are discussed in greater detail in the Centers for Disease Control and Prevention's web site on adult immunization updated annually [44].

## Conclusion

As stated previously, the purpose of the PHE is for health promotion and screening of disease risk factors and subclinical illness. Three driving factors for the PHE is the belief that the exam detects subclinical illness, the belief that the annual exam is of proven value, and the fear of negative outcomes. The value of the long honored annual physical examination has been questioned and discredited [45]. In more than 25%, tests or procedures of unproven value were performed. Some have called for its abandonment. In its place, a more focused evidence-based exam has been advocated. The AHRQ recommended that, "Rather than perform a standardized comprehensive exam on all patients, clinicians need to individualize the visit to meet the specific needs of the patient" [6].

So how does a health-care provider compromise to meet the public's expectation and perceived value of the annual PHE? An evidence-based checklist of recommendations such as discussed in this chapter should provide a health-care provider an outline to fill the potential void resulting from abandoning the annual PHE and perceived value. Dr. Reinhart indicated in his letter to the editor that there are "probably very few of us, at any age, who would not be candidates for at least some health advice, such as on diet, exercise, or substance use or abuse. It also seems logical to believe that at least to some degree, repetition of heath advice may have cumulative value." [46] Lastly, better patient adherence may lead to better health outcomes. A major factor promoting adherence is the doctor–patient relationship or rapport with a physician. The annual PHE is an extremely valuable building block in achieving such rapport [3].

## References

1. Oboler SK, Prochazka AV, Gonzales R, et al. Public Expectations and Attitudes for Annual Physical Examinations and Testing. Ann Intern Med. 2002;136:652–9.
2. Prochazka AV, Lundahl K, Pearson W, et al. Support of evidence-based guidelines for the annual physical examination: a survey of primary care providers. Arch Intern Med. 2005;165:1347–52.
3. Mehrotra A, Zaslavsky AM, Ayanian JZ. Preventive health examinations and preventive gynecological examinations in the United States. Arch Intern Med. 2007;167:1876–83.

4. U.S. Agency for Healthcare Research and Quality Healthy Men Home. Available at http://www.ahrq.gov/healthymen. Accessed 15 Aug 2011.
5. USPSTF recommendation for adults. Available at: http://www.uspreventiveservicestaskforce.org/adultrec.htm. Accessed 1 Aug 2011.
6. Guide to Clinical Preventive Services, 2010–2011: recommendations of the U.S. Preventive Services Task Force. AHRQ Publication No. 10-05145. Rockville, MD: Agency for Healthcare Research and Quality; August 2010. Available at http://www.ahrq.gov/clinic/pocketgd1011/. Accessed 1 Sept 2011.
7. USPSTF A and B recommendations. Available at: http://www.uspreventiveservicestaskforce.org/uspstf/uspsabrecs.htm. Accessed 1 Sept 2011.
8. Lloyd-Jones D, Adams R, Carnethon M, et al. Heart Disease and Stroke Statistics—2009 Update A Report From the American Heart Association Statistics Committee and Stroke Statistics Subcommittee. Circulation. 2009;119:e21–181.
9. The Seventh Report of the Joint National Committee on Prevention, Detection, Evaluation, and Treatment of High Blood Pressure (JNC 7). Available at http://www.nhlbi.nih.gov/guidelines/hypertension. Accessed 21 Aug 2011.
10. Centers for Disease Control and Prevention (CDC). Disparities in screening for and awareness of high blood cholesterol: United States, 1999–2002. Morb Mortal Wkly Rep. 2005;54:117–9.
11. Expert Panel on Detection, Evaluation, and Treatment of High Blood Cholesterol in Adults. Executive Summary of the Third Report of the National Cholesterol Education Program (NCEP) Expert Panel on Detection, Evaluation, and Treatment of High Blood Cholesterol in Adults (Adult Treatment Panel III). JAMA. 2001;285:2486–97.
12. American Diabetes Association. Executive summary: standards of medical care in diabetes—2010. Diabetes Care. 2010;33:S11–61.
13. Centers for Disease Control and Prevention (CDC). Overweight and obesity. Available at http://www.cdc.gov/obesity/data/adult.html. Accessed 15 Aug 2011.
14. Flegal HM, Carroll MD, Ogden CL, et al. Prevalence and trends in obesity among US adults, 1999–2008. JAMA. 2010;303:235–41.
15. Finkelstein EA, Trogdon JG, Cohen JW, et al. Annual medical spending attributable to obesity: payer- and service-specific estimates. Health Affairs. 2009;28(5):w822–31.
16. U.S. Preventive Services Task Force. Screening for obesity in adults. Available at http://www.uspreventiveservicestaskforce.org/uspstf/uspsobes.htm. Accessed 1 Sept 2011.
17. Kochanek KD, Xu J, Murphy SL, et al. Deaths: preliminary data for 2009. National Vital Statistics Reports, vol 59, no. 4, 16 Mar 2011.
18. National Cholesterol Education Program. Third Report of the Expert Panel on Detection, Evaluation, and Treatment of High Blood Cholesterol in Adults (Adult Treatment Panel III). http://hp2010.nhlbihin.net/atpiii/calculator.asp?usertype=prof. Accessed 1 Sept 2011.
19. U.S. Preventive Services Task Force. Aspirin for the prevention of cardiovascular disease. Available at http://www.uspreventiveservicestaskforce.org/uspstf/uspsasmi.htm. Accessed 1 Aug 2011.
20. U.S. Preventive Services Task Force. Screening for abdominal aortic aneurysm. Available at http://www.uspreventiveservicestaskforce.org/uspstf/uspsaneu.htm. Accessed 1 Aug 2011.
21. Maciosek MV, Solberg LI, Coffield AB, Edwards NM, Goodman MJ. Colorectal cancer screening: health impact and cost effectiveness. Am J Prev Med. 2006;31:80–9.
22. Levin B, Lieberman DA, McFarland B, et al. Screening and Surveillance for the Early Detection of Colorectal Cancer and Adenomatous Polyps, 2008: A Joint Guideline From the American Cancer Society, the US Multi-Society Task Force on Colorectal Cancer, and the American College of Radiology. Gastroenterology. 2008;134:1570–95.
23. Centers for Disease Control and Prevention. HIV prevalence estimates—United States, 2006. Morb Mortal Wkly Rep. 2008;57(39):1073–6.
24. Marks G, Crepaz N, Janssen RS. Estimating sexual transmission of HIV from persons aware and unaware that they are infected with virus in the USA. AIDS. 2006;20:1447–50.
25. U.S. Preventive Services Task Force. Screening for HIV. Available at http://www.uspreventiveservicestaskforce.org/uspstf/uspshivi.htm. Accessed 1 Sept 2011.
26. Centers for Disease Control and Prevention. Revised recommendations for HIV testing of adults, adolescents, and pregnant women in health-care settings. Morb Mortal Wkly Rep. 2006;55(14):RR-1–17.
27. U.S. Preventive Services Task Force. Counseling and interventions to prevent tobacco use and tobacco-caused disease in adults and pregnant women. Available at: http://www.uspreventiveservicestaskforce.org/uspstf09/tobacco/tobaccors2.htm. Accessed 1 Sept 2011.
28. U.S. Preventive Services Task Force. Screening for syphilis infection. Available at http://www.uspreventiveservicestaskforce.org/uspstf/uspssyph.htm. Accessed 1 Sept 2011.
29. U.S. Preventive Services Task Force. Screening and behavioral counseling interventions in primary care to reduce alcohol misuse. Available at http://www.uspreventiveservicestaskforce.org/uspstf/uspsdrin.htm.
30. U.S. Preventive Services Task Force. Screening for depression in adults. Available at http://www.uspreventiveservicestaskforce.org/uspstf/uspsaddepr.htm.
31. U.S. Preventive Services Task Force. Behavioral counseling to prevent sexually transmitted infections. Available at http://www.uspreventiveservicestaskforce.org/uspstf/uspsstds.htm.
32. U.S. Preventive Services Task Force. Routine aspirin or nonsteroidal anti-inflammatory drugs for the primary prevention of colorectal cancer. Available at

http://www.uspreventiveservicestaskforce.org/uspstf/uspsasco.htm. Accessed 1 Sept 2011.
33. U.S. Preventive Services Task Force. Screening for testicular cancer. Available at http://www.uspreventiveservicestaskforce.org/uspstf/uspstest.htm. Accessed 1 Sept 2011.
34. American Cancer Society. Testicular cancer. Available at http://www.cancer.org/Cancer/TesticularCancer/DetailedGuide/testicular-cancer-detection. Accessed 1 Sept 2011.
35. U.S. Preventive Services Task Force. Routine vitamin supplementation to prevent cancer and cardiovascular disease. Available at http://www.uspreventiveservicestaskforce.org/uspstf/uspsvita.htm. Accessed 1 Sept 2011.
36. U.S. Preventive Services Task Force. Screening for carotid artery stenosis. Available at http://www.uspreventiveservicestaskforce.org/uspstf/uspsacas.htm. Accessed 1 Sept 2011.
37. U.S. Preventive Services Task Force. Screening for peripheral arterial disease. Available at http://www.uspreventiveservicestaskforce.org/uspstf/uspspard.htm. Accessed 1 Sept 2011.
38. Qureshi AI, Alexandrov AV, Tegeler CH, Hobson II RW, Dennis Baker J, Hopkins LN. American Society of Neuroimaging. Guidelines for screening of extracranial carotid artery disease: a statement for healthcare professionals from the multidisciplinary practice guidelines committee of the American Society of Neuroimaging; cosponsored by the Society of Vascular and Interventional Neurology. J Neuroimaging. 2007;17:19–47.
39. Society for Vascular Surgery. SVS position statement on vascular screenings. Available at http://www.vascularweb.org/about/positionstatements/Pages/svs-position-statement-on-vascular-screening.aspx. Accessed 30 Sept 2011.
40. U.S. Preventive Services Task Force. Screening for coronary artery disease. Available at http://www.uspreventiveservicestaskforce.org/uspstf/uspsacad.htm. Accessed 1 Sept 2011.
41. Centers for Disease Control and Prevention. Recommended adult immunization schedule—United States, 2011. Morb Mortal Wkly Rep. 2011;60(4).
42. Centers for Disease Control and Prevention. HPV and men—fact sheet. Available at http://www.cdc.gov/std/hpv/stdfact-hpv-and-men.htm. Accessed 1 Aug 2011.
43. Centers for Disease Control and Prevention. Prevention of herpes zoster. Morb Mortal Wkly Rep. 2008;57(05):1–30.
44. Centers for Disease Control and Prevention. Adult immunization schedule. Available at http://www.cdc.gov/vaccines/recs/schedules/adult-schedule.htm. Accessed 1 Oct 2011.
45. Chacko KM, Anderson RJ. The annual physical examination: important or time to abandon? Am J Med. 2007;120:581–3.
46. Reinhart D. Annual physical examination: necessary or needless? Ann Intern Med. 2003;138(5):W–W48.

# Clinical Testing of Endothelial Function in Erectile Dysfunction

2

Titte R. Srinivas and Mark S. Segal

## Introduction

The healthy endothelium is a monolayer of relatively simple appearing cells that was regarded in the past as a mere semipermeable barrier lining the vasculature. The importance of endothelial function in the physiology of erection is highlighted by the work of Ignarro and colleagues who defined the role of nitric oxide (NO) in the relaxation of the smooth muscle of human corpus cavernosum tissue [1]. Endothelial dysfunction has been increasingly recognized as a precursor of or accompaniment of cardiovascular events and is associated with numerous cardiovascular risk factors [2]. Initial studies of endothelial function in humans measured the response of epicardial coronary arteries to infused acetylcholine; a technique clearly not applicable to repeated study especially in those with no indications for angiography [3]. In more recent years, the availability of noninvasive techniques that measure endothelial function has allowed testing of this critical aspect of cardiovascular health to be applied at the bedside. Using such a technique, a homeostatic phenotype may be described as one that is characterized by preserved flow-mediated dilatation and an antithrombotic antiproliferative antioxidant and anti-inflammatory diathesis. A dysfunctional phenotype would be characterized by impaired flow-mediated dilatation and a prothrombotic and inflammatory tendency [4–6]. These techniques are gaining ground in the clinical arena in that endothelial dysfunction precedes the development of atherosclerotic plaque, allowing earlier intervention [5].

In this chapter, we review endothelial physiology pertinent to erectile dysfunction and techniques that can be used to measure endothelial function in the clinic. We review key studies that have studied endothelial dysfunction in ED and articulate a framework for its application in clinical practice and clinical investigation.

T.R. Srinivas, MD (✉)
Department of Nephrology and Hypertension, Glickman Urologic and Kidney Institute, Cleveland Clinic, 9500 Euclid Avenue Q7, Cleveland, OH 44195, USA
e-mail: SRINIVT@ccf.org

M.S. Segal, MD, PhD
Division of Nephrology, Hypertension and Transplantation, University of Florida, Gainsville, FL, USA

## Physiologic Considerations

The microarchitecture of the corpora is composed of a mass of smooth muscle (trabecular network), which contains a network of endothelial lined vessels (lacunar spaces). Penile tumescence leading to erection is dependent on the increased flow of blood into the lacunar network of the corpora cavernosa and the complete relaxation of arteries and corporal smooth muscle [7]. Subsequent compression of the trabecular smooth muscle against the fibroelastic tunica albuginea causes

D.A. Shoskes (ed.), *Urological Men's Health: A Guide for Urologists and Primary Care Physicians*, Current Clinical Urology, DOI 10.1007/978-1-61779-900-6_2,
© Springer Science+Business Media New York 2012

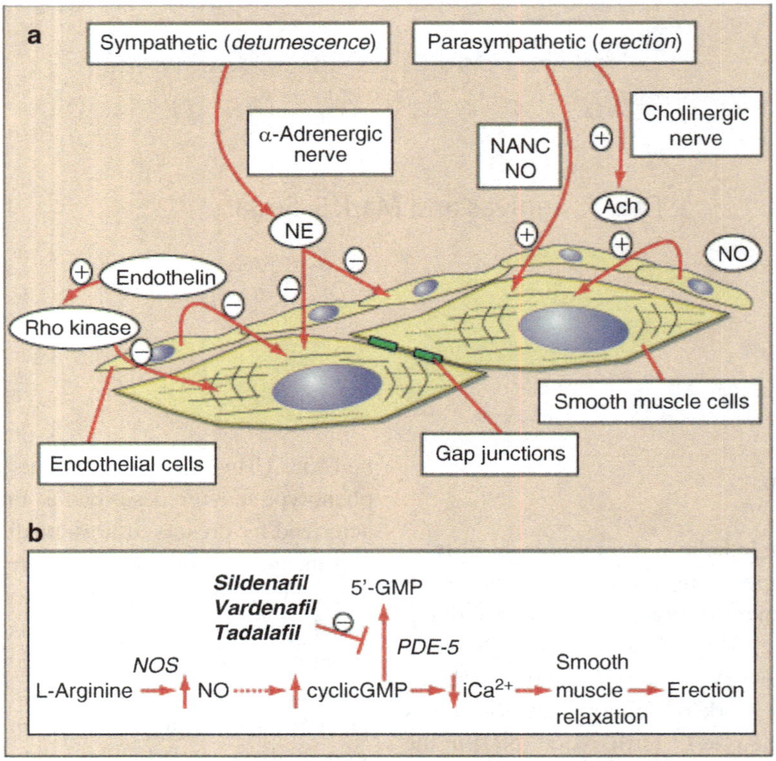


**Fig. 2.1** Tumescence is accomplished by vasodilatation of the corporal vascular network. Detumescence is initiated by vasoconstriction in the vascular network. As shown in *panel A* of figure above, the primary mediators of corporal vasodilatation are nitric oxide (NO), which is elaborated through the action of nonadrenergic noncholinergic nerves (NANC) and acetylcholine (Ach) that serves the cholinergic neural pathway. Vasocontsrictor pathways are subserved by nonadrenergic (alpha receptor) neural pathways and pathways that involve endothelin via rho-kinase (GMP, Guanosine monophosphate; PDE-5, phosphodiesterase 5; iCa2+, ionised calcium;NOS, nitric oxide synthase;

passive closure of the emissary veins and accumulation of blood in the corpora cavernosa [7]. In the presence of a full erection and a competent valve mechanism, the corpora become noncompressible cylinders from which blood cannot escape [7]. Neural influences on smooth-muscle tone are critical to the initiation and maintenance of erection [7]. The corporal smooth muscle cell in turn interacts with its endothelial cell covering (Fig. 2.1). Nitric oxide (NO) induces vascular relaxation, promotes an erection, and is antagonized by endothelin-1 (ET-1), which promotes constrictive responses through rho-kinase-mediated pathways [2, 7]. NO is synthesized from L-arginine by NO synthase and is also released from nonadrenergic noncholinergic autonomic nerves to act postsynaptically on smooth muscle cells, relaxing them. NO increases the production of cyclic 3′,5′ guanosine monophosphate (cyclic GMP), which induces relaxation of the corporal smooth muscle [2]. Cyclic GMP is gradually broken up by phosphodiesterase type 5 (PDE-5). Inhibitors of PDE-5 such as sildenafil, vardenefil, and tadalafil maintain erections by reducing the breakdown of cyclic GMP. However, if there is a primary reduction in the production of NO, PDE-5 inhibitors will be ineffective as these drugs facilitate but do not initiate the initial cascade leading to smooth muscle relaxation [2]. In addition to NO, vasoactive prostaglandins (PGE1, PGF2α) are synthesized within the cavernosal tissue and increase cyclic AMP levels, which also lead to smooth muscle relaxation in the corpora [2]. Detumescence is effected by smooth muscle contraction and is mediated by noradrenergic sympathetic neural influence on postsynaptic alpha-adrenergic receptors and endothelin released by the endothelium [7].

## Measurement of Endothelial Function

The first description of noninvasive measurement of endothelial function by flow-mediated dilatation appeared in 1992 [5]. Measurement of FMD was accomplished by measuring the diameter of the brachial artery by ultrasound before and after increasing shear stress induced by reactive hyperemia [5]. The dilatation of the artery in this instance reflects for the most part, the effect of NO release from the endothelium in the artery. Arterial diameter change averages 10% and a physiologic response entails an increase in flow greater than 1.5 times the flow at baseline [5]. More recently, the availability of finger plethysmographic equipment allows measurement of endothelial function in the clinic without the need for ultrasonography [4, 6].

Vascular health (compliance; stiffness) can also be measured using plethysmographic devices by measurements such as the augmentation index (AI) [8].

We review the technique and interpretation of noninvasive measurement of endothelial and vascular health in the ED clinic. We also summarize recent studies that have applied the endothelial function measurement in the study of ED.

## Practical Considerations

FMD is highly susceptible to factors that may impact vascular function transiently affect vascular function but not necessarily impact cardiovascular (atherosclerotic events) risk. These include food intake (especially fatty meals), intercurrent viral illness, circadian variability, caffeine, and cigarette smoking [4, 5]. Stressors such as noise can also impair the response through sympathetic nervous system impairment of vasorelaxation [4]. As such, it is preferable that endothelial function testing be carried out in a quiet room with minimal ambient light [6]. Subjects are tested early in the morning after and overnight fast except for water or a decaffeinated unsweetened drink [6].

## Ultrasound-Based Measurement of Flow-Mediated Dilatation

High-resolution ultrasound is used to image brachial artery diameter using a 7.5 MHz linear array transducer at rest and 1 min after reactive hyperemia is induced by occluding blood flow with a blood pressure cuff inflated to 60 mm Hg above systolic blood pressure [9]. Commercially available software (Brachial Analyzer; Medical Imaging Applications, Iowa City, IA) can be used to measure brachial artery diameter offline. FMD is calculated as the percent change in brachial diameter from the resting state [100(hyperemic diameter at 60 s − resting diameter)/resting diameter] [9]. Doppler flow at rest and after occlusion is calculated after correction for angle of insonation and integration of wave forms to quantify mean resting and hyperemic flow velocities [9].

Ultrasound-based measurement of flow-mediated dilation is noninvasive, repeatable, and reproducible, reflects clinically relevant physiology, and has been used in serial studies of disease reversibility [4, 5, 10]. Brachial artery FMD has also been correlated with coronary circulatory findings [11].

The major disadvantages to widespread clinical applicability of brachial artery FMD are the need for relatively expensive equipment, specialized training, and operator-dependent technique [4]. Despite guidelines that attempt standardization of the performance and interpretation of brachial artery FMD testing, its widespread clinical use has been limited by the above [4].

The recent availability of finger plethysmographic techniques to measure reactive hyperemia and vascular stiffness has added another tool whereby the clinician can interrogate vascular health [4].

## Assessment of Vascular Function Using Digital Plethysmography

Pulse amplitude tonometry (PAT) involves the measurement of digital pulse amplitude using a finger plethysmographic device [6]. Endothelial vasomotor function can be tested after reactive hyperemia by PAT (RH-PAT). Measurement of digital RH-PAT is carried out by quantifying arterial volume under resting conditions and during a condition of shear stress and resultant hyperemia that is primarily NO mediated. This measurement is carried out using a novel finger plethysmograph that takes the form of a longitudinal socket in the form of a split thimble that is closed off at its proximal end (Fig. 2.2) [4, 6]. The probe has an internal membrane that is surrounded by a rigid outer wall and is pressurized to provide a uniform field over the distal index finger by applying a near-diastolic external pressure. This application of near-diastolic pressure unloads arterial wall tension and increases the signal-to-noise ratio. Control of systemic influences is achieved by simultaneous measurement of the PAT signal without RH in the contralateral fingertip [4] (Fig. 2.3).

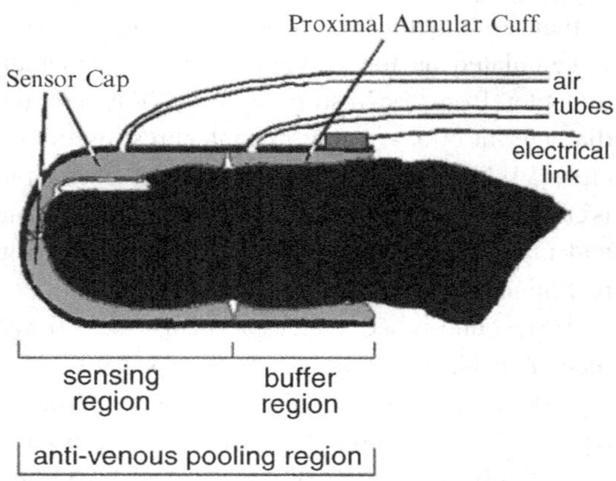


**Fig. 2.2** Cutaway diagram illustrating the EndoPAT device sensor. A pressurized cuff wherein pressure is near diastolic unloads the vascular wall and provides a seal for finger plethysmography. This near-diastolic pressure minimizes signal-to-noise ratio

The distal fingertip is a major site of sympathetic alpha-adrenergic vasoconstrictor activity and plays an important role in circulatory regulation. Endogenous NO-mediated vasorelaxation is particularly prominent in the AV anastomoses in human fingertips [4].

Studies using the RH-PAT technique have shown impaired endothelial function in children with type 1 diabetes mellitus and impaired responses in patients with coronary microvascular dysfunction [4, 8]. Reversibility of peripheral vascular endothelial dysfunction using interventions such as bioflavonoids has been demonstrated using RH-PAT [12].

In a cross-sectional study that examined RH-PAT in the Framingham Heart Study, impaired endothelial function tracked with traditional risk factors. While brachial artery FMD evaluates reactive hyperemia in larger conduit vessels, RH-PAT measurements interrogate the microvasculature. A subsequent study conducted

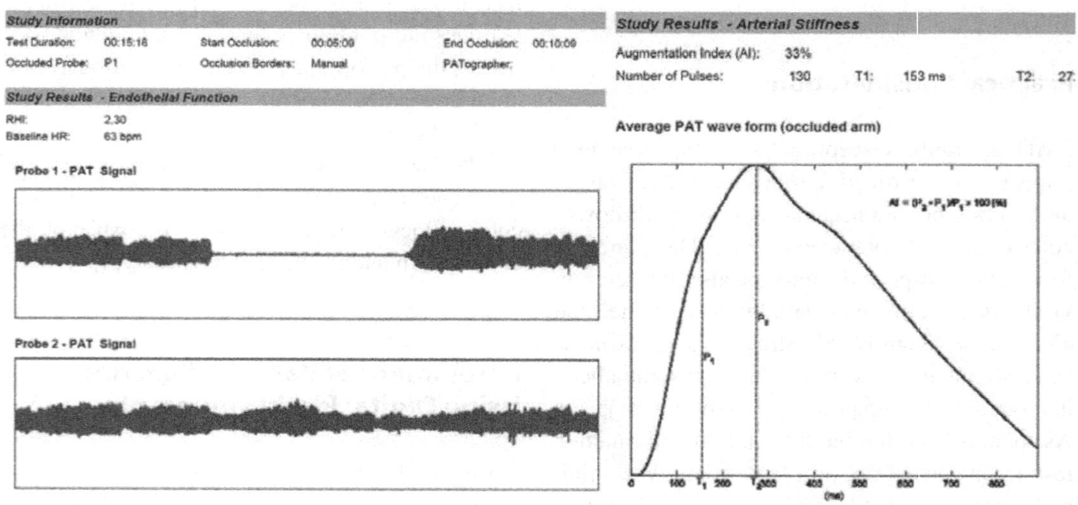


**Fig. 2.3** *Left panel* shows PAT tracing at baseline and with induction of reactive hyperemia. The *right panel* shows a stiffened artery with an increased augmentation index (AI). The reactive hyperemia index is normal

in the Framingham Heart Study cohort compared brachial artery FMD with RH-PAT responses. In that study, RH-PAT ratio was not associated with brachial FMD in multivariate models that included data from concurrently tested patients. The prevalence of abnormal brachial FMD but not RH-PAT was associated with advancing age and systolic blood pressure. Increasing BMI was associated with abnormal brachial FMD and with abnormal RH-PAT. Correlates of abnormal RH-PAT included lower systolic blood pressure, increasing total/high density lipoprotein cholesterol ratio, diabetes, smoking, and lipid-lowering medication; lipid-lowering medication effect likely reflective of indication bias. Thus, brachial FMD and RH-PAT may provide information that distinguishes the function of conduit versus smaller digital blood vessels.

We briefly describe the technique of obtaining measures of reactive hyperemia using the Endo-PAT 2000 device (Itamar Medical Ltd., Caesarea, Israel). The Endo-PAT 2000 consists of two finger-mounted probes with inflatable latex air cushions in a rigid external case (see above and Fig. 2.3). Pulsatile changes in fingertip volume are sensed by a pressure transducer and transferred to software in a personal computer wherein the signal is band pass-filtered (0.3–30 Hz), amplified, displayed, and stored.

RH-PAT studies must be performed with the patient in the supine position and both hands at the same level in a comfortable thermoneutral environment. The test arm wherein RH-PAT measurements will be obtained should preferably be the nondominant arm). The probe placed on the same digit on the contralateral hand is used to obtain measurements that are used as the control. RH-PAT probes are usually placed on the index finger but digits III and IV may be used; the same digit on each hand should be used for test and control. The fingers adjacent to the finger with the probe should be isolated from the probe finger using supplied soft sponge rings. Continuous pulse volume recordings can then be initiated. After a 10-min period of baseline recording and equilibration, arterial blood flow to the test arm is occluded by inflating a blood pressure cuff to 60 mmHg above systolic pressure. This 5-min occlusion of the brachial artery allows the creation of a downstream hyperemic response. In some cases, complete occlusion may not be achieved and the device alerts the operator who can increase cuff pressure to produce complete occlusion. After the 5-min occlusion, the blood pressure cuff is deflated and PAT recording is continued for a further 5 min. It is common for subjects to complain of pain and discomfort at this juncture, and it is important that they be alerted of this phenomenon so that arms continue to be held still. Each segment of the PAT testing must be measured using a stopwatch with a countdown timer function. RH-PAT data are then analyzed with the computer in an operator-independent manner.

The extent of RH, the RH-PAT index or RHI is calculated as the ratio of the average amplitude of the PAT signal over a 1-min time interval that begins 1-min after cuff deflation (post-occlusion) and divided by the average amplitude of the PAT signal in the 3.5-min period that precedes cuff deflation (baseline). The software normalizes RH-PAT readings obtained from the study arm to those obtained from the control arm to correct for effects of systemic changes. An RH-PAT index below 1.35 is associated with a sensitivity of 80% and a specificity of 85% in identifying patients with coronary endothelial dysfunction (Fig. 2.3).

For research purposes, especially if repeat measures or between group comparisons are being carried out, it is recommended that raw values of RH-PAT index be used in analyses as a continuous variable as this may help maintain smaller sample sizes.

The Endo-PAT 2000 machine also yields a measure of arterial stiffness, the augmentation index (AI). This is calculated automatically by analyzing the waveform of the PAT signal averaged from multiple recordings obtained during the baseline period. The AI is calculated automatically as the ratio between the amplitude difference between the two systolic peaks and the amplitude of the first peak [$AI(\%) = 100 \times ((P2 - P1)/P1)$]. The larger the AI value, the stiffer the arterial system (Fig. 2.4). Negative values may be obtained in younger subjects with compliant vascular systems wherein the first peak is higher (Fig. 2.5).

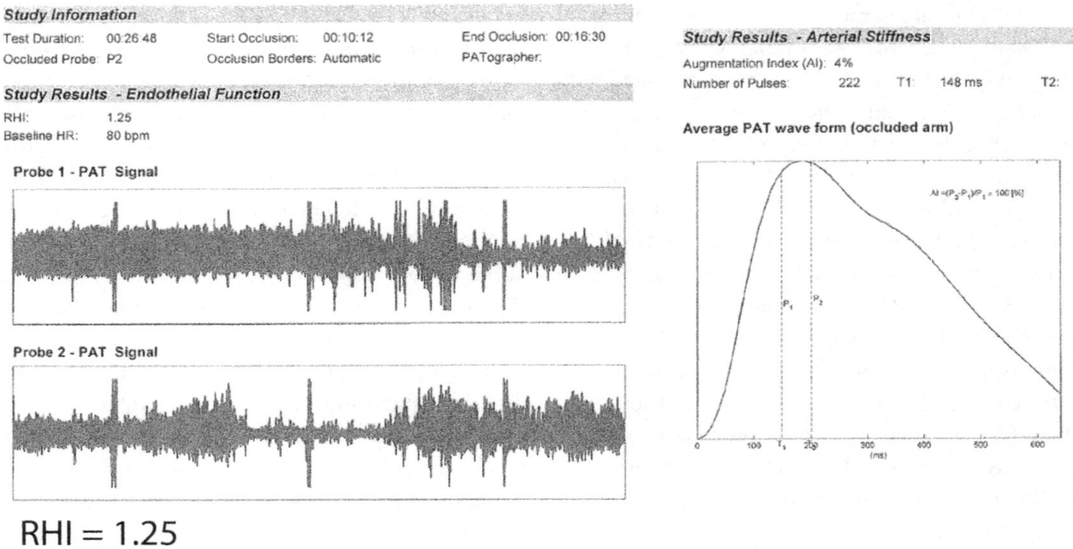


**Fig. 2.4** *Left panel* shows a normal reactive hyperemia response. *Right panel* shows a pulse wave tracing from an artery with preserved compliance as reflected in a negative value for the augmentation index

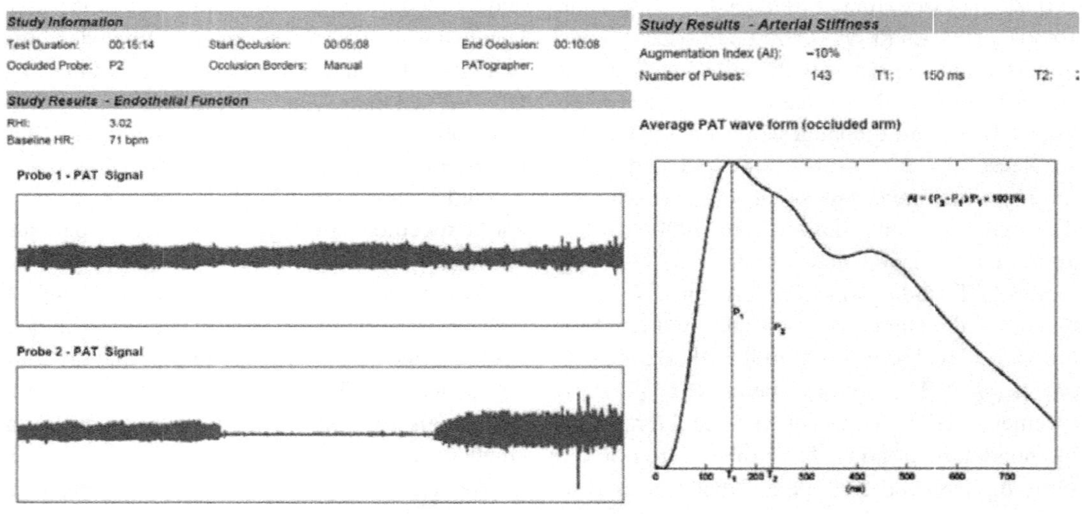


**Fig. 2.5** *Left panel* depicts an abnormal reactive hyperemia response with an RHI of 1.25. The *right panel* depicts a relatively stiff artery with a positive value for the augmentation index

## Other Biomarkers of Endothelial Health

In addition to traditional cardiovascular risk factors, recent studies point toward the dynamic role f endothelial repair and injury in determining the net state of health of the vasculature. Populations of circulating endothelial cells (CECs) and endothelial progenitor cells (EPCs) can be identified using cell surface markers and their numbers in circulating blood can be measured by flow cytometry [13, 14]. Increased numbers of EPCs and CECs correlate with increased burden of vascular pathology and disease. Such correlations have been observed in chronic kidney disease, hypertension, systemic lupus erythematosus, atherosclerotic cardiovascular disease, and hemodialysis patients [13, 14].

## Endothelial Function and Cardiovascular Risk in Erectile Dysfunction

It is now known that coronary risk factors in middle-aged men predict subsequent development of ED. It has also been noted that almost two thirds of men with angiographically proven coronary artery disease had symptomatic ED in the preceding 3 years. New onset ED in men aged 40–49 years has been associated with a 50-fold increase in the incidence of coronary artery disease and/or sudden death in the subsequent 10 years (Inman). Penile systolic velocity is inversely correlated with ischemic heart disease and ED is associated with coronary calcification at a younger age. As such ED has been termed "penile angina." Brachial artery FMD has been noted to be lower in men with ED. ED is also highly correlated with components of the metabolic syndrome, increased C-reactive protein, and an increased ratio of total cholesterol to HDL-cholesterol. Obesity is strongly associated with ED and this association is likely mediated by the cardiovascular risk associated with obesity. The prevalence of ED is almost threefold higher in men with hypertension and the incidence of ED rises with the duration and severity of hypertension.

As is now well recognized, obesity may be modifiable by lifestyle interventions. That lifestyle factors may play a role in erectile dysfunction and is supported by some experimental evidence. Esposito et al. conducted a randomized single-blind trial in 110 obese men with documented ED without diabetes, hypertension, or hyperlipidemia and assigned 55 men to the intervention group achieve a weight loss of 10% or more of total body weight through reduced caloric intake and increased levels of physical activity. The control group ($n=55$) was given general information about healthy food choices and exercise. The duration of follow-up was 2 years, the primary outcome measure being the international index of erectile function (IIEF) score. The mean IIEF score improved in the intervention group from 13.9 to 17 ($p<0.001$) but remained stable in the control group going from 13.5 at baseline to 13.6 at 2 years ($p=0.89$). In multivariate analyses, changes in body mass index, physical activity, and C-reactive protein were independent correlates of changes in IIEF score.

La Vignera et al. studied the effects of aerobic physical activity on endothelial function in middle-aged patients with erectile dysfunction [15]. Fifty patients with ED aged 48–62 years underwent 150 min/week of moderate intensity physical activity. Twenty age-matched patients with ED who did not consent to the exercise protocol were used as controls. All patients were evaluated the IIEF-5 questionnaire, penile color Doppler, and blood concentration of EPCs. Higher numbers of circulating EPCs are associated with endothelial dysfunction and vascular events in several populations. After 3 months, the exercise group showed a significant improvement in IIEF score, Doppler measurements, and EPC numbers [15].

Taken together, the two studies summarized above suggest that lifestyle modification impacts ED and cardiovascular risk with measurable changes in markers of endothelial function.

This then brings up the question of what the correlates of endothelial function measurements using techniques such as RH-PAT are in men with vasculogenic ED.

Aversa et al. recently published results of a study examining the clinical applicability of PAT and RH-PAT to the diagnostic investigation of endothelial dysfunction in men with ED. A total of 40 patients underwent diagnostic evaluation for ED, which included penile duplex ultrasound (PDU), PAT, and RH-PAT. A control group of 30 patients without ED was chosen. Based on PDU peak systolic velocity (PSV), cutoff values of 35 cm/s patients were further divided into vascular ($n=30$) and nonvascular ($n=10$) ED etiologies. Controls were further subdivided based on the presence or absence of vascular risk factors. Mean RH-PAT values did not differ significantly between patients and controls ($p=0.56$). This relationship was independent of the presence of vascular risk factors. The AI was significantly higher in men with ED compared to the controls ($p<0.0001$). Higher values of AI were associated with lower PSVs ($r^2=-0.72$; $p<0.0001$). The authors concluded that an increased AI but not impaired RH-PAT is associated with ED independent of traditional vascular risk factors and suggested that AI as a marker of vascular health may precede endothelial dysfunction. However, it is important to note at this juncture that endothelial dysfunction or a heightened alpha-adrenergic tone may be associated with vasospasm and a functional dynamic stiffening of arteries. It should also be noted that in this study, the mean body mass index in the group with ED was 25 in both the patients and controls. As such, this population may not represent those examined in other studied that included obese subjects with multiple cardiovascular risk factors who may have manifest endothelial dysfunction at the time of study. Moreover, the sample size was small. Nevertheless, the presence of an early marker of vascular stiffness, a higher AI in those with ED in this study highlights the role of examining vascular health in men with ED.

## Applying Endothelial Function Testing in the Clinic

The availability of noninvasive measures of endothelial function with RH and vascular stiffness by AI adds a new dimension to traditional evaluation of ED in the clinic.

We suggest that in addition to the traditional history and physical examination that are routine in the evaluation of ED, a comprehensive evaluation for cardiovascular risk factors such as obesity, hyperlipidemia, insulin resistance, and a careful smoking history be obtained.

In addition to these measures, measurement of RH-PAT and AI adds measurable dimensions of vascular health to the overall clinical picture. These measurements at baseline may be useful for risk stratification and may help underscore the critical need to effect lifestyle modifications in those with ED and vascular risk factors. At the time of this writing, it is not clear as to how repeat measures of endothelial function and AI can be used to monitor the success or failure of interventions on erectile dysfunction or cardiovascular risk factors. Small studies using antioxidants suggest that some measures of vascular stiffness measured in the radial artery may be modified favorably [12].

It is well known from the cardiovascular risk factor that interventions such as exercise and weight loss and attendant dietary modifications can improve endothelial dysfunction in young adults. A growing body of literature suggests that markers such as circulating EPCs reflect overall vascular health and the propensity to cardiovascular events. It is interesting that circulating EPC levels can be modified favorably in men with ED by both lifestyle and pharmacologic interventions [15, 16]. Whether these results can translate into clinical practice in patients with ED need further rigorous study.

## Conclusion

The availability of techniques to measure endothelial function and vascular health at the bedside in patients with ED offers numerous opportunities for refinement in diagnosis, risk stratification, treatment selection, and follow-up for these patients. Future studies will need to address measures of vascular health in the context of well-designed studies that examine both diagnostic and therapeutic strategies.

## References

1. Rajfer J, Aronson WJ, Bush PA, Dorey FJ, Ignarro LJ. Nitric oxide as a mediator of relaxation of the corpus cavernosum in response to nonadrenergic, noncholinergic neurotransmission. N Engl J Med. 1992;326(2):90–4.
2. Meldrum DR, Gambone JC, Morris MA, Meldrum DA, Esposito K, Ignarro LJ. The link between erectile and cardiovascular health: the canary in the coal mine. Am J Cardiol. 2011;108(4):599–606.
3. Ludmer PL, Selwyn AP, Shook TL, et al. Paradoxical vasoconstriction induced by acetylcholine in atherosclerotic coronary arteries. N Engl J Med. 1986; 315(17):1046–51.
4. Celermajer DS. Reliable endothelial function testing: at our fingertips? Circulation. 2008;117(19):2428–30.

5. Celermajer DS, Sorensen KE, Gooch VM, et al. Non-invasive detection of endothelial dysfunction in children and adults at risk of atherosclerosis. Lancet. 1992;340(8828):1111–5.
6. Rozanski A, Qureshi E, Bauman M, Reed G, Pillar G, Diamond GA. Peripheral arterial responses to treadmill exercise among healthy subjects and atherosclerotic patients. Circulation. 2001;103(16):2084–9.
7. McVary KT. Alterations in sexual function and reproduction. In: Fauci AS, editor. Harrison's principles of internal medicine. New York: McGraw Hill; 2008. p. 297–9.
8. Haller MJ, Silverstein JH, Shuster JJ. Correlation between radial artery tonometry- and fingertip tonometry-derived augmentation index in children with type 1 diabetes. Diab Vasc Dis Res. 2007;4(1):66.
9. Hamburg NM, Palmisano J, Larson MG, et al. Relation of brachial and digital measures of vascular function in the community: the Framingham heart study. Hypertension. 2011;57(3):390–6.
10. Woo KS, Chook P, Yu CW, et al. Effects of diet and exercise on obesity-related vascular dysfunction in children. Circulation. 2004;109(16):1981–6.
11. Rigo F, Pratali L, Palinkas A, et al. Coronary flow reserve and brachial artery reactivity in patients with chest pain and "false positive" exercise-induced ST-segment depression. Am J Cardiol. 2002;89(9):1141–4.
12. Fisher ND, Hughes M, Gerhard-Herman M, Hollenberg NK. Flavanol-rich cocoa induces nitric-oxide-dependent vasodilation in healthy humans. J Hypertension. 2003;21(12):2281–6.
13. Mohandas R, Segal MS. Endothelial progenitor cells and endothelial vesicles—what is the significance for patients with chronic kidney disease? Blood Purif. 2010;29(2):158–62.
14. Koc M, Bihorac A, Segal MS. Circulating endothelial cells as potential markers of the state of the endothelium in hemodialysis patients. Am J Kidney Dis. 2003;42(4):704–12.
15. La Vignera S, Condorelli R, Vicari E, D'Agata R, Calogero A. Aerobic physical activity improves endothelial function in the middle-aged patients with erectile dysfunction. Aging Male. 2011;14(4):265–72.
16. La Vignera S, Condorelli R, Vicari E, D'Agata R, Calogero A. Original immunophenotype of blood endothelial progenitor cells and microparticles in patients with isolated arterial erectile dysfunction and late onset hypogonadism: effects of androgen replacement therapy. Aging Male. 2011;14(3):183–9.

# Controversies and Opportunities for PSA Screening

3

Benjamin Cohen and Eric A. Klein

## Introduction

The use of serum prostate specific antigen (PSA) to screen for prostate cancer remains one of the major controversies in modern medicine, despite its wide use in the general population. The discoverer of PSA has maligned it publically as "the great prostate mistake" [1]. This negative press may be because of its limitations as an ideal screening test for prostate cancer. The ideal screening test is able to detect those with true disease at an early stage, where treatment can alter the course of and, ideally, cure the patient's disease. In addition, the best screening test provides prognostic information. Finally, the ideal screening test is cheap and cost effective. PSA screening for prostate cancer meets some of these criteria but falls short on many others. Despite these limitations, there are important ways PSA can be utilized in the diagnosis of prostate cancer. This chapter will review the controversies of PSA screening and the current and future opportunities of incorporating PSA measurements in prostate cancer screening.

B. Cohen, MD • E.A. Klein, MD(✉)
Glickman Urologic and Kidney Institute, Cleveland Clinic, 9500 Euclid Avenue, Q10-1, Cleveland, OH 44195, USA
e-mail: kleine@ccf.org

## Controversies

### Controversy #1: Data on the Benefits of PSA Screening Are Conflicting

One of the major criticisms surrounding the use of serum PSA measurements alone for the early detection of prostate cancer is that randomized trials have demonstrated conflicting results regarding the impact of screening on mortality. Recently, two highly publicized randomized controlled trials have attempted to answer the question of whether population-based PSA screening decreases the risk of mortality from prostate cancer. Both trials used a single PSA cut point to recommend and did not mandate prostate biopsy. The European Randomized Study of Screening for Prostate Cancer (ERSPC) was a multicenter, multinational study of screening in 182,160 men 50–74 years old [2]. A 20% reduction in the risk of prostate cancer deaths was observed among men screened with PSA compared to men who were not screened after 9 years of follow-up (2011 AUA update). However, overtreatment of prostate cancer was observed, noting that 1,410 men would need to be screened and 48 men would need to be treated to prevent one death from prostate cancer. This trial has been criticized for containing a number of methodological flaws. Screening practices in the seven countries in which patients were enrolled differed. In the control group, 20% of the men ultimately underwent PSA screening outside of the study protocol. In addition, 80% of men in

D.A. Shoskes (ed.), *Urological Men's Health: A Guide for Urologists and Primary Care Physicians*, Current Clinical Urology, DOI 10.1007/978-1-61779-900-6_3,
© Springer Science+Business Media New York 2012

the screening arm ultimately underwent PSA screening as planned. However, Hanley has suggested that the true reduction in mortality in the ERSPC is underestimated because of long lead times until prostate cancer death, estimating a potential benefit of >50% [3].

The prostate, lung, colon, and ovary trial organized by the National Cancer Institute was an RCT of PSA screening in 76,693 men [4]. This trial found no difference in prostate cancer mortality between men in the screened vs. the control groups after 7–10 years of follow-up. One of the confounding factors in the trial was that 44% of men had PSA screening prior to enrollment, likely culling out those with cancers that were potentially most lethal. Furthermore, there was an exceedingly increased rate of contamination in the control group with 52% of men undergoing off-study PSA screening, a higher PSA cutoff was used than is in common practice today, and biopsy was delayed in a significant number of participants. A post hoc analysis of the PLCO trial demonstrated a 44% reduction in mortality in the screening arm in those with no or minimal comorbidities [5].

The results of these two highly publicized trials contrast with those reported in the less publicized Goteborg randomized, population-based screening trial [6]. This trial demonstrated a relative risk reduction of 50% in the group that underwent PSA screening. The number needed to be screened was 293 and only 12 needed to be treated to prevent one prostate cancer-related death. There are likely several reasons why the results from this trial were more encouraging than those from the ERSPC and the PLCO. Men in the Goteborg study were younger with ages ranging from 50 to 64 years. In addition, follow-up was longer than that reported in the PLCO and ERSPC, with 77% of the patients having 14 years of follow-up. It has been shown that the median time from the diagnosis of prostate cancer to prostate cancer related death is over 13 years, so that one would not expect to see a mortality benefit until follow-up at 13 years had been reached. Analysis of the ERSPC demonstrated separation of mortality curves around 9 years of follow-up, and additional follow-up data from the ERSPC has demonstrated that at 12 years of follow-up, the number needed to treat to prevent a prostate cancer related mortality had decreased to 12 [7]. A published meta-analysis of screening suggested no benefit in mortality reduction, but the conclusions are based on the inclusion of two trials, which had significant flaws [8, 9].

## Controversy #2: There Is No Agreed Upon PSA Threshold at Which to Perform a Prostate Biopsy

Prostate cancers are heterogeneous, and thus the prognosis of prostate cancer may be highly variable. Serum PSA cannot distinguish among these forms of prostate cancer. Furthermore, no single PSA measurement exists at which prostate cancer is definitively diagnosed, and disagreement abounds regarding the PSA threshold at which to pursue a prostate biopsy. Historically, a serum PSA level >4 ng/ml prompted a physician to recommend a patient undergo prostate biopsy. Using data from the Prostate Cancer Prevention Trial (PCPT) in which all study participants underwent a transrectal prostate biopsy at the end of the study protocol, it was determined that a PSA level >4 ng/ml had specificity of 93% and sensitivity of 24% for detecting prostate cancer [10]. Therefore, the use of this cut point misses 76% of all prostate cancers. In addition, among men in the PCPT with PSA <4 ng/ml, 15% had high-grade cancer with a Gleason score of 7 or higher [11]. To further compound the problem, prostate cancer is not rare among men with serum PSA<4 ng/ml. In the PCPT cohort, of which the median age was 72 years, prostate cancer was detected on biopsy in 6.6% of men with PSA<0.5 ng/ml and in 27% of men with PSA 3.1–4 ng/ml [12]. The authors concluded that there is no single PSA cut point that achieves both high sensitivity and high specificity, and therefore that there is no "normal" level of PSA above which the presence of prostate cancer is certain nor one below which the risk of finding cancer is negligible [13].

### Controversy #3: The Current Use of PSA Screening Results in the Overdiagnosis of Harmless Cancers

Because screening using PSA cannot distinguish among prostate cancers with varying prognoses, reliance on PSA alone may result in overdetection and thus overtreatment of indolent disease. This can lead to unnecessary morbidity and adds an excessive financial burden. Indolent prostate cancer is common. Seventy percent of men in their 60s have latent prostate cancer on autopsy [14]. In men aged 60–64, PSA screening results in "overdiagnosis" in 10% of cancers in white men and 21% of cancers in black men, where overdiagnosis is defined as cancer that would not have caused morbidity or mortality during the patient's lifetime [15]. In the ERSPC, in which men were screened at 2- or 4-year intervals with biopsy thresholds ranging from 2.5 to 4 ng/ml, 43% of men who underwent radical prostatectomy were found to have cancer that was considered to be "minimal" [16]. Overdiagnosis is a legitimate concern and has led to efforts to improve the current screening paradigm (see "Opportunities" section, vide infra) and to more widespread use of active surveillance as a management strategy [17].

## Opportunities

Recognition of the limits of utilizing PSA for prostate cancer screening in the general population, there are opportunities to improve its use with the goal of reducing unneeded biopsies and minimizing the detection of indolent cancers. Recent work has demonstrated that PSA in combination with other risk factors can improve diagnostic accuracy, predict future prostate cancer risk, and possibly to improve our understanding of the biology of prostate cancer.

### Opportunity #1: Can Risk Assessment for Prostate Cancer Be Individualized?

PSA is not the only risk factor for prostate cancer; other well-established factors include age, race, and family history; abnormal DRE has been shown to be an independent risk factor and is usually considered an indication on its own for prostate biopsy [18]. Furthermore, a prior negative biopsy is associated with a decreased risk of prostate cancer. Data on these and other risk factors in the control arm of the PCPT, which included more than 9,000 men who were screened yearly for 7 years with DRE and PSA and then had an end of study biopsy, were used to develop a tool that predicts individual risk of prostate cancer. Now available online [19], the PCPT "risk calculator" was the first multivariable model that incorporates all the known predictive variables for prostate cancer and can generate a risk estimate tailored to an individual patient [20]. PCPT investigators have used their calculator to demonstrate that using PSA as a dichotomous variable and abnormal DRE as an independent indication for prostate biopsy results in recommendations for biopsy that are incongruent with a patient's actual risk of disease [11]. In addition to estimating an individual's risk of having prostate cancer, the risk calculator estimates the risk of having high-grade disease, a major advance that allows the clinician and the patient to decide together what the potential yield of a biopsy is, and defer or avoid biopsy if the risk of finding only indolent cancer is high. The advantage of a risk calculator approach over a PSA threshold approach for deciding on biopsy include capturing all of the information inherent in continuous variables (PSA, age), estimation of the risk of high-grade disease which can avoid both overdiagnosis and overtreatment, and flexibility to allow the incorporation of new predictive variables and biomarkers. Indeed, in addition to the six previously known variables that affect prostate cancer risk (age, race, PSA, DRE, family history, and prior biopsy), the current version of the calculator also includes BMI, PCA3, use of a 5-alpha reductase inhibitor, % free PSA and −2proPSA. One limitation of the PCPT risk calculator is that it does not perform well in all populations tested [21], emphasizing the need for a calculator derived from the local population in which it is used. Indeed, several other similar calculators derived from other populations, including the ERSPC, are also available online [22, 23]. All of the calculators also need improved performance at the low end of the risk scale [24], a limitation that is likely only to be addressed by the addition of new biomarkers.

## Opportunity #2: Can the Diagnostic Accuracy of PSA Be Improved?

Data from two randomized clinical trials have demonstrated that the sensitivity and specificity of PSA for detecting any prostate cancer and high-grade cancer can be improved by the use of a 5-alpha reductase inhibitor. In the placebo arm of the PCPT and using ROC analysis, the AUC of PSA for all outcomes was greater for those on finasteride: for detecting prostate cancer vs. no cancer, the AUCs were 0.757 and 0.681, respectively ($P<.001$); for detecting Gleason grade ≥7 vs. ≤6 or no cancer, the AUCs were 0.838 and 0.781, respectively ($P=0.003$); and for detecting Gleason grade ≥8 vs. ≤7 or no cancer, the AUCs were 0.886 and 0.824, respectively ($P=0.071$) [10]. In the REDUCE trial, a randomized trial that demonstrated a 23% reduction in risk of prostate cancer in men with a PSA of 2–10 and a prior negative biopsy, the final PSA level before biopsy and change from month 6 to final PSA level performed better for the diagnosis of Gleason score 7–10 tumors in men who received dutasteride vs. placebo (AUC 0.700 vs. 0.650, $P=0.0491$; and 0.699 vs. 0.593, $P=0.0001$, respectively) [25]. Increases in PSA were associated with a higher likelihood of biopsy detectable, Gleason score 7–10 and clinically significant (modified Epstein criteria) prostate cancer. REDUCE demonstrated similar declines in PSA from baseline to 6 months in men with or without cancer; subsequently, PSA declined slightly in those without cancer and rose in those with low- or high-grade cancer [25]. In a population of patients with symptomatic BPH, use of dutasteride resulted in an overall lower rate of biopsy and a higher likelihood of a positive biopsy compared to an agent (an alpha blocker) that does not affect PSA [26]. While widespread use of these agents has been limited by a debate over whether they make it easier to find high-grade cancers vs. actually induce them [27], the results of the PCPT and REDUCE clearly suggest that use of 5-alpha reductase inhibitors can improve the diagnostic accuracy of PSA.

## Opportunity #3: PSA Testing May Be Utilized to Predict Long-Term Prostate Cancer Risk

Given that the use of PSA has the potential to result in the detection of many indolent cancers, there is interest in directing screening efforts only at those at increased risk. A number of recent reports have helped elucidate the natural history of non-screen-detected prostate cancer and have improved our understanding of how PSA may be used to identify and screen only those at highest risk. Lilja demonstrated that a single PSA value in men in their 40s can predict lifetime risk of prostate cancer, with those under the population mean (about 0.7 ng/ml) having <10% risk, and increasing risk with higher PSAs [28]. Similar results were seen in the Baltimore Longitudinal Study of Aging, where PSA velocity in young men was able to predict for prostate cancer specific mortality 25 years later [29]. In the ERSPC, initial PSA at the time of screening was predictive of risk of prostate cancer, with a PSA<1 associated with a <5% chance of cancer over the next 14 years; those with a PSA between 1 and 2 had a 10% risk and those >2 at 25% risk [30]. These data clearly highlight the ability of PSA to predict lifetime risk of cancer, and should lead to an improved screening regimen by eliminating yearly screening in those who are at lowest risk. This would likely substantially reduce the number of unneeded biopsies and reduce overdiagnosis.

At the other end of the spectrum, Vickers performed a case–control study on 1,167 men in Sweden who provided archived frozen blood samples in 1981 at age 60 and who were closely followed for cancer or cancer-related death [31]. A majority of these men never underwent PSA screening. Given that PSA has been shown to be stable under these storage conditions, they were able to measure their PSA and correlate values at age 60 with eventual prostate cancer diagnosis or death. They discovered that 90% of fatal prostate cancers occurred in men with PSA concentrations in the top quartile. In addition, among men with concentrations less than or equal to the median PSA, the risk of prostate cancer death by age 85 was 0.5% and the risk of prostate cancer death was 0.2%. The authors suggest that half of men at age 60 may therefore be exempted from any form of prostate cancer screening. In a slightly different vein, several studies have shown that the risk of prostate cancer is low over the ensuing 4 years in a 60-year-old with a PSA < 1.5 [32, 33]. These data clearly suggest that intensive screening in men 60 or older with PSA below 1 or 1.5 is unnecessary.

## Opportunity #3: New Biomarkers

Several new markers already available or in clinical trials hold promise for improving the ability of current screening paradigms to detect clinically significant cancers. PCA3 is a noncoding mRNA that is specific for prostate cancer and can be reliably detected in a post-DRE urine sample [34]. A recent prospective trial in a screening population in Europe demonstrated that PCA3 score had a sensitivity of 64% and specificity of 76% and a significantly higher AUC compared to total PSA, PSA density, and % free PSA [35]. Other studies have suggested that PCA3 may be able to predict for disease aggressiveness, helping to decide who is a good candidate for active surveillance [36].

An isoform of free PSA, −2proPSA, also has improved accuracy over PSA in the detection of cancer. In a prospective trial from the EDRN, a multivariate model including serum −2proPSA had significant improvement (area under the curve, 0.76) over total and % free PSA [37]. This marker is still being developed in clinical trials. A fusion between the androgen-sensitive gene and TRMPSS2 and the ERG family of growth promoting genes can be detected in 50% of prostate cancers and appears to be a cancer-specific marker. In clinical trials, detection of TMPRSS2:ERG fusions in urine in combination with PCA3 improved the performance of the multivariate PCPT risk calculator in predicting cancer on biopsy [38]. In the biopsy cohorts, men in the highest and lowest of three TMPRSS2:ERG + PCA3 score groups had markedly different rates of cancer, clinically significant cancer by Epstein criteria, and high-grade cancer on biopsy. If confirmed by other trials, addition of this marker to current screening regimens should result in improved rates of detection of biologically significant cancers.

## Conclusion

PSA is the most sensitive way for detecting the presence or absence of prostate cancer. While PSA is prostate specific, its major limitation is the fact that it is not prostate cancer specific, so that many men who do not have cancer undergo biopsy needlessly. However, an improved screening paradigm is at hand with the incorporation of tools that predict individual risk, the use of agents that improve the diagnostic accuracy of PSA, recognition of the power of PSA to predict future risk, and the use of new biomarkers. With these tools, the risks associated with unneeded biopsy, overdiagnosis and overtreatment are likely to subside.

## References

1. http://www.nytimes.com/2010/03/10/opinion/10Ablin.html.
2. Schroder FH, Hugosson J, Roobol MJ, et al. Screening and prostate-cancer mortality in a randomized European study. N Engl J Med. 2009;360(13):1320–8.
3. Hanley JA. Mortality reductions produced by sustained prostate cancer screening have been underestimated. J Med Screen. 2010;17(3):147–51.
4. Andriole GL, Crawford ED, Grubb 3rd RL, et al. Mortality results from a randomized prostate-cancer screening trial. N Engl J Med. 2009;360(13):1310–9.
5. Crawford ED, Grubb 3rd R, Black A. Comorbidity and mortality results from a randomized prostate cancer screening trial. J Clin Oncol. 2011;29(4):355–61.
6. Hugosson J, Carlsson S, Aus G, et al. Mortality results from the Goteborg randomised population-based prostate-cancer screening trial. Lancet Oncol. 2010; 11(8):725–32.
7. Loeb S, Vonesh EF, Metter EJ, Carter HB, Gann PH, Catalona WJ. What is the true number needed to

screen and treat to save a life with prostate-specific antigen testing? J Clin Oncol. 2011;29(4):464–7.
8. Labrie F, Candas B, Cusan L, et al. Screening decreases prostate cancer mortality: 11-year follow-up of the 1988 Quebec prospective randomized controlled trial. Prostate. 2004;59(3):311–8.
9. Sandblom G, Varenhorst E, Rosell J, Löfman O, Carlsson P. Randomised prostate cancer screening trial: 20 year follow-up. BMJ. 2011;342:d1539.
10. Thompson IM, Chi C, Ankerst DP, et al. Effect of finasteride on the sensitivity of PSA for detecting prostate cancer. J Natl Cancer Inst. 2006;98(16):1128–33.
11. Thompson IM, Ankerst DP, Etzioni R, Wang T. It's time to abandon an upper limit of normal for prostate specific antigen: assessing the risk of prostate cancer. J Urol. 2008;180(4):1219–22.
12. Thompson IM, Ankerst DP, Chi C, et al. Operating characteristics of prostate-specific antigen in men with an initial PSA level of 3.0 ng/ml or lower. JAMA. 2005;294(1):66–70.
13. Thompson IM, Pauler DK, Goodman PJ, et al. Prevalence of prostate cancer among men with a prostate-specific antigen level < or =4.0 ng per milliliter. N Engl J Med. 2004;350(22):2239–46.
14. Sakr WA, Grignon DJ, Haas GP, Heilbrun LK, Pontes JE, Crissman JD. Age and racial distribution of prostatic intraepithelial neoplasia. Eur Urol. 1996;30(2):138–44.
15. Telesca D, Etzioni R, Gulati R. Estimating lead time and overdiagnosis associated with PSA screening from prostate cancer incidence trends. Biometrics. 2008;64(1):10–9.
16. Postma R, Schroder FH, van Leenders GJ, et al. Cancer detection and cancer characteristics in the European Randomized Study of Screening for Prostate Cancer (ERSPC)—Section Rotterdam. A comparison of two rounds of screening. Eur Urol. 2007;52(1):89–97.
17. Cooperberg MR, Carroll PR, Klotz L. Active surveillance for prostate cancer: progress and promise. J Clin Oncol. 2011;29(27):3669–76.
18. Patel AR, Klein EA. Risk factors for prostate cancer. Nat Clin Pract Urol. 2009;6(2):87–95.
19. http://deb.uthscsa.edu/URORiskCalc/Pages/uroriskcalc.jsp. Accessed 10/2011.
20. Thompson IM, Ankerst DP, Chi C, et al. Assessing prostate cancer risk: results from the Prostate Cancer Prevention Trial. J Natl Cancer Inst. 2006;98:529–34.
21. Vickers AJ, Cronin AM, Roobol MJ, et al. The relationship between prostate-specific antigen and prostate cancer risk: the Prostate Biopsy Collaborative Group. Clin Cancer Res. 2010;16(17):4374–81.
22. http://sunnybrook.ca/content/?page=OCC_prostateCalc. Accessed 10/2011.
23. http://www.prostatecancer-riskcalculator.com/via.html. Accessed 10/2011.
24. Nam RK, Kattan MW, Chin JL, et al. Prospective multi-institutional study evaluating the performance of prostate cancer risk calculators. J Clin Oncol. 2011;29(22):2959–64.
25. Andriole GL, Bostwick D, Brawley OW, et al. REDUCE Study Group: the effect of dutasteride on the usefulness of prostate specific antigen for the diagnosis of high grade and clinically relevant prostate cancer in men with a previous negative biopsy: results from the REDUCE study. J Urol. 2011;185(1):126–31.
26. Roehrborn CG, Andriole GL, Wilson TH, Castro R, Rittmaster RS. Effect of dutasteride on prostate biopsy rates and the diagnosis of prostate cancer in men with lower urinary tract symptoms and enlarged prostates in the Combination of Avodart and Tamsulosin trial. Eur Urol. 2011;59(2):244–9.
27. Theoret MR, Ning YM, Zhang JJ, Justice R, Keegan P, Pazdur R. The risks and benefits of 5α-reductase inhibitors for prostate-cancer prevention. N Engl J Med. 2011;365(2):97–9.
28. Lilja H, Ulmert D, Vickers AJ. Prostate-specific antigen and prostate cancer: prediction, detection and monitoring. Nat Rev Cancer. 2008;8(4):268–78.
29. Carter HB, Ferrucci L, Kettermann A, et al. Detection of life-threatening prostate cancer with prostate-specific antigen velocity during a window of curability. J Natl Cancer Inst. 2006;98(21):1521–7.
30. Bul M, van Leeuwen PJ, Zhu X, Schröder FH, Roobol MJ. Prostate cancer incidence and disease-specific survival of men with initial prostate-specific antigen less than 3.0 ng/ml who are participating in ERSPC Rotterdam. Eur Urol. 2011;59(4):498–505.
31. Vickers AJ, Cronin AM, Bjork T, et al. Prostate specific antigen concentration at age 60 and death or metastasis from prostate cancer: case-control study. BMJ. 2011;341:c4521.
32. Aus G, Damber JE, Khatami A, Lilja H, Stranne J, Hugosson J. Individualized screening interval for prostate cancer based on prostate-specific antigen level: results of a prospective, randomized, population-based study. Arch Intern Med. 2005;165(16):1857–61.
33. Crawford ED, Moul JW, Rove KO, Pettaway CA, Lamerato LE, Hughes A. Prostate-specific antigen 1.5–4.0 ng/mL: a diagnostic challenge and danger zone. BJU Int. 2011;108(11):1743–9. doi:10.1111/j.1464-410X.2011.10224 [Epub June 28, 2011].
34. Hessels D, Schalken JA. The use of PCA3 in the diagnosis of prostate cancer. Nat Rev Urol. 2009;6(5):255–61.
35. de la Taille A, Irani J, Graefen M, et al. Clinical evaluation of the PCA3 assay in guiding initial biopsy decisions. J Urol. 2011;185(6):2119–25.
36. Ploussard G, Durand X, Xylinas E, et al. Prostate cancer antigen 3 score accurately predicts tumour volume and might help in selecting prostate cancer patients for active surveillance. Eur Urol. 2011;59(3):422–9.
37. Sokoll LJ, Sanda MG, Feng Z, et al. A prospective, multicenter, National Cancer Institute Early Detection Research Network study of [−2]proPSA: improving prostate cancer detection and correlating with cancer aggressiveness. Cancer Epidemiol Biomarkers Prev. 2010;19(5):1193–200.
38. Tomlins SA, Aubin SM, Siddiqui J, et al. Urine TMPRSS2:ERG fusion transcript stratifies prostate cancer risk in men with elevated serum PSA. Sci Transl Med. 2011;3(94):94ra72.

# 4 A Phenotypic Approach to the Evaluation and Treatment of Men with Chronic Pelvic Pain Syndrome

Kiranpreet Khurana and Daniel A. Shoskes

## Introduction

Chronic prostatitis/chronic pelvic pain syndrome (CP/CPPS) is a common condition with an estimated prevalence between 5% and 16% [1]. About 5% of visits to U.S. urologists are for prostatitis symptoms [2]. Among ambulatory visits by men 18 years or older, prostatitis accounts for two million visits annually [3]. Prostatitis is a clinically challenging entity due to poor understanding of its etiology, symptoms, and appropriate treatment.

In 1995, the NIH, based on expert opinion, developed a new syndrome-based classification for prostatitis (Table 4.1). Category III prostatitis was defined as urologic pain in the pelvic area, for at least three out of the previous 6 months, in the absence of recurrent urinary tract infection or other urologic diagnosis causing the symptoms. The NIH classification included two subcategories under category III: IIIA, the inflammatory subtype, has leukocytes in expressed prostatic secretions, post-prostate massage urine, or semen; and IIIB, the noninflammatory subtype, does not have any leukocytes [4]. Up to now, there has been no clinical significance to this subclassification [5].

K. Khurana, MD • D.A. Shoskes, MD, MSc, FRCS(C)(✉)
Department of Urology, The Glickman Urologic and Kidney Institute, Cleveland Clinic, 9500 Euclid Avenue, Q10-1, Cleveland, OH 44195, USA
e-mail: dshoskes@mac.com

Multiple factors may play a role in the pathophysiology of CPPS including initial urinary tract infection, intra-prostatic urinary reflux [6], cytokines [7], pelvic floor spasm [8], bladder, prostate, seminal vesicle pathology [9], hereditary factors, hormonal imbalance, or psychological traits [10]. However, none of these factors has been determined as the sole cause in majority of cases. Rather a combination of these factors is likely contributing to CPPS and therefore therapy must likely be directed toward individual patient's clinical phenotype. Our current best understanding of the etiologies is illustrated in Fig. 4.1 [11].

Different types of treatments have been used to treat CPPS. These include α-blockers, antibiotics, hormonal therapy, anti-inflammatory medications, phytotherapy, antispasmodics, nonpharmacological therapies, and combination therapies [10, 11] (Table 4.2).

## Monotherapies for CPPS

### α-Blockers

α-Blockers have been used in CPPS to ameliorate factors associated with dysfunctional voiding, which predisposes to presumed intraprostatic reflux, inflammation, and pain [6]. α-Blockers improve outflow obstruction and may play a role in diminishing intraprostatic reflux [39]. In animal studies, α-blockers have shown an inhibitory effect on C-fiber afferents in the lumbosacral spi-

D.A. Shoskes (ed.), *Urological Men's Health: A Guide for Urologists and Primary Care Physicians*, Current Clinical Urology, DOI 10.1007/978-1-61779-900-6_4,
© Springer Science+Business Media New York 2012

nal cord, improving bladder capacity during the storage phase [40], decrease bladder contractions when injected intrathecally [41], and decrease neurogenic inflammation [42].

Several α-blockers have been studied with conflicting results. Some of the differences among randomized controlled trials (RCTs) include different α-blockers, populations, duration of therapies, and outcomes. These RCTs have had anywhere from 19 to 138 patients in the treatment group, with treatment duration from 6 to 24 weeks (Table 4.2). Cheah et al. included only those patients without prior exposure to α-blockers [20], whereas Tugcu et al. enrolled patients regardless of prior exposure [15]. Two RCTs did not report whether patients had prior exposure [12, 17].

While most of the smaller RCTs have had positive results, two of the biggest trials did not support routine use of α-blockers [13, 16]. Alexander et al. studied the effect of 6 weeks of tamsulosin on total National Institutes of Health-Chronic Prostatitis Symptom Index (NIH-CPSI) [16]. There was no significant benefit of an α-blocker on total NIH-CPSI scores. Some of the drawbacks of this trial were that patients had long-standing symptoms and had prior exposure

**Table 4.1** NIH classification of prostatitis syndromes

| | NIH classification of prostatitis syndromes |
|---|---|
| Category I | Acute bacterial prostatitis |
| Category II | Chronic bacterial prostatitis—recurrent urinary tract infection with bacteria from a prostatic source |
| Category IIIA | Chronic prostatitis/chronic pelvic pain syndrome, inflammatory |
| Category IIIB | Chronic prostatitis/chronic pelvic pain syndrome, noninflammatory |
| Category IV | Asymptomatic inflammatory prostatitis |

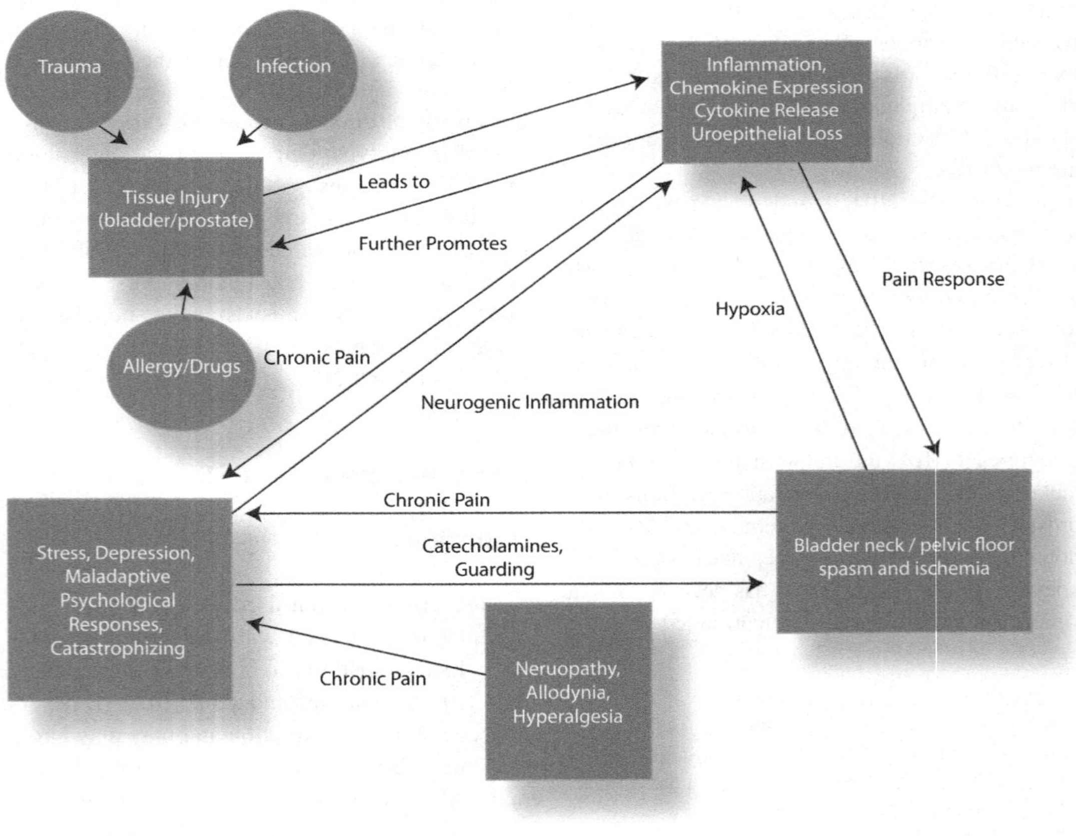


**Fig. 4.1** Multifactorial etiology of chronic pelvic pain syndrome

**Table 4.2** Summary of clinical studies for therapies in CPPS

| Therapy | No. of patients | Duration of therapy (weeks) | Outcome | Publication |
|---|---|---|---|---|
| *α-Blockers* | | | | |
| Alfuzosin | 19 (alfuzosin)<br>21 (placebo) | 24 | SSI in NIH-CPSI total scores | Mehik et al. [12] |
| Alfuzosin | 138 (alfuzosin)<br>134 (placebo) | 12 | No SSI in NIH-CPSI total scores | Nickel et al. [13] |
| Doxazosin | 30 (doxazosin)<br>30 (placebo) | 12 | SSI in IPSS and pain scores | Evliyaoglu et al. [14] |
| Doxazosin | 30 (doxazosin)<br>30 (placebo) | 24 | SSI in NIH-CPSI total scores | Tugcu et al. [15] |
| Tamsulosin | 49 (tamsulosin)<br>49 (placebo) | 6 | No SSI in NIH-CPSI total scores | Alexander et al. [16] |
| Tamsulosin | 27 (tamsulosin)<br>30 (placebo) | 6 | SSI in NIH-CPSI total scores | Nickel et al. [17] |
| Tamsulosin | 46 (tamsulosin)<br>47 (placebo) | 24 | SSI in NIH-CPSI total scores | Chen et al. [18] |
| Terazosin | 39 (terazosin)<br>30 (placebo) | 12 | SSI in PSSI | Gul et al. [19] |
| Terazosin | 43 (terazosin)<br>43 (placebo) | 14 | SSI in NIH-CPSI total scores | Cheah et al. [20] |
| *Antibiotics* | | | | |
| Levofloxacin | 45 (levofloxacin)<br>35 (placebo) | 6 | No SSI in NIH-CPSI total scores | Nickel et al. [21] |
| Ciprofloxacin | 49 (ciprofloxacin)<br>49 (placebo) | 6 | No SSI in NIH-CPSI total scores | Alexander et al. [16] |
| Tetracycline hydrochloride | 24 (tetracycline)<br>24 (placebo) | 12 | SSI in NIH-CPSI total scores | Zhou et al. [22] |
| *Hormonal agents* | | | | |
| Finasteride | 31 (finasteride)<br>10 (placebo) | 52 | No SSI in IPSS and pain scores | Leskinen et al. [23] |
| Finasteride | 33 (finasteride)<br>31 (placebo) | 24 | No SSI in NIH-CPSI total scores | Nickel et al. [24] |
| Meparticin | 13 (meparticin)<br>13 (placebo) | 8 | SSI in NIH-CPSI total scores | De Rose et al. [25] |
| *Anti-inflammatory* | | | | |
| Rofecoxib | 49 (rofecoxib)<br>59 (placebo) | 6 | No SSI in NIH-CPSI total scores | Nickel et al. [26] |
| Pentosan polysulfate | 51 (pentosan)<br>49 (placebo) | 16 | No SSI in NIH-CPSI and CGI scores | Nickel et al. [27] |
| Zafirlukast | 10 (zafirlukast)<br>7 (placebo) | 4 | No SSI in NIH-CPSI total scores | Goldmeier et al. [28] |
| Prednisolone | 9 (prednisolone)<br>12 (placebo) | 4 | No SSI in NIH-CPSI and HADS scores | Bates et al. [29] |
| Celecoxib | 32 (celecoxib)<br>32 (placebo) | 6 | SSI in NIH-CPSI total scores | Zhao et al. [30] |

(continued)

**Table 4.2** (continued)

| Therapy | No. of patients | Duration of therapy (weeks) | Outcome | Publication |
|---|---|---|---|---|
| *Phytotherapy* | | | | |
| Quercetin | 15 (quercetin)<br>13 (placebo) | 4 | SSI in NIH-CPSI total scores | Shoskes et al. [31] |
| Pollen extract (Prostat/ Poltit) | 30 (extract)<br>28 (placebo) | 24 | SSI in pain/LUTS questions | Elist [32] |
| Cernilton N (pollen extract) | 70 (cernilton N)<br>69 (placebo) | 12 | SSI in NIH-CPSI total scores | Wagenlehner et al. [33] |
| *Neuroleptic* | | | | |
| Pregabalin | 217 (pregabalin)<br>104 (placebo) | 6 | No SSI in rate of 6-point decrease between groups<br>SSI in secondary outcome—NIH-CPSI total scores | Pontari et al. [34] |
| *Physical therapy* | | | | |
| Physical therapy | 23 (myofascial)<br>24 (global massage) | 12 | No direct comparison; no placebo<br>No SSI of myofascial therapy over global massage therapy | FitzGerald et al. [35] |
| *Combination therapy* | | | | |
| Ciprofloxacin + tamsulosin | 49 (Ciprofloxacin + tamsulosin)<br>49 (ciprofloxacin)<br>49 (tamsulosin)<br>49 (placebo) | 6 | No SSI in NIH-CPSI total scores | Alexander et al. [16] |
| α-Blocker, anti-inflammatory, muscle relaxant | 30 (α-blocker)<br>30 (α-blocker, anti-inflammatory, muscle relaxant)<br>30 (placebo) | 24 | No SSI in NIH-CPSI total scores for triple therapy | Tugcu et al. [15] |
| Doxazosin + levofloxacin | 29 (doxazosin + levofloxacin)<br>26 (doxazosin)<br>26 (levofloxacin) | 6 | SSI in NIH-CPSI total scores for levofloxacin vs. doxazosin, doxazosin vs. combination<br>No SSI in NIH-CPSI total scores of combination vs. levofloxacin | Jeong et al. [36] |
| Tamsulosin + levofloxacin | 42 (tamsulosin + levofloxacin)<br>42 (tamsulosin)<br>21 (levofloxacin) | 12 | SSI on NIH-CPSI scores with combination therapy | Ye et al. [37] |
| UPOINT directed combination therapy | 100 (UPOINT directed therapy) | 24 | 84 patients with 6-point decrease in NIH-CPSI total scores<br>Not compared to placebo | Shoskes et al. [38] |

*NIH-CPSI* National Institutes of Health-Chronic Prostatitis Symptom Index, *IPSS* International Prostate Symptom Score, *PSSI* Prostatitis Symptom Score Index, *CGI* Clinical Global Improvement assessment, *HADS* Hospital Anxiety and Depression Scale, *LUTS* lower urinary tract symptoms to α-blockers. Furthermore, the 2×2 trial design was not powered to show efficacy for each individual study arm. Therefore, another trial was designed to investigate α-blocker use in patients with shorter duration of symptoms and without prior exposure to this class of drugs [13]. There was still no clear benefit of treatment with an α-blocker.

## Antibiotics

Antibiotics are often used in patients with pelvic pain for presumed bacterial prostatitis despite negative cultures. Studies with antibiotics have shown that they are not more effective than placebo [16, 21]. An RCT studied the efficacy of levofloxacin for 6 weeks compared to placebo. Although patients did better in terms of total NIH-CPSI scores in both groups over time, there was no significant difference between groups [21]. Similarly, in an NIDDK-sponsored trial, ciprofloxacin was evaluated for efficacy and was not found to be superior to placebo [16]. In another trial from China, patients were treated with tetracycline hydrochloride and a benefit was shown over placebo [22]; however, these men did have evidence of nanobacteria, which are particles not found by conventional methods due to their size and biological characteristics.

## Hormonal Agents

Finasteride, a type II 5α-reductase inhibitor, has been used in patients with benign prostatic hypertrophy with improvement in lower urinary tract symptoms. This drug has also been investigated in patients with CPPS. Two randomized, placebo-controlled trials were conducted with patients receiving finasteride for 24 or 52 weeks [23,24]. Neither of these trials showed a statistically significant improvement over the placebo group. A different hormonal agent, mepartricin, which reduces serum estrogen levels and prostatic estrogen receptors in rats, has been shown to have beneficial effects in total NIH-CPSI scores in men with CPPS [25]. However, this was a small study of 26 Italian men, and these results have not been reproduced.

## Anti-Inflammatories

Anti-inflammatory medications have been used as a therapeutic option for CPPS with variable results. Cyclooxygenase-2 inhibitor, rofecoxib, given to patients for 6 weeks showed a trend toward total NIH-CPSI score improvement but the effect was not significantly better than placebo [26]. A study done in China with celecoxib demonstrated improvement but the benefit deteriorated in 2 weeks after finishing therapy [30]. Pentosan polysulfate sodium, a glycosaminoglycan drug used in interstitial cystitis, was evaluated in a randomized controlled trial, which showed no significant benefit in Clinical Global Improvement and total NIH-CPSI scores [27]. A small study from UK showed no benefit for zafirlukast, a leucotriene antagonist [28]. Similarly, another study evaluating the efficacy of prednisolone did not find any value in its use [29].

## Phytotherapy

Phytotherapy has been found to be of benefit to men with CPPS. Quercetin is a natural bioflavonoid found in fruits, vegetables, leaves, and grains. It is thought to help in CPPS because of its antioxidant and anti-inflammatory properties. In a randomized, double-blind, placebo-controlled trial, 15 and 13 men were given four-week therapy of quercetin and placebo, respectively [31]. Patients taking quercetin had a mean decrease in NIH-CPSI scores of 7.9 points compared to a decrease of 1.4 points in the placebo group ($P=0.003$). An improvement of at least 25% was seen in 67% of men in the treatment group vs. 20% of men in the placebo group. In another study, a pollen extract, *Prostat/Poltit*, containing 74 mg of highly defined extract of pollen from selected *Graminae* species was studied in men with CPPS [32]. Twenty-two out of 30 patients had improvement in pain and lower urinary tract symptoms on a symptom questionnaire compared to 10 out of 28 men in the placebo group. However, they did not use a standardized questionnaire. In an RCT, cernilton, a pollen extract, was found to be clinically and statistically significantly better than placebo [33]. A decrease of at least 25% or 6 points in total NIH-CPSI scores was seen in 70.6% and 50.0% of patients in the pollen extract and placebo group ($P=0.01$), respectively.

There is some evidence that absorption of quercetin from the GI tract is enhanced by the herbal sourced products papain and bromelain. For quercetin, we usually use Prosta-Q (Farr Labs, CA), which has both papain and bromelain or Q-Urol, which also has pollen extract.

## Neuroleptic

Pregabalin is commonly used for neuropathic pain. One RCT showed no statistically significant improvement in primary outcome of 6-point decrease in total NIH-CPSI scores between groups [34]. However, 47.2% vs. 35.8% patients had a 6-point decrease in treatment and placebo groups ($P=0.07$), respectively. There was a significant improvement in secondary outcome of total NIH-CPSI scores. A decrease of 6.6 points was seen in the pregabalin arm and 4.2 points in the placebo arm ($P=0.01$). However, 59% of the patients in the pregabalin arm experienced adverse effects, most being mild to moderate.

## Nonpharmacological Therapy

Nonpharmacological therapies, including prostate massage, pelvic floor therapy, myofascial trigger point release, and biofeedback, have an important role in CPPS. Myofascial trigger point release is a type of physical therapy which targets the taut bands or tender nodules that provide relief by therapeutic manipulation. Anderson et al. showed that myofascial trigger point release and paradoxical relaxation training had a moderate to marked improvement in symptoms in 72% of patients [43]. This therapy also resulted in improved sexual function, which is often found in men with CPPS [44]. Conduction of a randomized, double-blind, placebo-controlled trial is limited by the fact that sham therapy and blinding of both patients and operators is difficult. An NIH sponsored pilot study evaluated the feasibility of performing a larger trial by comparing myofascial release physical therapy and global therapeutic massage in 48 patients including men with CPPS or women with interstitial cystitis [35]. The study did show that it was feasible to conduct a larger trial. However, myofascial release physical therapy in men was not found to be superior to global therapeutic massage.

## Development and Utility of UPOINT

The understanding of CPPS has evolved since the NIH classification. The major barrier in treating men with CPPS is the heterogenous nature of this syndrome. The therapies discussed above have had minimal or no success because they target a single mechanism for every patient with CPPS, whereas each patient should be evaluated individually to assess the nature of symptoms, and then be treated appropriately.

In order to direct appropriate therapy, we have developed a 6-point clinical phenotyping system to evaluate patients with chronic urologic pelvic pain [45]. The clinical domains are *u*rinary symptoms, *p*sychosocial dysfunction, *o*rgan specific findings, *i*nfection, *n*eurologic/systemic, and *t*enderness of muscles, which produces the acronym UPOINT (Fig. 4.2). Each patient is evaluated clinically for involvement of each domain and symptom severity is assessed using the NIH-CPSI. This is followed by a multimodal therapeutic approach towards positive domains.

We have shown that there is a stepwise increase in the total NIH-CPSI score with increase in the number of positive domains. In addition, the number of positive domains also correlates with longer duration of symptoms [46, 47]. In a Swedish study, the correlation between the

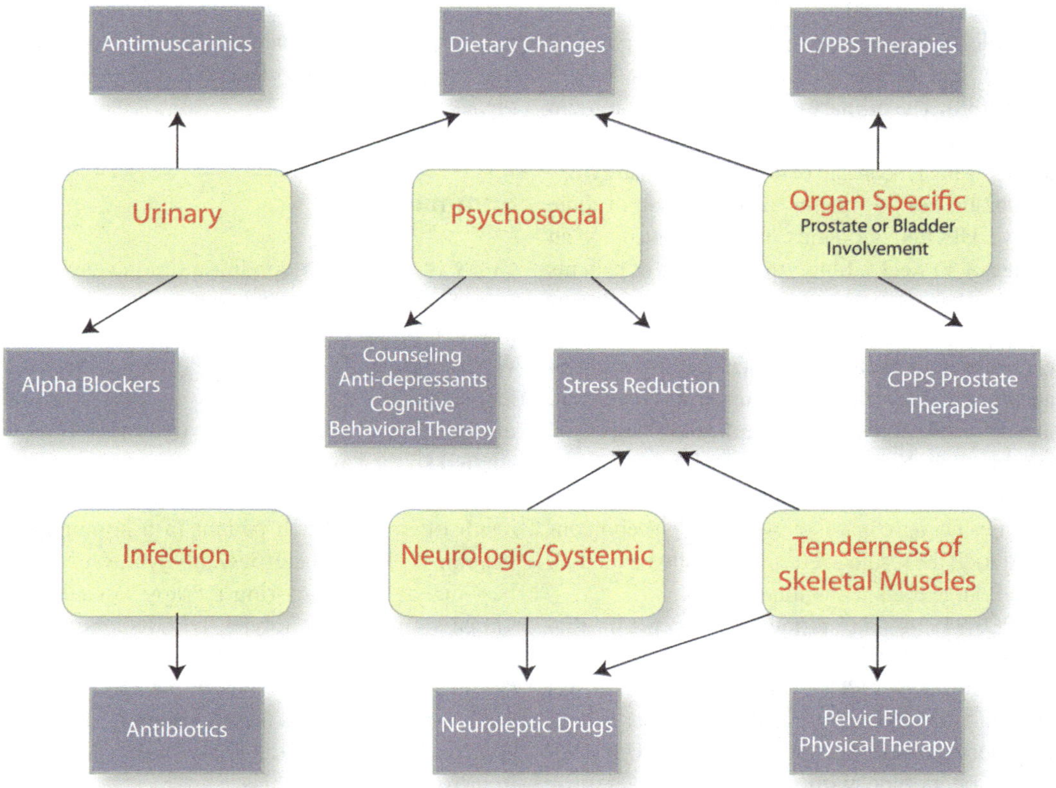


**Fig. 4.2** UPOINT domains and associated therapies

number of positive domains and NIH-CPSI was verified [48]. The UPOINT clinical phenotyping system may provide a useful and clinically relevant framework for multimodal therapy for the treatment of CPPS.

A European study evaluated the inclusion of a sexual dysfunction domain to the UPOINT clinical phenotyping system [49]. Nine hundred and thirty-seven men from Italy and 290 men from Germany with CPPS were retrospectively classified into a modified UPOINTS system (S = sexual dysfunction domain). The regular UPOINT system correlated well with symptom severity in the Italian but not in the German cohort. The modified clinical phenotyping system (UPOINTS) with an additional sexual dysfunction domain correlated significantly with NIH-CPSI scores in the German cohort.

This finding was further studied in a population of 100 patients at our institution [50]. Twenty-eight percent of men with CPPS were found to have bothersome erectile dysfunction. However, addition of the sexual domain decreased the correlation between the clinical phenotyping system and symptom severity. Total NIH-CPSI scores, pain subscores, and quality of life measures were unaffected by erectile dysfunction. Therefore, inclusion of a sexual domain did not appear to add value to in our patient population.

The development of UPOINT would have limited utility unless it actually improved treatment outcomes. A recent prospective study offered multimodal therapy based on the UPOINT phenotype (e.g., urinary: α-blocker or antimuscarinic; psychosocial: stress reduction/psychologic support; organ specific: quercetin; infection:

antibiotic; neurologic/systemic: amitriptyline or pregabalin; tenderness: pelvic floor physical therapy), and measured response after at least 6 months [38]. The primary endpoint was a minimum 6-point drop in total NIH-CPSI score. One hundred patients, with a mean age of 46 years, median symptom duration of 24 months, and a median of three positive UPOINT domains, were followed for an average of 50 weeks. Eighty-four percent of patients had at least a 6-point decrease in CPSI, with an average drop of 12 points. Fifty-one patients had a 50% or greater improvement in total CPSI while 84 patients had at least a 25% or greater improvement. All CPSI subscores were significantly improved from baseline. Number of positive domains, initial CPSI scores, and symptom duration did not predict outcome. Though this study was not a placebo-controlled trial, the results were significantly better than all prior large trials with monotherapy.

UPOINT is an attractive approach that simplifies treatment in patients with the challenging diagnosis of CPPS. An online resource has been made available for use by urologists, where one enters patient data and is given the UPOINT clinical phenotype with suggested therapies. A web-based algorithm is available at http://www.upointmd.com. The diagnostic criteria and typical therapies for each domain are summarized in Table 4.3. Again, each domain is categorized as positive or negative by clinical criteria, and for each positive domain therapy is offered. For example, a patient with urinary and organ specific may be treated with an α-blocker and quercetin while another with neurologic and tenderness may be treated with pregabalin and pelvic floor physical therapy.

## Summary

CPPS is a common condition among men with significant morbidity and impact on mental and physical measures of quality of life [51]. It provides a great diagnostic and therapeutic challenge, and is often a frustrating condition for both urologist and patient. Many treatment options studied so far have had minimal or no success in large trials. These negative outcomes are the result of treating each patient in a homogenous fashion. CPPS is a heterogenous syndrome that is best managed by tailoring therapy to each individual's clinical phenotype. UPOINT is a novel approach that stratifies patients to different domains based on their symptoms and is used to guide phenotypically directed therapy. In a prospective study, UPOINT has been found to improve patient outcomes.

## Future Plans

Further studies are needed to confirm our results in a multicenter and placebo-controlled trial. Due to the flexibility of UPOINT, future versions

**Table 4.3** Diagnostic criteria for UPOINT phenotypes and treatments

| Domain | Diagnostic criteria | Potential treatments |
|---|---|---|
| Urinary | Bothersome irritative or obstructive urinary symptoms<br>High postvoid residual | α-Blockers<br>Antimuscarinics |
| Psychosocial | Clinical depression<br>Catastrophizing (verbalized helplessness and hopelessness) | Psychologic or psychiatric counseling<br>Cognitive behavioral therapy |
| Organ specific (bladder or prostate) | Specific prostate tenderness<br>Hematospermia<br>Symptom relief with voiding | Quercetin (e.g. Prosta-Q)<br>Pollen extract (e.g. Q-Urol)<br>Pentosan polysulfate |
| Infection | Positive cultures of prostatic fluid in absence of UTI<br>Concomitant urethritis | Antibiotics |
| Neurologic/systemic | Pain outside pelvis<br>Systemic pain syndrome | Pregabalin<br>Amitriptyline |
| Tenderness | Pelvic floor spasm<br>Muscle trigger points | Pelvic physical therapy<br>Myofascial release |

will include modification of each domain, incorporation of disease biomarkers, and expansion of therapeutic choices. Moreover, the UPOINT system will play an important role in testing new therapies for CPPS. UPOINT is a promising clinical phenotyping system that provides precisely tailored therapy for patients who suffer from chronic pelvic pain syndrome resulting in improved outcomes.

## References


1. Schaeffer AJ. Epidemiology and demographics of prostatitis. Andrologia. 2003;35(5):252–7.
2. Schappert SM. National Ambulatory Medical Care Survey: 1991 summary. Vital Health Stat 13 1994;(116): 1–110.
3. Collins MM, Stafford RS, O'Leary MP, Barry MJ. How common is prostatitis? A national survey of physician visits. J Urol. 1998;159(4):1224–8.
4. Krieger JN, Nyberg Jr L, Nickel JC. NIH consensus definition and classification of prostatitis. JAMA. 1999;282(3):236–7.
5. Schaeffer AJ, Wendel EF, Dunn JK, Grayhack JT. Prevalence and significance of prostatic inflammation. J Urol. 1981;125(2):215–9.
6. Kirby RS, Lowe D, Bultitude MI, Shuttleworth KE. Intra-prostatic urinary reflux: an aetiological factor in abacterial prostatitis. Br J Urol. 1982;54(6):729–31.
7. Shahed AR, Shoskes DA. Correlation of beta-endorphin and prostaglandin E2 levels in prostatic fluid of patients with chronic prostatitis with diagnosis and treatment response. J Urol. 2001;166(5):1738–41.
8. Westesson KE, Shoskes DA. Chronic prostatitis/chronic pelvic pain syndrome and pelvic floor spasm: can we diagnose and treat? Curr Urol Rep. 11(4): 261–4.
9. Schaeffer AJ. Etiology and management of chronic pelvic pain syndrome in men. Urology. 2004;63(3 Suppl 1):75–84.
10. Anothaisintawee T, Attia J, Nickel JC, Thammakraisorn S, Numthavaj P, McEvoy M, et al. Management of chronic prostatitis/chronic pelvic pain syndrome: a systematic review and network meta-analysis. JAMA. 305(1):78–86.
11. Snow DC, Shoskes DA. Pharmacotherapy of prostatitis. Expert Opin Pharmacother. 11(14): 2319–30.
12. Mehik A, Alas P, Nickel JC, Sarpola A, Helstrom PJ. Alfuzosin treatment for chronic prostatitis/chronic pelvic pain syndrome: a prospective, randomized, double-blind, placebo-controlled, pilot study. Urology. 2003;62(3):425–9.
13. Nickel JC, Krieger JN, McNaughton-Collins M, Anderson RU, Pontari M, Shoskes DA, et al. Alfuzosin and symptoms of chronic prostatitis-chronic pelvic pain syndrome. N Engl J Med. 2008;359(25): 2663–73.
14. Evliyaoglu Y, Burgut R. Lower urinary tract symptoms, pain and quality of life assessment in chronic non-bacterial prostatitis patients treated with alpha-blocking agent doxazosin; versus placebo. Int Urol Nephrol. 2002;34(3):351–6.
15. Tugcu V, Tasci AI, Fazlioglu A, Gurbuz G, Ozbek E, Sahin S, et al. A placebo-controlled comparison of the efficiency of triple- and monotherapy in category III B chronic pelvic pain syndrome (CPPS). Eur Urol. 2007;51(4):1113–7; discussion 8.
16. Alexander RB, Propert KJ, Schaeffer AJ, Landis JR, Nickel JC, O'Leary MP, et al. Ciprofloxacin or tamsulosin in men with chronic prostatitis/chronic pelvic pain syndrome: a randomized, double-blind trial. Ann Intern Med. 2004;141(8):581–9.
17. Nickel JC, Narayan P, McKay J, Doyle C. Treatment of chronic prostatitis/chronic pelvic pain syndrome with tamsulosin: a randomized double blind trial. J Urol. 2004;171(4):1594–7.
18. Chen Y, Wu X, Liu J, Tang W, Zhao T, Zhang J. Effects of a 6-month course of tamsulosin for chronic prostatitis/chronic pelvic pain syndrome: a multicenter, randomized trial. World J Urol. 29(3):381–5.
19. Gul O, Eroglu M, Ozok U. Use of terazosine in patients with chronic pelvic pain syndrome and evaluation by prostatitis symptom score index. Int Urol Nephrol. 2001;32(3):433–6.
20. Cheah PY, Liong ML, Yuen KH, Teh CL, Khor T, Yang JR, et al. Terazosin therapy for chronic prostatitis/chronic pelvic pain syndrome: a randomized, placebo controlled trial. J Urol. 2003;169(2):592–6.
21. Nickel JC, Downey J, Clark J, Casey RW, Pommerville PJ, Barkin J, et al. Levofloxacin for chronic prostatitis/chronic pelvic pain syndrome in men: a randomized placebo-controlled multicenter trial. Urology. 2003;62(4):614–7.
22. Zhou Z, Hong L, Shen X, Rao X, Jin X, Lu G, et al. Detection of nanobacteria infection in type III prostatitis. Urology. 2008;71(6):1091–5.
23. Leskinen M, Lukkarinen O, Marttila T. Effects of finasteride in patients with inflammatory chronic pelvic pain syndrome: a double-blind, placebo-controlled, pilot study. Urology. 1999;53(3):502–5.
24. Nickel JC, Downey J, Pontari MA, Shoskes DA, Zeitlin SI. A randomized placebo-controlled multicentre study to evaluate the safety and efficacy of finasteride for male chronic pelvic pain syndrome (category IIIA chronic nonbacterial prostatitis). Br J Urol Int. 2004;93(7):991–5.
25. De Rose AF, Gallo F, Giglio M, Carmignani G. Role of mepartricin in category III chronic nonbacterial prostatitis/chronic pelvic pain syndrome: a randomized prospective placebo-controlled trial. Urology. 2004;63(1):13–6.
26. Nickel JC, Pontari M, Moon T, Gittelman M, Malek G, Farrington J, et al. A randomized, placebo controlled, multicenter study to evaluate the safety and

efficacy of rofecoxib in the treatment of chronic nonbacterial prostatitis. J Urol. 2003;169(4):1401–5.
27. Nickel JC, Forrest JB, Tomera K, Hernandez-Graulau J, Moon TD, Schaeffer AJ, et al. Pentosan polysulfate sodium therapy for men with chronic pelvic pain syndrome: a multicenter, randomized, placebo controlled study. J Urol. 2005;173(4):1252–5.
28. Goldmeier D, Madden P, McKenna M, Tamm N. Treatment of category III A prostatitis with zafirlukast: a randomized controlled feasibility study. Int J STD AIDS. 2005;16(3):196–200.
29. Bates SM, Hill VA, Anderson JB, Chapple CR, Spence R, Ryan C, et al. A prospective, randomized, double-blind trial to evaluate the role of a short reducing course of oral corticosteroid therapy in the treatment of chronic prostatitis/chronic pelvic pain syndrome. Br J Urol Int. 2007;99(2):355–9.
30. Zhao WP, Zhang ZG, Li XD, Yu D, Rui XF, Li GH, et al. Celecoxib reduces symptoms in men with difficult chronic pelvic pain syndrome (Category IIIA). Braz J Med Biol Res. 2009;42(10):963–7.
31. Shoskes DA, Zeitlin SI, Shahed A, Rajfer J. Quercetin in men with category III chronic prostatitis: a preliminary prospective, double-blind, placebo-controlled trial. Urology. 1999;54(6):960–3.
32. Elist J. Effects of pollen extract preparation Prostat/Poltit on lower urinary tract symptoms in patients with chronic nonbacterial prostatitis/chronic pelvic pain syndrome: a randomized, double-blind, placebo-controlled study. Urology. 2006;67(1):60–3.
33. Wagenlehner FM, Schneider H, Ludwig M, Schnitker J, Brahler E, Weidner W. A pollen extract (Cernilton) in patients with inflammatory chronic prostatitis-chronic pelvic pain syndrome: a multicentre, randomised, prospective, double-blind, placebo-controlled phase 3 study. Eur Urol. 2009;56(3):544–51.
34. Pontari MA, Krieger JN, Litwin MS, White PC, Anderson RU, McNaughton-Collins M, et al. Pregabalin for the treatment of men with chronic prostatitis/chronic pelvic pain syndrome: a randomized controlled trial. Arch Intern Med. 170(17):1586–93.
35. FitzGerald MP, Anderson RU, Potts J, Payne CK, Peters KM, Clemens JQ, et al. Randomized multicenter feasibility trial of myofascial physical therapy for the treatment of urological chronic pelvic pain syndromes. J Urol. 2009;182(2):570–80.
36. Jeong CW, Lim DJ, Son H, Lee SE, Jeong H. Treatment for chronic prostatitis/chronic pelvic pain syndrome: levofloxacin, doxazosin and their combination. Urol Int. 2008;80(2):157–61.
37. Ye ZQ, Lan RZ, Yang WM, Yao LF, Yu X. Tamsulosin treatment of chronic non-bacterial prostatitis. J Int Med Res. 2008;36(2):244–52.
38. Shoskes DA, Nickel JC, Kattan MW. Phenotypically directed multimodal therapy for chronic prostatitis/chronic pelvic pain syndrome: a prospective study using UPOINT. Urology 75(6):1249–53.
39. Roehrborn CG. Alfuzosin: overview of pharmacokinetics, safety, and efficacy of a clinically uroselective alpha-blocker. Urology 2001;58(6 Suppl 1):55–63; discussion 63–4.
40. Yokoyama O, Yusup A, Oyama N, Aoki Y, Tanase K, Matsuta Y, et al. Improvement of bladder storage function by alpha1-blocker depends on the suppression of C-fiber afferent activity in rats. Neurourol Urodyn. 2006;25(5):461–7.
41. Sugaya K, Nishijima S, Miyazato M, Ashitomi K, Hatano T, Ogawa Y. Effects of intrathecal injection of tamsulosin and naftopidil, alpha-1A and -1D adrenergic receptor antagonists, on bladder activity in rats. Neurosci Lett. 2002;328(1):74–6.
42. Geppetti P, Nassini R, Materazzi S, Benemei S. The concept of neurogenic inflammation. Br J Urol Int. 2008;101(Suppl 3):2–6.
43. Anderson RU, Wise D, Sawyer T, Chan C. Integration of myofascial trigger point release and paradoxical relaxation training treatment of chronic pelvic pain in men. J Urol. 2005;174(1):155–60.
44. Anderson RU, Wise D, Sawyer T, Chan CA. Sexual dysfunction in men with chronic prostatitis/chronic pelvic pain syndrome: improvement after trigger point release and paradoxical relaxation training. J Urol. 2006;176(4 Pt 1):1534–8; discussion 8–9.
45. Shoskes DA, Nickel JC, Rackley RR, Pontari MA. Clinical phenotyping in chronic prostatitis/chronic pelvic pain syndrome and interstitial cystitis: a management strategy for urologic chronic pelvic pain syndromes. Prostate Cancer Prostatic Dis. 2009;12(2): 177–83.
46. Nickel JC, Shoskes D, Irvine-Bird K. Clinical phenotyping of women with interstitial cystitis/painful bladder syndrome: a key to classification and potentially improved management. J Urol. 2009;182(1): 155–60.
47. Shoskes DA, Nickel JC, Dolinga R, Prots D. Clinical phenotyping of patients with chronic prostatitis/chronic pelvic pain syndrome and correlation with symptom severity. Urology 2009;73(3):538–42; discussion 42–3.
48. Hedelin HH. Evaluation of a modification of the UPOINT clinical phenotype system for the chronic pelvic pain syndrome. Scand J Urol Nephrol. 2009; 43(5):373–6.
49. Magri V, Wagenlehner F, Perletti G, Schneider S, Marras E, Naber KG, et al. Use of the UPOINT chronic prostatitis/chronic pelvic pain syndrome classification in European patient cohorts: sexual function domain improves correlations. J Urol. 2010;184(6):2339–45.
50. Samplaski MK, Li J, Shoskes DA. Inclusion of erectile domain to UPOINT phenotype does not improve correlation with symptom severity in men with chronic prostatitis/chronic pelvic pain syndrome. Urology. 2011;78(3):653–8.
51. McNaughton Collins M, Pontari MA, O'Leary MP, Calhoun EA, Santanna J, Landis JR, et al. Quality of life is impaired in men with chronic prostatitis: the Chronic Prostatitis Collaborative Research Network. J Gen Intern Med. 2001;16(10):656–62.

# Recurrent Urinary Tract Infections in Men

5

Stacey C. Carter, Mya E. Levy, and Scott I. Zeitlin

## Introduction

A urinary tract infection (UTI) refers to an infection of the bladder (cystitis), the upper urinary tract (pyelonephritis), and may (incorrectly) be used to describe asymptomatic bacteriuria. These types of infections are much less common in men than in women due to anatomical differences in urethral length, lower incidence of periurethral colonization, and antibacterial substances found in prostatic fluid [1]. Thus, men who acquire these types of infections require special consideration and workup. In this chapter, we will discuss the management of recurrent UTIs in men as well as prostatitis and urethritis.

Risk factors for UTIs include urinary stasis secondary to bladder outlet or upper tract obstruction, neurogenic bladder (bladder malfunction secondary to pathology of the nervous system), instrumentation of the urinary tract including catheterizations, procedure related manipulation such as cystoscopy, prostate biopsy, bacterial prostatitis, and urolithiasis. Additionally, men exhibit signs and symptoms of a UTI when they suffer from prostatitis and urethritis. Prostatitis may occur secondary to seeding from ascending bacteria from the urethra or reflux of infected urine into the prostatic ducts. Urethritis is generally thought to be caused by bacteria acquired through sexual relations, such as Chlamydia or Gonorrhea.

The lifetime prevalence of a man having 1–2 UTIs is 10,341 per every 100,000 men [2]. The initial workup for first time UTIs includes a thorough history with specific attention to their lower urinary tract symptoms (LUTS), a physical including an examination of the penis, scrotum, and the prostate, urinalysis, urine culture, and sensitivities. However, men with recurrent UTIs may require a more in-depth investigation. The lifetime prevalence of men who acquire three or more UTIs is 3,348 men per every 100,000 men [2]. If no obvious cause is identified on initial workup, the patient may require further evaluation including measurement of urinary flow (uroflowmetry) and post-void residual, more extensive imaging or physiologic testing, such as renal ultrasound, CT scan, cystoscopy, urodynamics, or nuclear renal scan.

In this chapter, we will focus on the evaluation and management of recurrent infections of the urinary tract in men.

## Urinary Tract Infections

A UTI refers to an infection of the urinary system, which may involve the lower urinary tract (cystitis) alone, or in conjunction with the upper

S.C. Carter, MD • M.E. Levy, MD
Department of Urology, David Geffen School of Medicine at UCLA, Los Angeles, CA, USA

S.I. Zeitlin, MD (✉)
Department of Urology and OB/GYN, David Geffen School of Medicine at UCLA, VA Greater Los Angeles Healthcare System, 2080 Century Park East #1407, Los Angeles, CA 90067, USA
e-mail: szeitlin@ucla.edu

D.A. Shoskes (ed.), *Urological Men's Health: A Guide for Urologists and Primary Care Physicians*, Current Clinical Urology, DOI 10.1007/978-1-61779-900-6_5,
© Springer Science+Business Media New York 2012

urinary tract (pyelonephritis). An uncomplicated UTI is one that occurs in a woman without associated risk factors for infection. A complicated UTI is defined as one that occurs in:

- Men
- Immunosuppressed patients (i.e., diabetes mellitus, HIV, on steroids or chemotherapy)
- Pregnancy
- Pediatric populations
- Setting of indwelling catheters or stents
- Urinary obstruction
- Renal insufficiency
- Urolithiasis

Bacterial entry into the urinary system is most frequently caused by periurethral bacteria ascending into the urinary tract. Hematogenous, lymphatogenous, and direct extension from surrounding organs are less common modes of bacterial seeding. The best host defense against this bacterial entry is to maintain an unobstructed urinary flow allowing washout of this ascending bacteria. Urine itself has natural defenses against pathogens, including Tamm-Horsfall glycoprotein that inhibits bacterial adhesion and the local immune response to pathogens that initiates both cellular and humoral-mediated immunity and maintains an osmolality and pH that is unfavorable to bacterial survival [3]. The definitive diagnosis of a UTI is made with a urine culture collected from midstream voided sample showing greater than $10^5$th CFU/mL in the absence of symptoms or $10^2$th CFU/mL with symptoms [4]. Presumptive diagnosis of a UTI may be made prior to urine culture results with evidence of a positive urinalysis in the setting of symptoms. Elements of a urinalysis that suggest the presence of a UTI are [5]:

- *Pyuria*: >5 WBCs/high power field. This is the most valuable test, as it is present in nearly all men with a UTI. It also may imply, however, evidence of an obstruction or chronic inflammation in the absence of an infection.
- *Leukocyte esterase*: When WBCs are present in the urine, they release this enzyme. This is also a nonspecific marker of inflammation, and can be positive in the setting of a chronic indwelling Foley catheter without a positive culture.
- Bacteria.
- *Nitrite positivity*: Many bacteria (*Escherichia coli*, *Klebsiella*, *Enterobacter*, *Serratia*, *Proteus*, *Staphylococcus*, *Pseudomonas*) convert nitrate to nitrite during protein metabolism using an enzyme called nitrate reductase.

Common symptoms of a UTI include:

- Dysuria
- Hematuria
- Suprapubic or pelvic discomfort
- Frequency
- Urgency
- Cloudy or foul-smelling urine
- Systemic signs of fever, chills, or sepsis indicate involvement of the upper urinary tract

The majority of community-acquired UTIs are caused by *E. coli*, with most others caused by Enterobacteriaceae (including *Proteus*, *Klebsiella*), *Enterococc*i, or coagulase-negative *Staphylococcus*. Nosocomial infections are also most commonly caused by *E. coli*, as well as *Pseudomonas*, *Klebsiella*, *Enterobacter*, *Citrobacter*, *Morganella*, *Staphylococcus aureus*, and *Candida* [6]. Targeted antibiotic therapy should be directed toward bacterial sensitivities with careful selection of an appropriate duration of treatment. Inappropriate choice and duration of treatment of UTIs can lead to increased bacterial resistance or persistent infection. Recurrent and complicated infections are more likely to be caused by organisms resistant to oral antibiotics that are commonly used to treat uncomplicated infections because they are likely to be overutilized [7]. This is particularly important in patients with asymptomatic bacteriuria, defined as a positive urine culture in the absence of symptoms. This is common in patients with chronic indwelling catheters, stents, or on intermittent catheterization, and becomes a challenge to the physician to determine whether there is a need for antibiotic treatment. The management of these specific patients will be discussed in a later section in the chapter.

Most of the literature published regarding length and type of treatment is based on data from women with uncomplicated UTIs. This has been extrapolated by physicians in order to treat men with UTIs, and thus there is no good consensus regarding the appropriate duration of treatment. For men with no concomitant risk factors a short course of targeted antibiotics is usually sufficient. For infections in the setting of obstruction, stones, or underlying comorbidities, a longer course is often recommended [8].

Choice of antibiotic therapy should be directed toward culture sensitivities. However, these are often not available for 48 h. Choice of empiric antibiotics depends on a variety of factors including whether or not the UTI is community or hospital acquired, underlying patient comorbidities, and severity of the infection. As antimicrobial resistance increases, physicians must change their choice of empiric antibiotic therapy. For uncomplicated infections, trimethoprim–sulfamethoxazole (TMP–SMZ) is traditionally used; however, its efficacy has somewhat declined as resistant strains of common uropathogens develop [9].

Fluoroquinolones are commonly used in men, and have a broad spectrum of activity, especially against gram-negative bacteria. For this reason they are being used more frequently for empiric treatment of both uncomplicated and complicated infections; however, this is contributing to an overall trend in resistance toward this class of antibiotics [10].

Distinction should be made between persistent infection and recurrent infection. A persistent UTI is one that is treated with antibiotic therapy; however, the bacteria persist due to incomplete eradication. Recurrent UTIs are those that resolve with antibiotic therapy; however, the urinary tract is re-seeded with the same or a different type of bacteria. Common risk factors for persistent UTIs include urinary stasis or obstruction, fistulas, urolithiasis, indwelling ureteral stents or catheters, and bacterial prostatitis. Preventing persistent UTIs requires accurate identification of the source of untreated bacteria followed by complete and targeted treatment. As a general rule, prevention of recurrent UTIs is aimed at treating the underlying cause of the infection and addressing risk factors that place the patient at higher risk for re-infection. Risk factors for recurrent UTIs in men include:

- Urinary obstruction and/or stasis
  - Bladder outlet obstruction
  - Urinary retention
  - Upper tract obstruction
  - Vesicoureteral reflux
  - Diverticulae
- Urolithiasis
- Immunocompromised state
  - Diabetes mellitus, HIV
  - Steroids or chemotherapy

The workup and management of these risk factors is discussed below.

## Lower Urinary Tract

In men, a common etiology of lower UTIs is urinary stasis or a foreign body (i.e., a stone or catheter) in the urinary tract. As such, investigation for an anatomical obstruction or dysfunction at any point along the entire urinary system should be pursued in men with recurrent UTIs.

### Bladder Outlet Obstruction and Urinary Stasis

Bladder outlet obstruction increases the risk of UTIs due to urinary stasis that occurs from inability to completely empty the bladder. Common causes of bladder outlet obstruction include benign prostatic hyperplasia (BPH), bladder neck contractures, urethral strictures, meatal stenosis, or severe phimosis. Additionally, urinary stasis may be caused by neurogenic bladder secondary to peripheral or central nervous system dysfunction. The workup should be aimed at identifying the anatomic or physiologic cause of the obstruction [11].

#### Signs and Symptoms

Development of LUTS is often the first sign that a patient is not completely emptying his bladder. These include:

- Frequency
- Urgency
- Nocturia

- Hesitancy
- Weak or intermittent stream
- Sensation of incomplete emptying

Men also may present initially with evidence of a UTI, impaired renal function, or hydronephrosis.

## Evaluation

Men with these symptoms should be assessed with measurement of uroflowmetry and post-void residual and digital rectal exam to evaluate the size and consistency of the prostate gland. A urinalysis and culture should also be collected using a voided midstream sample [12]. Post-void residual may be assessed in the clinic with an ultrasound bladder scan. Large post-void residuals put the patient at increased risk of infection and may indicate the presence of outlet obstruction. Low flow rates and elevated PVRs are not specific for obstruction, and may also be evident in patients with a neurogenic or dysfunctional bladder [13].

## Management

In the face of obstruction in the setting of LUTS or UTI, initial management is aimed at behavioral changes and medical therapy in addition to antibiotic treatment of the UTI. The patient should be counseled on the technique of double voiding to better empty his bladder, instructed to limit caffeine, alcohol, and oral fluid intake prior to bedtime. If post-void residual is greater than 180 mL or if there is evidence of hydronephrosis or impaired renal function, the patient may require decompression of the bladder with an indwelling Foley catheter or be instructed on clean intermittent catheterization (CIC) [14]. Initial medical therapy is typically an alpha-adrenergic antagonist that acts to relax the smooth muscle around the bladder neck, prostate capsule, and prostatic urethra so that voiding is facilitated [15]. Again, should there be evidence of infection, antibiotic treatment should be directed toward bacterial sensitivities. The goal for treatment duration should be the shortest course of antibiotics needed to fully eradicate the infection. After completion of the antibiotic treatment, follow-up urine culture should be obtained to confirm eradication.

If medical and behavioral management is unsuccessful in relieving the patient's LUTS or if he develops recurrent UTIs, further workup and treatment may be indicated. Cystoscopy gives a survey of the entire urethra for an anatomical outlet obstruction such as stricture disease, or potentially obstructing prostatic lobes. If no obstructing structures are identified in the setting of urinary retention, urodynamics may be helpful to evaluate for an outlet obstruction, element of neurogenic, or defunctionalized bladder, or voiding dysfunction.

If a urethral stricture is identified on cystoscopy, this should be dilated, incised, or treated open (see chapter on management of strictures). Once the stricture is treated, the patient may be reevaluated to see whether his retention and symptoms have improved. If the prostate is shown to be occlusive, then surgical options should be considered. Alternative options for relieving a bladder outlet obstruction in patients who are not surgical candidates include indwelling Foley catheter, suprapubic tube, or CIC [16].

Patients with urinary retention who have risk factors for neurogenic bladder, such as Parkinson's disease, spinal cord injury or surgery, prior pelvic surgery, multiple sclerosis, or other central or peripheral nerve pathology should be assessed with urodynamics [17]. Evidence of detrusor sphincter dysynergia (failure of the sphincter to relax while the bladder contracts) is a contraindication to transurethral resection of the prostate, and the patient's urinary retention requires nonoperative management. These patients often require CIC, indwelling Foley catheter, or a suprapubic tube for relief of their urinary stasis [18].

Once the cause of urinary stasis is identified and treated, follow-up should focus on evaluating for relief of symptoms and cessation of the cycle of infection. If the symptoms do not improve and the man continues to have recurrent UTIs once the obstruction is relieved, then further workup for another inciting cause should be pursued.

Cystoscopy may reveal a foreign body or lesion in the bladder or urethra such as a tumor, stone, or diverticulum which could serve as a nidus for a recurrent infection. If these are identified, they should be treated appropriately. Once removed, the patient should be evaluated to confirm resolution of the infection.

## Catheters or Device-Associated UTIs

Patients with indwelling catheters increase their risk of developing bacteriuria at a rate of 5–10% per day, and all have bacteriuria once the catheter has been in place for 1 week. The most common hospital acquired bacteremia is attributed to UTIs in the setting of indwelling catheters, with a mortality of approximately 10% [19]. The organisms most often identified with catheter-associated UTIs are *E. coli*, *Candida*, *Pseudomonas*, *Enterococcus*, and *Proteus* [20]. Catheters, in addition to other foreign bodies in the urinary tract such as ureteral stents, nephrostomy tubes, or other medical devices, can serve as an entry for bacteria into the urinary system. The urinary tract may become colonized with bacteria, resulting in repeatedly positive urine cultures with, or without, symptoms. Catheters and other foreign bodies develop a biofilm, or bacterial colonization on an extracellular matrix. This bacteria is often resistant to antibiotic treatment alone, and must be removed or exchanged for complete treatment [21].

A recent systematic review compared a silver alloy-coated catheter to the standard uncoated catheter. The data is limited; however, it indicates that silver alloy-coated catheters offer an advantage in preventing catheter-associated UTIs when used for a short term in hospitalized adults [22].

If a patient develops symptoms of a UTI when these types of catheters are in the urinary system, treatment should be directed toward microbial sensitivities. Urine should be collected from a voided sample or from a newly placed catheter so as to not contaminate the specimen with bacteria colonized on the already indwelling catheter. Current data does not recommend antibiotic treatment unless there is a planned procedure or operation that requires sterile urine. For symptomatic patients, or those who require sterile urine for a planned procedure or operation, a 10- to 14-day course of antibiotics with antibiotics directed toward culture results is indicated.

Data indicates that CIC has a lower risk of infection than a suprapubic tube, which in turn has a lower risk of infection than an indwelling urethral catheter for long-term use [23]. Evaluating the best option for each individual patient includes assessment of their manual dexterity, their overall body habitus, and their personal preference in terms of what best fits their lifestyle. If all precautions are taken to prevent recurrent symptomatic UTIs in patients with indwelling catheters, and oral antibiotic therapy proves unsuccessful, intravesical antibiotic solutions may be instilled directly into the bladder in an attempt to eradicate the offending organisms. The most common solution is 480 mg gentamicin sulfate into 1 L of sterile water with instillation of 30 $cm^3$ into the bladder [24].

As a general rule, temporary catheters or stents should be placed with aseptic technique, maintain a closed drainage system, and be removed as soon as possible from the urinary tract. It is recommended that chronic indwelling Foley catheters, suprapubic tubes, and nephrostomy tubes be exchanged once monthly [25]. Standard indwelling ureteral stents should be exchanged once every 3 months. Medical devices implanted near the urinary tract system, such as penile prostheses and artificial urinary sphincters can function as a source for recurrent infection, particularly if there is an area of erosion so that it is exposed to the urinary tract. For patients with these devices in the absence of another source, the workup should include thorough inspection with cystourethroscopy to ensure that no area of erosion or drainage is present. If this is indentified, the device should be surgically removed.

## Prophylaxis

Certain antibiotic regimens can be used for UTI prophylaxis. It is important to note, however, the difference between prophylaxis and suppression. Prophylactic therapy is administered for infections that have been treated with complete resolution of the bacteria. Suppressive therapy is when medication is given to suppress bacteria that cannot be fully eradicated. Surgical prophylaxis is when an antibiotic is administered for a short duration before and after a surgical procedure. If a patient has recurrent UTIs, it is often useful to administer a low dose of antibiotic to help prevent the recurrent episodes. Common regimens include:

- TMP–SMZ 40/200 mg qday
- Nitrofurantoin 50 or 100 mg qday
- Ciprofloxacin 250 mg qday
- Cephalexin 250 mg qday

The use of prophylactic antibiotics in patients with indwelling catheters is not recommended, as colonization is common and antibiotic use encourages the development of bacterial resistance [26].

## Upper Urinary Tract

Recurrent UTIs involving the upper urinary tract (kidneys, renal pelvis, and ureters) stem from:

- Ascending infections from the lower urinary tract
- Anatomic abnormalities—intrinsic and extrinsic
- Foreign objects—such as stones or implanted devices

Regarding ascending infections from the lower urinary tract, please refer to the section—*Lower urinary tract*, as management and prevention of the underlying etiology is discussed at length. Anatomic abnormalities encompass any of the following including reflux from the bladder, fistulous tracts, or narrowing anywhere along this tract—including the ureterovesical or ureteropelvic junction, ureters, or renal infundibulae. Additionally, intrinsic causes may be congenital, primary urothelial malignancies, or scarring. Recurrent infections secondary to congenitally anomalous upper urinary tract generally present in children [27, 28] and are a rare consideration in the adult male patient who has no remote history of UTIs. Extrinsic causes are varied, and encompass compression from any surrounding organ, vessel or fluid collection, as well as inflammation, fibrosis or surrounding malignancy. This narrowing results in obstruction, urinary status, and eventual infection. Foreign objects such as stones may cause obstruction but may initially serve as a nidus for infection and then a platform for the formation of a biofilm [29]. Less commonly, one may have recurrent infections of the upper urinary tract secondary to hematogenous seeding. If no genitourinary etiology is identified, and there is a high incidence of suspicion for systemic causes, an echocardiogram may be indicated to rule out a cardiac source. Consultation with an internal medicine specialist should be considered.

### Signs and Symptoms

Similar to lower UTIs, patients often present with irritative voiding symptoms. More common to upper tract infections are

- High fevers/chills
- Leukocytosis
- Nausea
- Vomiting
- Decreased appetite
- Flank pain
- Costovertebral angle tenderness

This pain associated with the upper tract may be due to the primary infection and inflammation of the tissue as well as distention from obstruction of the tract [30].

### Workup

As with all clinical investigations, a complete history and physical exam should be performed. This history should include inquiry of:

- Childhood UTIs
- Kidney stones and or the passage of stones
- Malignancies
- Abdominal or pelvic radiation
- Intra-abdominal surgery or trauma
- Instrumentation
- Implanted devices

Physical exam should be thorough, with close attention to percussion of the back to identify any costovertebral angle tenderness. Laboratory tests should include urine analysis, urine culture, complete blood count (CBC), and basic metabolic panel. Upper tract infections will demonstrate similar findings on urine analysis as lower tract infections but also may have white blood cell (WBC) casts and proteinuria [31, 32]. If uncompensated obstruction is present or there is severe pyelonephritis, one may have elevated creatinine, and leukocytosis.

Imaging is often helpful in the diagnosis of upper tract etiology. Techniques used commonly are:

- Ultrasound
- X-ray of kidneys, ureter, and bladder (KUB)
- CT KUB/urogram
- MRI urogram
- Ureteropyeloscopy
- Fluoroscopy—pyelogram
- Nuclear renogram

Ultrasound of the kidneys and bladder is a safe and relatively inexpensive way to identify gross abnormalities such as hydronephrosis or large kidney lesions. More specific imaging is generally warranted if the etiology of the recurrent infections is not elucidated by history and physical. Moreover, imaging is often crucial to comprehensive treatment planning. If nephrolithiasis is highly suspected, a noncontrast CT scan is sufficient for definitive localization of the stones. If a known device such as a ureteral stent is the suspected culprit, a simple KUB may be sufficient for localization and confirmation. Generally, a CT urogram, a contrast study with delayed images taken when contrast is secreted into the upper urinary tract, is excellent for elucidation of upper urinary tract pathology. This study should not be performed in patients with iodine contrast allergy, and renal insufficiency (GFR < 30 mL/min/1.73 $m^2$). For individuals with GFR between 30 and 60 mL/min/1.73 $m^2$, reduced iodine contrast loads should be considered [33]. An alternative to CT urogram is MR urogram, which does not involve ionizing radiation or iodinated contrast media. Similar to CT contrast studies, some level of impairment is tolerated, but a GFR < 30 mL/min/1.73 $m^2$ may not be sufficient to excrete the gadolinium contrast, and in addition these individuals are at increased risk of nephrogenic systemic sclerosis [33, 34].

If the above imaging techniques have resulted in an incomplete evaluation, more invasive diagnostics may be required. Direct visualization of the upper urinary tract can be conducted by endoscopic means using ureteropyeloscopy. Sampling of urine as well as biopsies can be taken at this time for further investigation of the infection or possible malignancy. Concurrent with ureteroscopy, one also can perform fluoroscopic delineation of the anatomy with a pyelogram. These more invasive approaches are often linked with interventions, which will be further outlined in the management portion of this section.

Appropriate treatment for the underlying pathology may depend on whether or not residual kidney function is present on the affected side. Should minimal function remain secondary to chronic obstruction, attempting directed treatments may be less successful than a simple nephrectomy. Determination of remaining kidney function can be performed with a nuclear renogram. This study is performed by intravenous injection of a radioisotope, which is subsequently filtered and secreted by the kidneys. The amount of isotope secreted is analyzed and allows one to quantify split kidney function, and relative obstruction. Common radioisotopes utilized for assessing kidney function, and presence of possible obstruction are MAG3 (Technetium-99 m mercaptoacetyltrigylcine), DTPA (Technetium-99 m diethylenetriamine pentaacetic acid), and DMSA (Technetium-99 m dimercaptosuccine acid) [35].

## Management

Treatment of recurrent upper tract UTIs first and foremost involves proper antibiotic selection and duration, as well as confirmation of resolution with repeat urine analysis and urine culture [36]. Medical management of urosepsis initially takes precedence over definitive treatment of the upper tract lesion; however in the setting of complete obstruction or abscess, antibiotic penetration will be zero and medical therapy will only treat the systemic infection in the blood. Emergent and or temporizing interventions are often needed in the acute setting as a means to allow for complete treatment of the active infection. Measures include placement of ureteral stents or percutaneous nephrostomy tubes for ureteral obstruction, percutaneous drainage of abscesses, or in extreme circumstances nephrectomy for emphysematous pyelonephritis or xanthogranulomatous pyelonephritis [37, 38]. When the upper tract is involved, antibiotic therapy should be tailored to the individual, but treatment course should be for a minimum of 14 days [39–41]. After resolution of active infection and medical stabilization of the patient, definitive treatments can be undertaken.

## Anatomic Abnormalities—Intrinsic and Extrinsic

Optimal treatment for obstruction of the upper urinary tract is accomplished through the use of techniques, which directly alleviate the narrowing in a permanent fashion. In individuals that are poor surgical candidates temporizing measures such as ureteral stents or percutaneous nephrostomy tubes may be a reasonable and necessary alternative [42]. Stents may obstruct with extrinsic compression, or may not pass if the stricture is too complete. Under these circumstances, a nephrostomy tube may be preferred [43]. For individuals with chronic obstruction unrelated to urolithiaisis, metal stents are a more durable and successful alternative [44]. Additionally, these stents allow for less frequent exchanges in comparison with their plastic counterparts. If any of these is utilized, they should be exchanged at regular intervals that are recommended by the device manufacturer.

For individuals who are surgical candidates, the following techniques can be used for treatment:

- Ureterovesical reflux (most commonly seen in children) [45, 46]:
  - Ureteroneocystostomy (ureteral reimplant)—open vs. laparoscopic
  - Subureteric injection of bulking agent (Deflux® dextranomer/hyaluronic acid copolymer)—endoscopic
  - Nephrectomy—if minimal to no renal function of ipsilateral side
- Intrinsic Ureteral strictures/UPJ or UVJ obstruction, infundibular stenosis [47–49]:
  - Endoscopic balloon dilation
  - Endoscopic Laser incision
  - Open or laparoscopic repair
  - Partial nephrectomy (infundibular stenosis)
  - Nephrectomy—if minimal to no renal function
- Fistulae—ureteroenteric [50]:
  - Ureterolysis
  - Ureteroureterostomy—if involved ureter cannot be isolated
  - Nephrectomy—if minimal to no renal function
  - Bowel resection—if indicated in the setting of malignancy or inflammatory bowel disease

When upper tract obstruction or a fistulous tract is identified, the presence of malignancy or inflammatory bowel disease should be considered and ruled out. If a primary urothelial cancer is identified through diagnostic means, surgical excision with nephroureterectomy should be considered. With extrinsic lesions, after resection, fluoroscopic pyelogram can be performed to determine whether there is persistence of obstruction [51].

## Foreign Objects

When the presence of a foreign object is the cause of recurrent infection, efforts should be made toward removal and future prevention. Common upper tract foreign objects include nephrolithiasis and implanted devices for the treatment of upper tract obstruction, such as ureteral stents and percutaneous nephrostomy tubes. In the setting of nephrolithiasis, initial management should be geared toward treatment of the acute infection and medical stabilization if upper tract obstruction or sepsis is present. Attention should then be directed toward complete removal of the stone(s), and prevention and treatment of an underlying metabolic abnormality. Methods at definitive removal of stones should not be attempted until one has confirmation of sterilization of urine due to the significant risk of bacteremia and sepsis. The techniques used for stone removal will depend on the location and size [52]. Small stones may be amenable to medical expulsion with alpha blockers and

**Table 5.1** Stone composition, metabolic abnormalities and associated conditions

| Stone composition | Predisposing conditions | Metabolic abnormality | Prevention strategies |
|---|---|---|---|
| Calcium oxalate<br>Calcium phosphate | Primary hyperparathyroidism<br>Medullary sponge kidney<br>Distal (type 1) renal tubular acidosis | Hypercalciuria<br>Hyperoxaluria<br>Hypocitraturia<br>Alkaline pH<br>Dehydration | Decreased Na<br>Oral hydration<br>Potassium citrate<br>Thiazide<br>Parathyroidectomy (hyperparathyroidism) |
| Uric acid | Hyperuricosuria | Acid urine, pH<6 | Allopurinol |
| Struvite | UTI—chronic urease producing bacterial colinization | Alkaline urine | Urine acidification |
| Cystine | Cystinuria | Acid urine | Urine alkalization |

aggressive oral hydration alone. If large stones are present, or the patient has failed a reasonable trial of passage, the following are different techniques that urologists utilize for stone elimination [52, 53]:

- Endoscopic removal, laser lithotripsy—small stones, generally in the ureter
- Extracorporal shock wave lithotripsy—small stones in the kidney, renal pelvis
- Percutaneous nephrolithotomy—large stones/staghorn calculi, in the kidney, renal pelvis

Should multiple stones be found, prevention of future stone formation should be targeted according to stone composition and underlying metabolic abnormalities. Over 70% of urinary tract stones contain calcium [54]. Basic strategies at prevention include aggressive oral hydration and decreased sodium intake. In the case of multiple stones or recurrent formation, further metabolic workup may be indicated in the form of a 24-h urine collection [55]. See Table 5.1 for common stones formed, as well as associated metabolic abnormalities and treatment prevention strategies [55].

Temporizing methods for elimination of upper tract obstruction may include placement of ureteral stents or nephrostomy tubes. These techniques employ the placement of inert tubes into the body, which with increased time may lead to biofilm formation, stone encrustation, and recurrent UTIs. As a result, if placed, the underlying cause of obstruction should be treated expeditiously, and if chronic diversion is needed, the device should be exchanged strictly according to the manufacturer's recommendations.

## Prostatitis

Quite prevalent, prostatitis accounts for approximately 8% of ambulatory urologic visits as documented by the National Ambulatory Medical Care Surveys [56]. Prostatitis is a broad clinical term used to describe conditions of inflammation, infection, and/or pain associated with the prostate gland. In 1995, the NIH constructed a classification scheme to organize the different pathology encompassed [57]. Please see Fig. 5.1 for the detailed description of the four categories. As outlined, prostatitis is a term used with conditions of the prostate that are related both to infectious etiology and to those which are not. The remainder of the chapter will primarily focus on signs and symptoms, workup, and management of types I and II prostatitis as they relate to recurrent UTIs. These two categories are the only two specifically associated with infectious etiology. More specifically, type II prostatitis is the most common cause of recurrent UTI in the adult male patient, and accounts for 10–15% of all prostatitis patients [58–60].

## Prostatitis Classification [57]

### Signs and Symptoms

Acute bacterial prostatitis (type I) is the least common form [60]. Associated signs and symptoms may include irritative voiding symptoms (frequency, urgency, and dysuria), hesitancy, acute urinary retention, localized pain to the

| NIH Category | Alternate Terminology | Description | Prostatic Fluid |
|---|---|---|---|
| I | Acute Bacterial Prostatitis | Acute bacterial infection | (massage contraindicated) |
| II | Chronic bacterial prostatitis | Chronic prostate infection | + bacteria, + WBC |
| IIIa | Chronic pelvic pain syndrome: inflammatory | Pelvic pain with Prostate inflammation w/out infection | - bacteria, + WBC |
| IIIb | Chronic pelvic pain syndrome: noninflammatory | Pelvic pain without Prostate inflammation/w/o infection | - bacteria, - WBC |
| IV | Asymptomatic inflammatory prostatitis | Incidentally detected | +/- bacteria, +/- bacteria |

**Fig. 5.1** Prostatitis classification

perineum, genitals, suprapubic, and inguinal regions as well as painful ejaculation. In most cases, systemic signs and symptoms may be associated including fevers, chills, nausea, vomiting, elevated WBC count, and in severe cases sepsis involving potential hemodynamic instability.

Individuals with type II prostatitis may have similar symptoms as those with type I, including the irritative voiding symptoms as outlined above. Generally, systemic signs of severe infection are not present. They often report recurrent, symptomatic episodes as well as recurrent UTIs, urethritis, or epididymitis.

## Workup

The diagnosis of bacterial prostatitis is largely accomplished with complete history and physical exam. Close attention to both will allow one to rule out noninfectious causes in most cases. The history should focus on frequency and time course of previous prostate infections, as well as risk factors for bacterial introduction into the prostate gland, which include [61–63]:

- Phimosis
- UTI
- Unprotected anal intercourse
- Acute epididymitis
- Condom or indwelling urethral catheter drainage
- Endoscopic transurethral surgery

Physical exam should be thorough with great attention given to the digital rectal exam. Abdominal exam may reveal suprapubic tenderness and or a full bladder if associated urinary retention is present. An infected prostate on exam may feel tender and be associated with a fever.

Often individuals with chronic bacterial prostatitis have a benign physical exam. If a chronic infection is suspected, the diagnostic gold standard is the "Meares–Stamey Four-glass" urine collection method [63]. This technique allows the examiner to isolate the anatomic location of the contributing infection. One should not perform a DRE prior to collection as it may contaminate the initial sample. The following outlines the appropriate collection technique, and the associated anatomic area targeted for culture:

- First 10 mL of voided bladder specimen (VB-1)—urethra
- Midstream urine (VB-2)—bladder
- Prostate massage is performed, and expressed prostate secretions (EPS) collected—prostate
- First 10 mL voided after prostate massage (VB-3)—prostate

Anything more than a gentle DRE should be avoided in patients with acute bacterial prostatitis as a simple voided specimen will generally be positive for bacteria and there can be an increased risk of bacteremia. With chronic bacterial prostatitis, there will be a minimum of 10× greater presence of bacteria in EPS or VB-3 vs. VB-2.

A simpler version of the four-glass technique involves the two-glass technique, which has 91% sensitivity and specificity to the four-glass technique [64, 65]. Utilizing this method, one collects a pre- and post-massage specimen. The post-massage specimen should only include the first 10 $cm^3$ of voided urine. Alternatively, a urethral swab plus post-massage specimen may be used, and has demonstrated high specificity and sensitivity to the two-glass technique [64, 66]. The latter techniques are favored by these authors.

Alternative diagnostic measures including imaging, cystoscopy, biopsy, and physiologic testing in the form of urodynamics are not routinely utilized. Imaging such as prostate ultrasound or pelvic MRI may be helpful if abscess or prostatic calculi, or ejaculatory duct obstruction is suggested [67–70].

### Management

Historically, prostate massage was the primary therapy for chronic bacterial prostatitis. Antibacterial therapy is now the standard of care for both acute and chronic bacterial prostatitis [64, 71–74]. If an underlying cause such as an indwelling Foley catheter is present, efforts to improve infection control should be employed, such as surgical management of urinary obstruction, suprapubic tube placement, or every 3–4 weeks clean exchanges of the Foley catheter.

The cornerstone of diagnosis and direction of treatment involves fluid culture—either urine or expressed prostate secretions. Typical pathogens associated are *E. coli*, as well as other common bacteria that are colonized in the gastrointestinal tract such as *Enterococci*, *Pseudomonas aeruginosa*, *Serratia*, *Klebsiella*, *Proteus*, *Staphylococcus*, and *Enterobacter aerogenes* [60, 69, 75–77]. Antibiotic selection should be tailored to specific bacteria cultures as well as to antibiotic sensitivities.

Antibiotic penetrance into the prostate is compromised secondary to the strong prostatic epithelial cell lipid membrane. As a result, lipophilic antibiotics are recommended that are able to more readily penetrate the prostate. Antibiotics which fit this criteria are fluoroquinolones, TMP–SMZ, clindamycin, erythromycin, and doxycycline [74, 77, 78]. Severe infection with associated sepsis requires hospitalization with acute medical management. Should a patient have urinary retention with associated prostatitis, one should not place a urethral Foley catheter but consider placement of suprapubic tube to avoid urethral manipulations and further bacterial seeding. For individuals with recurrent or chronic infection, a longer course of culture-specific antibiotics is indicated. Treatment may take up to 2–4 months, but quinolone therapy for 4 weeks is equal or superior to TMP/SMX therapy for 12 weeks. The quinolones used for 4 weeks each in these studies were Cipro 500 mg po bid, Norfloxacin 400 mg po bid, and Levaquin 500 mg po qday [60, 78–81]. Should recurrence take place, a suppressive antibiotic regimen should be employed, using a lower dose of culture sensitive antibiotic (TMP–SMX single strength one tab daily or ciprofloxacin 250 mg po qdaily), and continued for a minimum of 6 months [60].

Surgical resection of the prostate may be considered in patients with associated infected prostatic calculi and prostatic abscesses. The use of transrectal ultrasound and drainage of an abscess is now more practical than a transurethral approach [82]. With transurethral instrumentation, the risk of seeding is extremely high and this is a last resort when one's incidence of suspicion for infected stones refractory to antibiotic treatment or prostate abscess is suspected.

## Urethritis

Urethritis is the inflammation of the urethra, which may include infectious or noninfectious causes. Young, sexually active men are at the highest risk for infectious urethritis, as the most common bacterial sources are Gonorrhea and Chlamydia, which are transmitted via sexual contact. Risk factors for noninfectious urethritis include prior catheterizations, urethral stones, strictures, or lesions. For both etiologies, dysuria, or painful urination with burning during or just after urination, is the most common presenting symptom. In this section, we will discuss the symptoms, workup and management of urethritis.

## Signs and Symptoms

While the most common presenting symptom is dysuria, men often present with purulent discharge or pruritis, as well as nonspecific general LUTS such as frequency and urgency. Profuse purulent discharge suggests a diagnosis of gonococcal urethritis while scant or clear discharge is more often associated with nongonococcal urethritis. Diagnosis should not be made on symptoms alone, as it is important to note that 40% of patients with urethritis are asymptomatic at presentation. Patients with recurrent urethritis may develop obstructive voiding symptoms, as they are at higher risk for developing urethral strictures.

## Workup

As with any infection, the first step toward diagnosis is a thorough history and physical exam. A sexual history should be taken, with attention to any unprotected intercourse or multiple partners. Physical exam should include a thorough GU exam, with particular attention to any urethral discharge. A direct sample of the urethra or urine collected from the first 30–40 $cm^3$ of the voided stream should be obtained and sent for analysis. This ensures that a sample of cells from the urethra is collected. There are a variety of diagnostic modalities that can detect Gonorrhea, including culture on Thayer–Martin agar, microscopy, or DNA analysis. Evidence of leukocyte esterase in the urinalysis supports the diagnosis of urethritis, although it is a nonspecific finding for this condition. Culturing the specimen is convenient for many labs and is relatively inexpensive. Also, it allows for reporting of specificities of the bacteria, which is useful for resistant organisms. However, the test takes 48 h of turn over time and the low sensitivity produces many false-negative results [83]. For this reason, the CDC recommends using nucleic acid amplification test (NAAT) for diagnosis of Gonorrhea and Chlamydia [84]. While the cost of this test is higher, the sensitivity is much improved. In symptomatic men, the diagnosis can be made easily in the laboratory using microscopy. By simply analyzing a sample of the urethral fluid (collected with cotton swab 2–3 cm from the meatus) under a microscope, the diagnosis can be made with visualization of gram-negative diplococcic. The sensitivity and specificity of this test drops off, however, if the patient is asymptomatic. Other organisms responsible for urethritis include [85]:

- *Mycoplasma genitalium*
- *Mycoplasma hominis*
- *Ureaplasma urealyticum*
- *Trichomonas vaginalis*
- Herpes simplex virus
- Adenovirus

Along with *Chlamydia trachomatis*, these comprise the subset of urethritis referred to as nongonococcal urethritis. These are often not tested for on initial presentation, although should be considered if the infection persists after treatment. Imaging is not indicated in the workup for urethritis unless the patient has a history of recurrent infections and obstructive voiding symptoms, which would put him at risk for urethral stricture disease. In this event, a retrograde urethrogram would be useful.

## Management

Antibiotic treatment for urethritis should be directed at pathogen-specific disease. However, given that close to 40% of patients who are diagnosed with Gonorrhea are also co-infected with Chlamydia, the current CDC guidelines recommend treating for both infections, even if the *C. trachomatis* assay is negative at presentation. Gonococcal urethritis can be treated with ceftriaxone IM or oral Cefixime. Nongonococcal urethritis can be treated with Doxycycline 100 mg po bid for 1 week, or azithromycin 1 g po for one dose. Alternative regimens include erythromycin, levofloxacin, or ofloxacin. If the infection does not resolve, ensure that the patient's sexual partners have been evaluated and treated. Consider testing specifically for the other causes of urethritis, such as trichomonas, ureaplasma, mycoplasma, or herpes [86].

## Conclusion

Men with recurrent UTIs present a dilemma for the primary care physician as well as the urologist. Generally speaking, a recurrent UTI in a man is a sign that there is an anatomic abnormality or dysfunction at some point along the urinary tract. Investigation is aimed at identifying and then treating this abnormality. The cornerstone of treatment is appropriate antibiotic choice, which should be directed toward bacterial sensitivities. After the treatment course is completed, confirmation of resolution should be obtained with negative cultures. To prevent further recurrence, correction of the underlying cause of the bacterial entry into the urinary system should be investigated and appropriately managed.

## References


1. Schaeffer AJ. Role of vaginal colonization in urinary tract infections. Adv Exp Med Biol. 1999;462:339.
2. National Health and Nutrition Examination Survey III, 1988–1994.
3. Sobel JD. Pathogenesis of urinary tract infection: role of host defenses. Infect Dis Clin North Am. 1997;11:531.
4. Platt R. Quantitative definition of bacteriuria. Am J Med. 1983;75(1B):44–52.
5. Patel HD. Can urine dipstick testing for urinary tract infection at point of care reduce laboratory workload? J Clin Pathol. 2005;6(1):18–31.
6. Wilson ML. Laboratory diagnosis of urinary tract infections in adult patients. Clin Infect Dis. 2004;38(8):1150–8.
7. Miller LG. Treatment of uncomplicated urinary tract infections in an era of increasing antibicrobial resistance. Mayo Clin Proc. 2004;79(8):2048–53.
8. Wagenlehner FM. Hospital-acquired urinary tract infections. J Hosp Infect. 2000;46:171.
9. Brown PD. Prevalence and predictors of trimethoprim-sulfamethoxazole resistance among uropathogenic *Escherichia coli* isolates in Michigan. Clin Infect Dis. 2002;34:1061.
10. Karaca Y. Co-trimoxazole and quinolone resistance in *Escherichia coli* isolated from urinary tract infections over the last 100 years. Int J Antimicrob Agents. 2005;26(1):75–7.
11. Heyns CF. Urinary tract infection associated with conditions causing urinary tract obstruction and stasis, excluding urolithiasis and neuropathic bladder. World J Urol. 2011 [July 1; Epub ahead of print].
12. Thorpe A. Benign prostatic hyperplasia. Lancet. 2003;361(9366):1359–67.
13. Takeda M. Diagnosis and treatment of voiding symptoms. Urology. 2003;62(5):11–9.
14. May M. Post-void residual urine as a predictor of urinary tract infections—is there a cutoff in asymptomatic men? J Urol. 2009;181(6):2540–4.
15. O'Leary MP. Lower urinary tract symptoms/benign prostatic hyperplasia: maintaining symptom control and reducing early complications. Urology. 2003;62 (3 Suppl 1):15–23.
16. Zivan I. New modality for treatment of resistant anstamotic strictures after radical prostatectomy: UroLume Urethral stent. J Endourol. 2001;15(8):869–71.
17. Jepsen JV. Comprehensive patient evaluation for benign prostatic hyperplasia. Urology. 1998;51(Suppl 4A):13–8.
18. Blaivas JG. Obstructive uropathy in the male. Urol Clin North Am. 1996;23(3):373–84.
19. Gould CV. Guideline for prevention of catheter-associated urinary tract infections, 2009. Infect Control Hosp Epidemiol. 2010;31:319.
20. Schaberg DR. Nosocomial bacteriuria: a prospective study of case clustering and antimicrobial resistance. Ann Intern Med. 1980;93(3):420–4.
21. Kass EH. Entry of bacteria into the urinary tracts of patients with inlying catheters. N Engl J Med. 1957;256(12):556.
22. Schumm K. Types of urethral catheters for management of short-term voiding problems in hospitalized adults. Neurourol Urodyn. 2008;27(8):738–46.
23. Horgan AFB. Acute urinary retention. Comparison of suprapubic and urethral catheterization. Br J Urol. 1992;70:149–51.
24. Warren JW. Antibiotic irrigation and catheter-associated urinary-tract infections. N Eng J Med. 1978; 299:570.
25. Burton DC. Trends in catheter-associated urinary tract infections in adult intensive care units—United States, 1990–2007. Infect Control Hosp Epidemiol. 2011; 32(3):748–56.
26. Clarke SA. Are prophylactic antibiotics necessary with clean intermittent catheterization? A randomized controlled trial. J Pediatr Surg. 2005;40:568–71.
27. Johnston JH. The pathogenesis of hydronephrosis in children. B J Urol. 1969;41:724–34.
28. Johnston JH. Pelvic hydronephrosis in children: a review of 219 personal cases. J Urol. 1977;117(1):97–101.
29. Anderson GG. Intracellular bacterial biofilm-like pods in urinary tract infections. Science. 2003; 301(5629):105–7.
30. Bass PF. Urinary tract infections. Prim Care. 2003; 30(1):41–61.
31. Pollock HM. Laboratory techniques for detection of urinary tract infections and assessment of value. Am J Med. 1983;75(1B):79–84.
32. Pfaller MA. Laboratory evaluation of leukocyte esterase and nitrite tests for the detection of bacteriuria. J Clin Microbiol. 1985;21(5):840–2.

33. Silverman SG. What is the current role of CT urography and MR urography in the evaluation of the urinary tract? Radiology. 2009;250(2):309–23.
34. Leyendecker JR. MR urography: techniques and clinical applications. Radiographics. 2008;28(1):23–46.
35. Sfakianakis GN. A renal protocol for all ages and all indications: mercapto-acetyl-triglycine (MAG3) with simultaneous injection of furosemide (MAG3-F0): a 17-year experience. Semin Nucl Med. 2009;39(3):156–73.
36. Roberts JA. Management of pyelonephritis and upper urinary tract infections. Urol Clin North Am. 1999;26(4):753–63.
37. Chen MT. Percutaneous drainage in the treatment of emphysematous pyelonephritis: 10-year experience. J Urol. 1997;157(5):1569–73.
38. Eastham J. Xanthogranulomatous pyelonephritis: clinical findings and surgical considerations. Urology. 1994;43(3):295–9.
39. Nickel JC. The management of acute pyelonephritis in adults. Can J Urol. 2001;8 Suppl 1:29–38.
40. Bader MS. Management of complicated urinary tract infections in the era of antimicrobial resistance. Postgrad Med. 2010;122(6):7–15.
41. Ramakrishnan K. Diagnosis and management of acute pyelonephritis in adults. Am Fam Physician. 2005; 71(5):933–42.
42. Barton DP. Percutaneous nephrostomy and ureteral stenting in gynecologic malignancies. Obstet Gynecol. 1992;80(5):805–11.
43. Plesinac-Karapandzic V. Percutaneous nephrostomy in the management of advanced and terminal-stage gynecologic malignancies: outcome and complications. Eur J Gynaecol Oncol. 2010;31(6):645–50.
44. Benson A. Metal ureteral stent for benign and malignant ureteral obstruction. J Urol. 2011;185(6):2217–22.
45. Pichler R. Endoscopic treatment of vesicoureteral reflux using dextranomer/hyaluronic acid copolymer in children: results of postoperative follow-up with real-time 3D sonography. Urol Int. 2011 [Aug 24; Epub ahead of print].
46. Sung J. Surgical management of vesicoureteral reflux in children. Pediatr Nephrol. 2011 [Jun 22; Epub ahead of print].
47. Corcoran AT. Management of benign ureteral strictures in the endoscopic era. J Endourol. 2009; 23(11):1909–12.
48. Rassweiler JJ. Ureteral reimplantation for management of ureteral strictures: a retrospective comparison of laparoscopic and open techniques. Eur Urol. 2007;51(2):512–22.
49. Salehipour M. Open dismembered tubularized flap pyeloplasty: an effective and simple operation for treatment of ureteropelvic junction obstruction. Urol Int. 2006;76(4):345–7.
50. Chang JH. Uretero-enteric fistula. Br J Urol. 1998; 81(1):162–3.
51. Hyams ES. Malignant extrinsic ureteral obstruction: a survey of urologists and medical oncologists regarding treatment patterns and preferences. Urology. 2008; 72(1):51–6.
52. Wolf JS. Treatment selection and outcomes: ureteral calculi. Urol Clin North Am. 2007;34(3):421–30.
53. Pearle MS. Prospective randomized trial comparing shock wave lithotripsy and ureteroscopy for management of distal ureteral calculi. J Urol. 2001;166(4): 1255–60.
54. Gault MH. Relationship of frequency, age, sex, stone weight and composition in 15,624 stones: comparison of results for 1980 to 1983 and 1995 to 1998. J Urol. 2000;164(2):302–7.
55. Johri N. An update and practical guide to renal stone management. Nephron Clin Pract. 2010;116(3): c159–71.
56. McNaughton-Collins M. How common is prostatitis? A national survey of physician visits. J Urol. 1998;159(4):1224–8.
57. Krieger JN. NIH consensus definition and classification of prostatitis. JAMA. 1999;282(3):236–7.
58. Wagenlehner FM. Fluoroquinolone antimicrobial agents in the treatment of prostatitis and recurrent urinary tract infections in men. Curr Urol Rep. 2004;5(4):309–16.
59. Schaeffer AJ. Prevalence and significance of prostatic inflammation. J Urol. 1981;125(2):215–9.
60. Weidner W. Chronic prostatitis: a thorough search for etiologically involved microorganisms in 1,461 patients. Infection. 1991;19 Suppl 3:S119–25.
61. Van Howe RS. Circumcision and infectious diseases revisited. Pediatr Infect Dis. 1998;17(1):1–6.
62. Berger RE. Etiology and manifestations of epididymitis in young men: correlations with sexual orientation. J Infect Dis. 1987;155(6):1341–3.
63. Meares Jr EM, Stamey TA. Bacteriologic localization patterns in bacterial prostatitis and urethritis. Invest Urol. 1968;5(5):492–518.
64. McNaughton Collins M. Diagnosing and treating chronic prostatitis: do urologists use the four-glass test? Urology. 2000;55(3):403–7.
65. Nickel JC. How does the pre-massage and post-massage 2-glass test compare to the Meares–Stamey 4-glass test in men with chronic prostatitis/chronic pelvic pain syndrome? J Urol. 2006;176(1):119–24.
66. Magri V. Microscopic and microbiological findings for evaluation of chronic prostatitis. Arch Ital Urol Androl. 2005;77(2):135–8.
67. Doble A. Ultrasonographic findings in prostatitis. Urol Clin North Am. 1989;16:763–72.
68. Berger RE. Bacteria in the prostate tissue of men with idiopathic prostatic inflammation. J Urol. 1997; 157(3):863–5.
69. Nickel JC. Bacterial localization in antibiotic-refractory chronic bacterial prostatitis. Prostate. 1993; 23(2):107–14.
70. Schaeffer AJ. Overview summary statement. Diagnosis and management of chronic prostatitis/chronic pelvic pain syndrome (CP/CPPS). Urology. 2002;60 Suppl 6:1–4.

71. Bergman B. On the relevance of gram-positive bacteria in prostatitis. Infection. 1994;22 Suppl 1:S22.
72. De la Rosette JJ. Diagnosis and treatment of 409 patients with prostatitis syndromes. Urology. 1993; 41(4):301–7.
73. Nickel JC. Prostatitis: myths and realities. Urology. 1998;51(3):362–6.
74. Becopoulos T. Acute prostatitis: which antibiotic to use first. J Chemother. 1990;2(4):244–6.
75. Stamey TA. Pathogenesis and treatment of urinary tract infections. Baltimore: Williams & Wilkins; 1980. p. 343–429.
76. Meares Jr EM. Acute and chronic prostatitis: diagnosis and treatment. Infect Dis Clin North Am. 1987;1(4): 855–73.
77. Neal DE Jr. In: Nickel JC, editor. Textbook of prostatitis. Oxford: ISIS Medical Media; 1999. p. 279–284.
78. Nickel JC. Prostatitis: evolving management strategies. Urol Clin North Am. 1999;26(4):743–51.
79. Schaeffer AJ. The efficacy of norfloxacin in the treatment of chronic bacterial prostatitis refractory to trimethoprim-sulfamethoxazole and/or carbenicillin. J Urol. 1990;144(3):690–3.
80. Bundrick W. Levofloxacin versus ciprofloxacin in the treatment of chronic bacterial prostatitis: a randomized double-blind multicenter study. Urology. 2003; 62(3):537–41.
81. Koff W. Clinical trial comparing lomefloxacin and ofloxacin in the treatment of chronic bacterial prostatis. Rev Bras Med. 1996;53:88–91.
82. Granados EA. Prostatic abscess: diagnosis and treatment. J Urol. 1992;148(1):80–2.
83. Koumans EH. Laboratory testing for *Neisseria gonorrhoeae* by recently introduced nonculture tests: a performance review with clinical and public health considerations. Clin Infect Dis. 1998;27(5):1171–80.
84. Van Dyck E. Detection of *Chlamydia trachomatis* and *Neisseria gonorrhoeae* by enzyme immunoassay, culture, and three nucleic acid amplification tests. J Clin Microbiol. 2001;39(5):1751–6.
85. Deguchi T. Mycoplasma genitalium: another important pathogen of nongonococcal urethritis. J Urol. 2002;167(3):1210–7.
86. Centers for Disease Control and Prevention. Updated recommended treatment regimens for gonococcal infections and associated conditions—United States 2007.

# Evaluation and Medical Management of BPH and LUTS in Men

6

Bilal Chughtai, Richard Lee, Matthew Hall, and Alexis E. Te

## Introduction

Voiding symptoms impair health-related quality of life (QoL). In males, lower urinary tract symptoms (LUTS) is typically attributed to benign prostatic hyperplasia (BPH). Approximately, half of men above the age of 40 will develop a histological diagnosis of BPH [1]. Of these patients, about half will develop LUTS [2]. The histological diagnosis of BPH increases with age [3]. Treatments for BPH are aimed at improving subjective symptoms, preventing disease progression, and improving QoL. First-line therapy is usually medical, with surgical therapy usually reserved for medication failure or complications (Table 6.1).

B. Chughtai, MD
Department of Urology, Weill Cornell Medical Center, 525 East 68th Street, Suite F9W, Box 261, New York, NY 10065, USA
e-mail: bic9008@med.cornell.edu

R. Lee, MD
Department of Urology, Weill-Cornell Medical College of Cornell University, New York, NY, USA

M. Hall, MD, BS
Physician, Department of Urology, Mount Sinai School of Medicine, New York, NY, USA
e-mail: Matthew.Hall@mssm.edu;

A.E. Te, MD (✉)
Department of Urology, Weill Cornell Medical Center, Brady Prostate Center and Urodynamic Laboratory, New York Presbyterian-Cornell, 1300 York Avenue, F9 West, Box 261, New York, NY 11030, USA
e-mail: aet2005@med.cornell.edu

## Assessment of Male LUTS

Any patient assessment should begin with a thorough history and physical examination. The medical history should include any causes that may lead to bladder dysfunction including cerebral vascular accidents, previous surgical procedures, and history of prostate disease. It is equally important to review medications, for example, diuretics that impact urinary symptoms. The physical examination should also include a prostate exam to evaluate size and the presence of nodules and a focused neurologic examination, which assesses a patient's mental status, ambulatory status, lower extremity neuromuscular function, and anal sphincter tone. A urinalysis should be performed to screen for blood and infection. Bladder cancer, carcinoma in situ of the bladder, urethral strictures, and stones can also produce LUTS in aging men. Urine cytology may be obtained in patients with irritative symptoms and risk factors. PSA testing should follow the American Urological Association (AUA) guidelines and is most appropriate for patients likely to have a natural life span greater than 10 years and in whom the known presence of prostate cancer would change management. Even though there is not a direct correlation between degree of BPH symptoms and flow rate, serum PSA correlates with prostate volume in the absence of cancer [4–7]. In addition, serum PSA and prostate volume may predict worsening symptoms or need for surgery [4]. Furthermore, urinary symptoms should be assessed with a validated instrument

D.A. Shoskes (ed.), *Urological Men's Health: A Guide for Urologists and Primary Care Physicians*, Current Clinical Urology, DOI 10.1007/978-1-61779-900-6_6,
© Springer Science+Business Media New York 2012

**Table 6.1** List of medications for BPH

| | |
|---|---|
| *Alpha blockers* | |
| | Alfuzosin |
| | Doxazosin |
| | Tamsulosin |
| | Terazosin |
| | Silodosin |
| *5ARI* | |
| | Dutasteride |
| | Finasteride |
| *Alpha blocker and 5ARI* | |
| | Dutasteride and tamsulosin |
| *Anticholinergics* | |
| | Darifenacin |
| | Fesoterodine |
| | Oxybutynin |
| | Oxybutynin XL |
| | Tolterodine |
| | Tolterodine LA |
| | Trospium |
| | Solifenacin |
| *Anticholinergic patches* | |
| | Oxybutynin transdermal |
| *PDE-5 inhibitors* | |
| | Tadalafil |
| | Sildenafil |
| | Vardenafil |

such as the International Prostate Symptom Score (IPSS). Objective parameters such as maximum urinary flow (Qmax) via uroflow and postvoid residual (PVR) can also be measured (Fig. 6.1). Cystoscopy should be included in the evaluation when there is a history of previous lower urinary tract surgery, stricture disease, or during a hematuria workup. The utilization of urodynamics is case dependent in order to confirm the presence of outflow obstruction, bladder contractility, and bladder compliance.

## Treatment Options

### Observation

Patients who are mildly symptomatic, defined as a score 7 or less on the IPSS questionnaire can often be observed. These patients should be counseled about behavioral modifications including fluid restriction, timed voiding and double voiding. Also, patients with moderate symptoms (8–19 points) who are not bothered by their symptoms can be observed as well. These patients should be monitored for recurrent infection, bladder stones, urinary retention, refractory hematuria, or renal dysfunction.

### Phytotherapy

Saw palmetto is a commonly used over-the-counter supplement for LUTS due to BPH. In a placebo-controlled study using saw palmetto extract, it failed to show any improvement in any urinary parameter or subjective parameter measured after a 12-month treatment period [8]. In addition, no guidelines, either AUA or European Association of Urology, supports its use.

### Alpha Blockers

There are three subtypes of $\alpha_1$ adrenergic receptors that have been identified, $\alpha_{1a}$, $\alpha_{1b}$, and $\alpha_{1d}$. $\alpha_{1a}$ receptors have been shown to mediate prostatic smooth-muscle contraction [9]. Alpha blockers decrease bladder outlet resistance provided by urethral smooth and possibly striated sphincter tone to alleviate LUTS [10, 11]. As a class, alpha blockers have a side effect profile that includes orthostatic hypotension and dizziness [12]. The prostate-specific alpha blockers result in retrograde ejaculation. All medications in this class should be stopped prior to cataract surgery for fear of floppy iris syndrome.

### Nonselective Alpha Blockers

#### Prazosin

In a study by Kirby et al., 80 patients were randomized in a double-blind parallel study with prazosin 2 mg bid vs. placebo [13]. Patients in the prazosin arm showed a significant improvement in Qmax with a reduction in the mean number of voids from 10.0 to 7.9 voids/24 h. The efficacy was confirmed by Chapple et al. in a 12-week placebo-controlled study of 93 BPH patients that demonstrated improvements in Qmax [14].

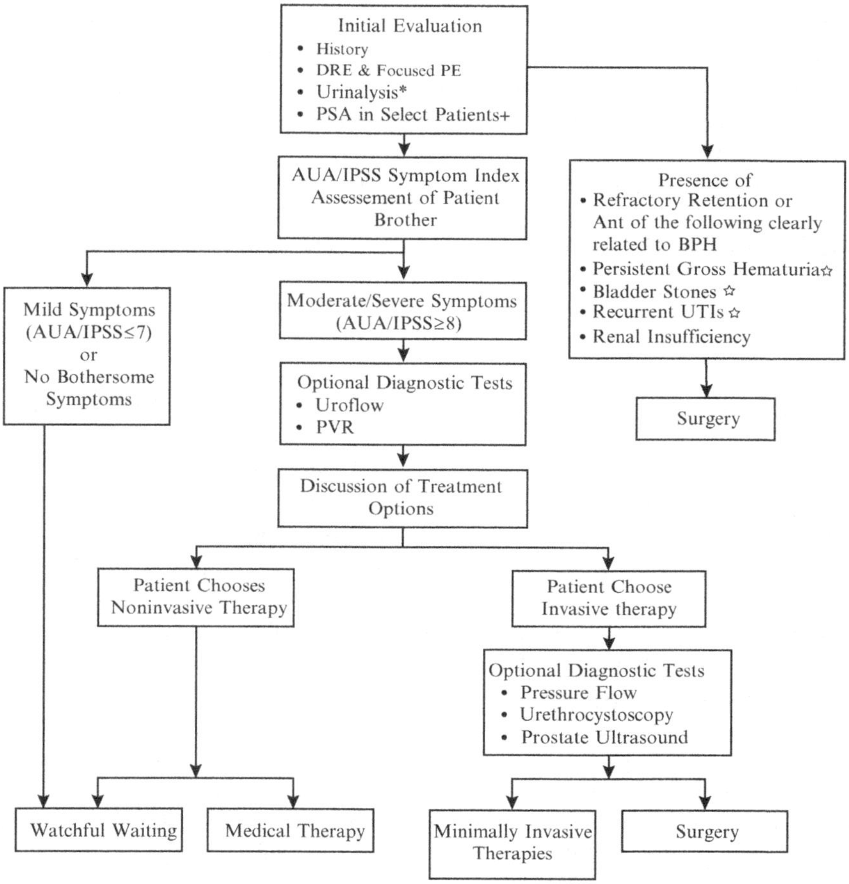


* In patients with clinically significant prostatic bleeding, a course of a 5-alpha reductase inhibitor may be used. If bleeding persists, tissue ablative surgery is indicated.

✧ Patients with at least a 10-year life expectancy for whom knowledge of the presence of prostate would change management or patients for whom the PSA measurement may change the management of voiding symptoms.

☆ After exhausting other therapeutic options.

✧ Some diagnostic tests are used in predicting response to therapy. Pressure-flow studies are most useful in men prior to surgery.

AUA, American Urological Association; DRE, digital rectal exam; IPSS, International Prostate Symptoms Score; PE, physical exam; PSA, prostate-specific antigen; PVR, postvoid resodual urine; UTI, urinary tract infection.

**Fig. 6.1** AUA guidelines BPH diagnosis and treatment. *Reprinted with permission from Benign Prostatic Hyperplasia (revised 2010). McVary, K.T., Roehrborn, C.G., Avins, A.L., Barry, M.J., Bruskewitz, R.C., Donnell, R.F., Foster, Jr., H.E., Gonzalez, C.M., Kaplan, S.A., Penson, D.F., Ulchaker, J.C., Wei, J.T.: American Urological Association Guideline: Management of Benign Prostatic Hyperplasia (BPH) Revised, 2010. American Urological Association Education and Research, Inc., © 2010. http://www.auanet.org/content/guidelines-and-quality-care/clinical-guidelines.cfm?sub=bph*

## Terazosin and Doxazosin

Terazosin and doxazosin are daily dosed with a $t_{1/2}$ of 12 and 22 h, respectively. Multiple studies have demonstrated the efficacy of terazosin [15]. In a study by Lepor et al., 285 men with LUTS due to BPH were randomized to placebo vs. 2, 5, or 10 mg terazosin daily over a 12-week double-blind treatment period [16]. The authors found a statistically significant, dose-dependent improvement in Qmax (1.9 ml/s, $P<0.001$) in the 10 mg treatment group. A greater incidence of postural hypotension was noted in the 5 mg group compared to placebo, although the overall incidence of syncope was less than 0.5%. Doxazosin has also been studied in multiple randomized controlled trials [17–19]. In a study of 100 males who underwent a 16-week double-blind, dose titration trial up to 8 mg of doxazosin. Improvements in Qmax were 2.2 ml/s ($P<0.01$), in addition, treatment groups were superior to placebo in patient and investigator assessments of LUTS associated with BPH [18].

## Selective Alpha Blockers

### Tamsulosin

In order to increase the efficacy of this class of medications while reducing side effects, the concept of receptor selectivity has propelled a newer generation of α-adrenergic antagonists. These medications would theoretically relax prostatic smooth muscle while avoiding the systemic side effects, such as orthostatic hypotension, dizziness, nasal congestion, and fatigue. Two phase III trials studied the selective $\alpha_{1a}$ blocker, tamsulosin. Lepor, in a multicenter study, randomized 756 patients to receive tamsulosin at 0.4 or 0.8 mg vs. placebo over 13 weeks [20]. Statistically significant improvements were noted in both tamsulosin groups compared to placebo as measured by Qmax (1.75 and 1.78 ml/s vs. 0.52 ml/s, $P<0.001$) and AUA symptom score (−8.3 and −9.6 vs. −5.5, $P<0.001$). Although there was a correlation between number of side effects and dose escalation, the overall rate of serious adverse events was low (1–2%). Narayan and Tewari looked at tamsulosin in 735 patients at similar doses over a 13-week period [21]. Similar to the Lepor study, they noted a 25% improvement in American Urological Association Symptom Score (AUASS) and a ≥30% improvement in Qmax compared to placebo. The incidence of orthostatic hypotension was low in the 0.8-mg/day group (2), the 0.4-mg/day group (1), and in the placebo group (0).

### Alfuzosin

Alfuzosin was the second selective alpha-blocker introduced for treating BPH. There were three randomized, double-blind, placebo-controlled trials which comprised the analysis by Roehrborn et al. [22]. A total of 955 patients were randomized to alfuzosin 10 mg vs. placebo over 12 weeks. Alfuzosin significantly improved Qmax by 2.3 ml/s vs. 1.1 ml/s ($P<0.001$) and mean IPSS by −6.0 vs. −4.2 ($P<0.005$) irrespective of prostate size. There were no significant changes in blood pressure and sexual side effects were rare (0.6%).

### Silodosin

Silodosin is a newer selective $\alpha_{1a}$ blocker. In a Phase III study by Kawabe et al. of 457 men with objectively diagnosed BPH in 88 Japanese centers were randomized to receive silodosin 4 mg twice daily, tamsulosin 0.2 mg once daily, or placebo, for 12 weeks. The change in the mean IPSS ± SD total IPSS for silodosin, tamsulosin, and placebo groups were −8.3 ± 6.4, −6.8 ± 5.7, and −5.3 ± 6.7 points. Also, the change in QoL from baseline was −1.7, −1.4 and −1.1 in the silodosin, tamsulosin, and placebo groups, respectively; silodosin showed a significant improvement in the QoL score vs. placebo. Silodosin gave a significantly better symptom relief in patients with severe symptoms (IPSS > 20) than did placebo (−12.4 vs. −8.7). With regard to secondary outcome measures, Qmax improved in all groups, with no significant difference observed between groups. The most common adverse event in the silodosin group was abnormal ejaculation, which occurred more often in the silodosin than in the tamsulosin group (22.3% vs. 1.6%) [23].

The urodynamic effects of silodosin were evaluated by Yamanishi et al. The authors found significant increases in Qmax and maximal bladder capacity while detrusor overactivity disappeared or improved in 40% and 35% of patients, respectively [24]. Pressure/flow studies showed significant decrease in detrusor opening pressure, detrusor pressure at Qmax, bladder outlet obstruction index (BOOI), and Schafer's linear passive urethral resistance relation obstructive class.

In the largest 12-week, parallel-group, multicenter, double-blind, placebo-controlled studies study performed by Marks et al., 923 patients were randomized to silodosin or placebo. After 0.5 weeks, patients achieved significant improvement in total IPSS that was sustained to week 12 ($P<0.0001$). Mean change from baseline in peak urinary flow rate (ml per second) 2–6 h after initial dose was greater ($P<0.0001$) with silodosin and remained consistently greater. The most common adverse event was retrograde ejaculation (silodosin 28.1%, placebo 0.9%). Proportions of patients with orthostatic hypotension were similar for silodosin (2.6%) and placebo (1.5%) [25].

### Naftopidil

Naftopidil, a new selective alpha blocker, targets $\alpha_{1d}$, in pharmacological studies shows increased frequency within the bladder compared to the a1a subtype within the prostatic urethra. This is the reason it has greater impact on overactive bladder symptoms [26]. It has limited study in America with no randomized, placebo-controlled trials. In a Cochrane review of five trials ($n=419$), naftopidil showed a mean IPSS improvement similar to low-dose tamsulosin (0.2 mg/day) (8.4 points vs. 8.9 points), although symptom improvement was not significantly different between high-dose (75 mg/day) and low-dose (25 mg/day) naftopidil groups. Qmax increment was significantly higher with high doses compared with low-dose naftopidil groups (1.2 ml/s vs. 0.2 ml/s). Patients reported improved symptom scores as well as improved QoL. Few adverse drug effects were reported, which were mild [27].

## 5-Alpha Reductase Inhibitors (5ARIs)

BPH growth is an androgen-dependent process [28, 29]. Reducing prostate volume through surgical castration dates back to the nineteenth century. More recently, various medications have been utilized to block androgen synthesis and effectiveness, such as GnRH analogues, progestational agents, as well as antiandrogens [30–34]. 5ARIs were developed to block the conversion of testosterone to dihydrotestosterone, thus reducing prostate volume in order to decrease bladder outlet obstruction. The two commonly used medications are finasteride and dutasteride, the former which competitively inhibits 5-alpha reductase type 2 and the latter of which inhibits both subtypes. The side effects include erectile dysfunction, reduced libido, and decreased ejaculate volume in 5–10% of patients, and breast enlargement and tenderness may occur in 1–2% of patients [35].

### Finasteride

In 1992, the North American Finasteride Trial of 895 men, finasteride was administered at 1 and 5 mg vs. placebo given once daily over 12 months [36]. Patients treated with 5 mg demonstrated a 22% (1.6 ml/s) increase in Qmax, and a 19% (−13 cm$^3$) decrease in prostate volume. Patients treated with either dose of finasteride demonstrated a significantly higher incidence of decreased libido, impotence, and ejaculatory disorders. A multicenter Scandinavian study of 707 patients, randomized to 5 mg finasteride vs. placebo for 24 months, confirmed the results of the North American Finasteride Trial. Again, patients on the finasteride arm had increased Qmax and reduction in prostate volume while having increased rates of sexual dysfunction [37]. The PROWESS study had 3,270 men randomized to finasteride vs. placebo, also showing improvement in, Qmax (+1.5 ml/s), prostate volume (−15.3%), and total symptom score (−3.2) over 24 months, with greater improvement seen in symptom scores for men with larger prostates (−3.2 vs. −1.3 for placebo, $P=0.053$) [38]. In the 3 years follow-up to the North American and International Finasteride Studies, Stoner et al. showed lasting changes of finasteride over placebo in Qmax by 2.3 ml/s, prostate volume by 27% [39]. One of the largest trials to date, with the longest follow-up is the Proscar Long-term Efficacy and Safety Study (PLESS) [40]. In this 4-year double-blind, trial of 3,040 men randomized to finasteride daily vs. placebo, 69/1503 (5%) vs. 152/1513 (10%) men, respectively, underwent surgery for BPH; a risk reduction of 55%. The rate of acute urinary retention (AUR) was 3% in the finasteride group vs. 7% in the placebo group. Urinary flow rates increased by 0.2 ml/s in the placebo group vs. 1.9 ml/s in the finasteride arm ($P<0.001$). There was a statistically significant increase in the urinary flow rates of 1.9 ml/s vs. 0.2 ml/s ($P<0.001$) and a decrease in the symptom score of 3.3 vs. 1.3 ($P<0.001$) in the finasteride group and placebo group, respectively. Overwhelmingly, finasteride decreased symptoms score, episodes of AUR and the need for BPH surgery. Unfortunately, there was high dropout in both groups in this study due to treatment failures and adverse side effects.

## Dutasteride

Dutasteride unlike finasteride inhibits both types of 5-alpha reductase enzyme. In three clinical trials with a total of 4,325 men, BPH patients were randomized to 0.5 mg dutasteride daily or placebo. At 24 months, serum dihydrotestosterone was reduced from baseline by a mean of 90.2% (median −93.7%; $P<0.001$), and the total prostate and transition zone volumes were reduced by a mean of 25.7 and 20.4%, respectively ($P<0.001$). The IPSS was improved by as early as 3 months, with a reduction of 4.5 points (21.4%) at 24 months ($P<0.001$). The maximal flow rate improved significantly from 1 month ($P<0.01$), with an increase of 2.2 ml/s reported at 24 months ($P<0.001$). Similar to the finasteride studies, the risk reduction of AUR was 57% and the risk reduction of BPH surgery was 48% compared with placebo. A 2-year open-label extension study was offered to patients in these three trials, which reported improved AUA symptom score from 24 to 48 months (4.4 vs. 6.5) [41].

Overall, the use of 5ARIs has led to the ability to effectively reduce prostate volume, to lower the number of episodes of AUR, and decrease in the number of surgical treatments for BPH.

In a retrospective analysis, comparing the reduction of AUR and BPH-related surgeries between dutasteride and finasteride, dutasteride-treated patients experienced significantly lower rates of AUR as compared with finasteride-treated patients (12% vs. 14.7%, respectively; $P<0.004$). The risk for BPH-related surgeries was also significantly lower for dutasteride compared with finasteride (3.9% vs. 5.1%, respectively; $P<0.03$) [42].

## Antimuscarinics

Stimulation of the parasympathetic postganglionic muscarinic cholinergic receptors is in large part responsible for bladder contraction. Often, LUTS seen with bladder outlet obstruction due to BPH results in changes in detrusor function leading to overactivity. Both M2 and M3 muscarinic receptors have been identified in the human bladder, although M3 is thought to be the dominant receptor in detrusor contraction [43]. There has been reluctance to prescribe antimuscarinics to men with overactivity for fear of decreasing detrusor contractility in the setting of bladder outlet obstructing resulting in urinary retention. However, multiple trials have supported the safety and efficacy of these medications in treating men with BPH [44, 45].

Abrams et al. studied the safety and tolerability of tolterodine IR in men with both BOO and OAB. Patients underwent urodynamic before and after treatment. In this study, 222 men were randomized to tolterodine IR 2 mg twice daily or placebo for 12 weeks. Median treatment difference in Qmax and pdet @ Qmax were comparable. Tolterodine significantly reduced BOOI (−9 vs. 0; $P<0.02$), increased volume to first detrusor contraction (+59 ml: 95% CI 19–100; $P=0.0026$), and increased maximum cystometric capacity (+67 ml: 95% CI 25–103; $P<0.003$) compared to placebo. Change in PVR was significantly higher among patients treated with tolterodine (+25 ml) than placebo (0 ml; $P<0.004$). Moreover, patients with residuals more than 40% of capacity or had previous lower urinary tract surgery were excluded from this study [45].

In a study by Martin-Merino, the overall incidence of AUR in the study cohort (1,844) was 1.0 per 1,000 person-years, with the incidence rate increasing with age. The first 30 days of antimuscarinic use was associated with a relative risk of AUR of 8.3 (95% CI 4.8–14.2) and with longer term use (more than 30 days) the relative risk was 2.0 (95% CI 1.2–3.1). The relative risk of AUR was similar for low/medium and high antimuscarinic doses (relative risk 2.8 vs. 3.0, 95% CI 2.1–3.8 and 1.3–6.8, respectively). The relative risk of AUR was highest during early treatment for a urogenital indication (relative risk 14.2, 95% CI 6.8–29.6) [46]. Therefore, monitoring PVR after starting this medication is necessary.

# PDE-5 Inhibitors

Multiple epidemiologic studies have demonstrated a link between LUTS and sexual dysfunction [47–50]. There are four theories of etiology to explain this link mechanistically; the nitric oxide synthetase/nitric oxide (NOS/NO) cyclic-guanine monophosphate pathway, the Rho-kinase activation/endothelin pathway, the autonomic hyperactivity and metabolic syndrome hypothesis, pathophysiologic consequences of pelvic atherosclerosis [51, 52]. Based on the proposed link of LUTS and ED, multiple authors have studied the effects of various PDE-5 inhibitors on LUTS.

Sairam et al. first reported the use of on-demand sildenafil on LUTS in 112 men with ED [53]. At baseline, there was no relationship between the IPSS and IIEF. After treatment with sildenafil the IPSS and QoL scores improved; at 3 months, in all those who initially had severe LUTS became moderate, in 60% of those with moderate LUTS they became mild and in 18% of the mild group they became moderate. A similar study was performed by Mulhall et al. who reported the effect of 48 men with LUTS taking 100 mg on demand sildenafil [54]. The mean improvement in the EF domain score was 7 points ($P=0.01$). The mean improvement in the IPSS score was 4.6 points ($P=0.013$) and in QoL score was 1.4 points ($P=0.025$). In total, 60% of men improved their IPSS score, and 35% had at least a 4-point improvement in their score. In a study by Porst et al. reporting on tadalafil at escalating doses vs. placebo, improvements were seen in ED and IPSS scores with all doses over placebo, although no improvement was noted in Qmax [55].

The use of PDE-5 inhibitor is still experimental and should not be used routinely in the clinical setting. Long-term experience in patients with LUTS is still lacking.

## Combination Therapy

### Alpha Blocker with 5ARI

The Medical Therapy of Prostatic Symptoms (MTOPS) trial was the first to show the efficacy of combination therapy over monotherapy [56]. In a long-term (mean 4.5 years), double-blind trial of 3,047 men randomized to placebo, doxazosin, finasteride, and combination therapy, the overall clinical progression—defined as 4-point increase in AUA symptom score, AUR, urinary incontinence, renal insufficiency, or recurrent urinary tract infection—was significantly reduced by doxazosin (39% risk reduction, $P<0.001$) and finasteride (34% risk reduction, $P=0.002$), and with combination therapy (66% for the comparison with placebo, $P<0.001$) as compared with placebo. The risks of AUR and the need for invasive therapy were significantly reduced by combination therapy and finasteride but not by doxazosin. Doxazosin, finasteride and combination therapy each resulted in significant improvement in symptom scores, with combination therapy being superior to both doxazosin and finasteride alone.

The Combination of Avodart and Tamsulosin (CombAT) study of 4,844 men is the most extensive trial evaluating the efficacy of combination therapy of dutasteride and tamsulosin in patients with moderate to severe LUTS secondary to BPH and enlarged prostate (prostate volume>30 ml, PSA>1.5) [57]. This multicenter, randomized, double-blind study of 4,844 men revealed that combination treatment achieved significantly greater mean reductions in both voiding and storage symptoms than either monotherapy, at 24 months. Dutasteride alone was as effective as tamsulosin for control of storage symptoms, but provided significantly greater relief of voiding symptoms at 24 months out. At this point, combination therapy was more effective than monotherapy on voiding symptoms in men with prostate volumes between 30 and 42 $cm^3$. Moreover, combination therapy led to significant increases in patient reported, disease-specific QoL [58]. At 4 years, the CombAT study demonstrated that both arms with dutasteride had significant increase time to first AUR or BPH-related surgery compared to tamsulosin alone. The occurrence of drug-related adverse events was significantly greater in the combination group, but with similar withdrawal rates across the treatment groups. There was no difference in overall cardiovascular events [59].

Jeong et al. investigated the effect of discontinuation of 5AR inhibitor in patients on combination therapy [60]. Although 5AR in combination with alpha blockers decrease both prostate volume and symptoms, with cessation of 5AR inhibitor, the prostate gland enlarges and symptoms reoccur. They suggested that 5AR inhibitors should be prescribed indefinitely for severe symptoms or larger prostates.

## Alpha Blockers with Anticholinergics

Anticholinergic medications were first studied in the setting of de novo overactive bladder. Only later did they gain popularity in the setting of OAB in conjunction with BPH. In a study by Kaplan et al., 43 men with BPH and LUTS who had failed alpha-blocker therapy alone were given combination therapy with the addition of 4 mg tolterodine for 6 months [61]. Mean 24-h micturition frequency decreased from 9.8 to 6.3 voids and nocturia decreased from 4.1 to 2.9 episodes nightly. Significant changes were also seen in mean AUA symptom score (−6.1), the peak urinary flow rate (1.9 ml/s), and postvoid residual volume (−22 ml).

In a subsequent study, Kaplan et al. performed a randomized, double-blind, placebo-controlled study designed to evaluate the efficacy and safety of using an antimuscarinic agent alone or in conjunction with a alpha-blocker in the treatment of LUTS with both BPH and OAB symptoms [44]. This study is known as the TIMES (Tolterodine and Tamsulosin in Men With LUTS including OAB), of 879 men with moderate to severe LUTS were randomly assigned to receive placebo, 4 mg of tolterodine ER, 0.4 mg of tamsulosin, or both for 12 weeks. Of note, patients with evidence of BOO were excluded. Combination therapy resulted in a significant difference vs. placebo and vs. monotherapy in percentage of patient perceiving treatment benefit. Combination therapy was shown to improve diary variables such as urge incontinence, urgency episodes, nocturia episodes, and micturitions per night and per 24 h. Combination therapy demonstrated significant improvement in IPSS and QoL compared to placebo. Tolterodine ER showed only improvement in urge incontinence episodes, while tamsulosin only demonstrated significant benefit in frequency, incontinence episodes, and IPSS at 12 weeks. The most frequent adverse effects noted were dry mouth. Both Qmax and PVR between the four arms showed no statistically significant differences. All interventions were well tolerated. The incidence of AUR requiring catheterization was low (tolterodine ER plus tamsulosin, 0.4%; tolterodine ER, 0.5%; tamsulosin, 0%; and placebo, 0%).

In a study by Athanasopoulos et al. of 50 patients randomized to receive tamsulosin vs. combination therapy with tamsulosin plus tolterodine for 3 months was evaluated with urodynamics and QoL questionnaires. There was significant improvement in QoL scores, increased bladder capacity, decreased maximum unstable contraction pressure ($P=0.0004$), and increased volume at first unstable contraction in the combination group over the tamsulosin-only group [62].

In a meta-analysis from 5 randomized controlled trials and 15 observational studies, the total IPSS scores did not change with anticholinergic therapy, although the IPSS storage subscores, which constitute the majority of subjective bother, were improved [63]. This analysis confirmed the low incidence of AUR at 0.3% at 12 weeks. These studies demonstrate that in combination with alpha blockers, anticholinergics are safe and effective in treating OAB due to BPH.

## Alpha Blockers and PDE-5 Inhibitors

Combination therapy of alpha blocker and PDE-5 inhibitors for LUTS and ED is gaining interest due to increasing frequency of their utilization in the aging population. In a study by Kaplan et al., 62 men with previously untreated LUTS and ED were randomized to daily 25 mg sildenafil vs. 10 mg alfuzosin vs. combination therapy [64]. Combination therapy showed greater improvement in IPSS and IIEF scores over either monotherapy. The most common side effects included dyspepsia, dizziness, and flushing. Roehrborn et al. in a study of 1,058 men with BPH-related LUTS randomly allocated patients to receive 12-week, once daily treatment with placebo or tadalafil (2.5, 5, 10 or 20 mg) [65]. Significant improvement was seen in IPSS score as well as adverse effects seen with higher doses. Although subjective improvement was seen with medication, no change in Qmax was demonstrated. In a study by Stief et al. of 222 men with BPH and LUTS, patients on 10 mg vardenafil twice daily vs. placebo demonstrated improvement in IPSS score without significant change in Qmax or PVR [66]. Dmochowski et al. studied urodynamic parameters of 200 men randomized to 20 mg tadalafil vs. placebo over 12 weeks. There were improvements in IPSS score over placebo with no significant changes were seen in urodynamic parameters [67]. Tuncel et al. demonstrated that combination therapy of tamsulosin and sildenafil was not superior to monotherapy with tamsulosin in terms of voiding symptoms. The rate of improvement on IPSS for combination therapy at 40.1% and tamsulosin at 36.2% was similar and significantly greater than sildenafil monotherapy at 28.1% ($P<0.001$) [68]. Currently, PDE-5 inhibitors have not been approved for LUTS.

### Antimuscarinics and 5ARIs

Chung et al. showed the safety and efficacy of dutasteride and tolterodine ER in patients with OAB and LUTS refractory to dutasteride alone [69]. This open-label trial of 51 men with OAB and prostate size >30 g who failed monotherapy with dutasteride 0.5 mg for 6 months was given additional tolterodine, extended release 4 mg tabs for 3 months. Tolterodine significantly reduced frequency and urgency: 24-h micturition frequency (−3.2, $P<0.02$), OAB episodes (19.2%, $P<0.03$), severe OAB episodes (71.4%, $P<0.05$), and nighttime voiding (−0.9, $P<0.003$). IPSS decreased with dutasteride (19.3–14.3) and decreased again with addition of tolterodine to 7.1 ($P<0.001$). Storage symptoms decreased from 98 to 4.5 ($P<0.001$). PVR increased by 4.2 ml, Qmax decreased by 0.2 ml/s, and no patients went into retention. The side effects were minimal with one report of constipation due to tolterodine, one dry mouth on dutasteride, which increased to four with the addition of tolterodine. Two patients on dutasteride reported sexual side effects.

## Conclusion

There are currently multiple treatments available for BPH-related LUTS, including alpha-adrenergic receptor antagonists, 5ARIs, PDE-5 inhibitors and anticholinergics. It is important to approach each patient individually, focusing on history, physical examination, laboratory tests, imaging as well as urodynamics. As men age, BPH is often progressive as measured by symptoms and deterioration in urinary flow rate, increase in prostate size, and ultimately AUR and need for surgery. Assessment parameters (AUA symptom score, uroflowmetry, and prostate size) may help in identifying men at greater risk of progression who may benefit from more aggressive medical management using combination therapy. Excellent and widely accepted guidelines are available for the primary care provider to help in the assessment of men with male LUTS and BPH, and in choosing from a variety of treatment options. Patients with mild symptoms may be excellent for conservative treatment with behavioral therapy (timed voiding, fluid restriction). As symptom severity increases, patients will be candidates for one or a combination of currently available treatments.

## References


1. Roehrborn CG. Etiology, pathophysiology, epidemiology and natural history of benign prostatic hyperplasia. In: Wein AJ, Kavoussi LR, Novick AC, Partin AW, Peters CA, editors. Campbell's urology. 9th ed. Amsterdam: Elsevier.
2. Oishi K, Boyle P, Barry M. Epidemiology and natural history of benign prostatic hyperplasia. In: Fourth international consultation on benign prostatic hyperplasia. Plymouth: Plymbridge Distributors Ltd; 1998. p. 23.
3. Girman CJ. Natural history and epidemiology of benign prostatic hyperplasia: relationship among urologic measures. Urology. 1998;51:8.
4. Roehrborn CG. The utility of serum prostatic-specific antigen in the management of men with benign prostatic hyperplasia. Int J Impot Res. 2008;20 Suppl 3:S19.
5. Bohnen AM, Groeneveld FP, Bosch JL. Serum prostate-specific antigen as a predictor of prostate volume in the community: the Krimpen study. Eur Urol. 2007;51:1645.
6. Lieber MM, Jacobsen SJ, Roberts RO, et al. Prostate volume and prostate-specific antigen in the absence of prostate cancer: a review of the relationship and prediction of long-term outcomes. Prostate. 2001;49:208.
7. Roehrborn CG, Boyle P, Gould AL, et al. Serum prostate-specific antigen as a predictor of prostate volume in men with benign prostatic hyperplasia. Urology. 1999;53:581.
8. Bent S, Kane C, Shinohara K, et al. Saw palmetto for benign prostatic hyperplasia. N Engl J Med. 2006; 354:557.

9. Forray C, Bard J, Wetzel J, et al. The alpha 1-adrenergic receptor that mediates smooth muscle contraction in human prostate has the pharmacological properties of the cloned human alpha 1c subtype. Mol Pharmacol. 1994;1994:4.
10. Krane R, Olsson C. Phenoxybenzamine in neurogenic bladder dysfunction: I. A theory of micturition. J Urol. 1973;110:650.
11. Nordling J, Meyhoff H, Hald T. Sympatholytic effect on striated urethral sphincter. Scand J Urol Nephrol. 1981;15:173.
12. McNaughton-Collins M, Barry MJ. Managing patients with lower urinary tract symptoms suggestive of benign prostatic hyperplasia. Am J Med. 2005;118:1331.
13. Kirby RS, Coppinger SW, Corcoran MO, et al. Prazosin in the treatment of prostatic obstruction. A placebo-controlled study. Br J Urol. 1987;60:136.
14. Chapple CR, Christmas T, Milroy EJ. A 12-week placebo-controlled double-blind study of prazosin in the treatment of prostatic obstruction due to benign prostatic hyperplasia. BJU Int. 1992;70:285.
15. Kirby RS, Lepor H. Evaluation and nonsurgical management of benign prostatic hyperplasia. In: Wein AJ, Kavoussi LR, Novick AC, Partin AW, Peters CA, editors. Campbell's urology. 9th ed. Amsterdam: Elsevier.
16. Lepor H, Auerbach S, Puras-Baez A, et al. A randomized, placebo-controlled multicenter study of the efficacy and safety of terazosin in the treatment of benign prostatic hyperplasia. J Urol. 1992;148:1467.
17. Chapple C, Carter P, Christmas T, et al. A three-month double-blind study of doxazosin as treatment for benign prostatic obstruction. BJU Int. 1994;74:50.
18. Fawzy A, Braun K, Lewis GP, et al. Doxazosin in the treatment of benign prostatic hyperplasia in normotensive patients: a multicenter study. J Urol. 1995;154:105.
19. Gillenwater JY, Conn RL, Chrysant SG, et al. Doxazosin for the treatment of benign prostatic hyperplasia in patients with mild to moderate essential hypertension: a double-blind, placebo-controlled, dose–response multicenter study. J Urol. 1995;154:110.
20. Lepor H. Phase III multicenter placebo-controlled study of tamsulosin in benign prostatic hyperplasia. Tamsulosin Investigator Group. Urology. 1998; 51:892.
21. Narayan P, Tewari A. A second phase III multicenter placebo controlled study of 2 dosages of modified release tamsulosin in patients with symptoms of benign prostatic hyperplasia. United States 93-01 Study Group. J Urol. 1998;160:1701.
22. Roehrborn CG, Van Kerrebroeck P, Nordling J. Safety and efficacy of alfuzosin 10 mg once-daily in the treatment of lower urinary tract symptoms and clinical benign prostatic hyperplasia: a pooled analysis of three double-blind, placebo-controlled studies. BJU Int. 2003;92:257.
23. Kawabe K, Yoshida M, Homma Y. Silodosin, a new alpha1A-adrenoceptor-selective antagonist for treating benign prostatic hyperplasia: results of a phase III randomized, placebo-controlled, double-blind study in Japanese men. BJU Int. 2006;98:1019.
24. Yamanishi T, Mizuno T, Tatsumiya K, et al. Urodynamic effects of silodosin, a new alpha 1A-adrenoceptor selective antagonist, for the treatment of benign prostatic hyperplasia. Neurourol Urodyn. 2010;29:558.
25. Marks LS, Gittelman MC, Hill LA, et al. Rapid efficacy of the highly selective alpha1A-adrenoceptor antagonist silodosin in men with signs and symptoms of benign prostatic hyperplasia: pooled results of 2 phase 3 studies. J Urol. 2009;181:2634.
26. Malloy BJ, Price DT, Price RR, et al. Alpha1-adrenergic receptor subtypes in human detrusor. J Urol. 1998;160:937.
27. Garimella PS, Fink HA, Macdonald R, et al. Naftopidil for the treatment of lower urinary tract symptoms compatible with benign prostatic hyperplasia. Cochrane Database Syst Rev. 2009;CD007360.
28. Coffey D, Walsh P. Clinical and experimental studies of benign prostatic hyperplasia. Urol Clin North Am. 1990;17:461.
29. Shapiro E. Embryologic development of the prostate. Urol Clin North Am. 1990;17:487.
30. Cabot A. The question of castration for enlarged prostate. Ann Surg. 1896;24:265.
31. White J. The results of double castration in hypertrophy of the prostate. Ann Surg. 1895;22:1.
32. Caine M, Perlberg S, Gordon R. The treatment of benign prostatic hypertrophy with flutamide (SCH: 13521): a placebo-controlled study. J Urol. 1975; 114:564.
33. Donkervoort T, Zinner NR, Sterling AM, et al. Megestrol acetate in treatment of benign prostatic hypertrophy. Urology. 1975;6:580.
34. Schroeder FH, Westerhof M, Bosch RJ, et al. Benign prostatic hyperplasia treated by castration or the LH-RH analogue buserelin: a report on 6 cases. Eur Urol. 1986;12:318.
35. APG Committee. AUA guideline on management of benign prostatic hyperplasia. Chapter 1: diagnosis and treatment recommendations. J Urol. 2003;170(2 Pt 1):530.
36. Gormley GJ, Stoner E, Bruskewitz RC, et al. The effect of finasteride in men with benign prostatic hyperplasia. The Finasteride Study Group. N Engl J Med. 1992;327:1185.
37. Andersen J, Ekman P, Wolf H, et al. Can finasteride reverse the progress of benign prostatic hyperplasia? A two-year placebo controlled study. Urology. 1995;46:631.
38. Marberger M. Long-term effects of finasteride in patients with benign prostatic hyperplasia: a double-blind, placebo-controlled, multicenter study. Urology. 1998;51:677.
39. Stoner E. Three-year safety and efficacy data on the use of finasteride in the treatment of benign prostatic hyperplasia. Urology. 1994;43:284.
40. McConnell JD, Bruskewitz R, Walsh P, et al. The effect of finasteride on the risk of acute urinary retention and the need for surgical treatment among men with benign prostatic hyperplasia. Finasteride Long-Term Efficacy and Safety Study Group. N Engl J Med. 1998;338:557.
41. Roehrborn CG, Lukkarinen O, Mark S, et al. Long-term sustained improvement in symptoms of benign

prostatic hyperplasia with the dual 5alpha-reductase inhibitor dutasteride: results of 4-year studies. BJU Int. 2005;96:572.

42. Fenter TC, Davis EA, Shah MB, et al. Dutasteride vs finasteride: assessment of differences in acute urinary retention rates and surgical risk outcomes in an elderly population aged > or =65 years. Am J Manag Care. 2008;14:S154.
43. Anderson KE. Pharmacology of lower urinary tract smooth muscles and penile erectile tissues. Pharmacol Rev. 1993;45:253.
44. Kaplan SA, Roehrborn CG, Rovner ES, et al. Tolterodine and tamsulosin for treatment of men with lower urinary tract symptoms and overactive bladder: a randomized controlled trial. JAMA. 2006;296:2319.
45. Abrams P, Kaplan S, De Koning Gans HJ, et al. Safety and tolerability of tolterodine for the treatment of overactive bladder in men with bladder outlet obstruction. J Urol. 2006;175:999.
46. Martin-Merino E, Garcia-Rodriguez LA, Masso-Gonzalez EL, et al. Do oral antimuscarinic drugs carry an increased risk of acute urinary retention? J Urol. 2009;182:1442.
47. Li MK, Garcia LA, Rosen R. Lower urinary tract symptoms and male sexual dysfunction in Asia: a survey of ageing men from five Asian countries. BJU Int. 2005;96:1339.
48. Rosen R, Altwein J, Boyle P, et al. Lower urinary tract symptoms and male sexual dysfunction: the multinational survey of the aging male (MSAM-7). Eur Urol. 2003;44:637.
49. Rosen RC, Giuliano F, Carson CC. Sexual dysfunction and lower urinary tract symptoms (LUTS) associated with benign prostatic hyperplasia (BPH). Eur Urol. 2005;47:824.
50. Vallancien G, Emberton M, Harving N, et al. Sexual dysfunction in 1,274 European men suffering from lower urinary tract symptoms. J Urol. 2003;169:2257.
51. McVary K. Lower urinary tract symptoms and sexual dysfunction: epidemiology and pathophysiology. BJU Int. 2006;97 Suppl 2:23.
52. McVary KT, Rademaker A, Lloyd GL, et al. Autonomic nervous system overactivity in men with lower urinary tract symptoms secondary to benign prostatic hyperplasia. J Urol. 2005;174:1327.
53. Sairam K, Kulinskaya E, McNicholas TA, et al. Sildenafil influences lower urinary tract symptoms. BJU Int. 2002;90:836.
54. Mulhall JP, Guhring P, Parker M, et al. Assessment of the impact of sildenafil citrate on lower urinary tract symptoms in men with erectile dysfunction. J Sex Med. 2006;3:662.
55. Porst H, McVary KT, Montorsi F, et al. Effects of once-daily tadalafil on erectile function in men with erectile dysfunction and signs and symptoms of benign prostatic hyperplasia. Eur Urol. 2009;56:727.
56. McConnell JD, Roehrborn CG, Bautista OM, et al. The long-term effect of doxazosin, finasteride, and combination therapy on the clinical progression of benign prostatic hyperplasia. N Engl J Med. 2003;349:2387.
57. Becher E, Roehrborn CG, Siami P, et al. The effects of dutasteride, tamsulosin, and the combination on storage and voiding in men with benign prostatic hyperplasia and prostatic enlargement: 2-year results from the Combination of Avodart and Tamsulosin study. Prostate Cancer Prostatic Dis. 2009;12:369.
58. Barkin J, Roehrborn CG, Siami P, et al. Effect of dutasteride, tamsulosin and the combination on patient-reported quality of life and treatment satisfaction in men with moderate-to-severe benign prostatic hyperplasia: 2-year data from the CombAT trial. BJU Int. 2009;103:919.
59. Roehrborn CG, Siami P, Barkin J, et al. The effects of combination therapy with dutasteride and tamsulosin on clinical outcomes in men with symptomatic benign prostatic hyperplasia: 4-year results from the CombAT study. Eur Urol. 2010;57:123.
60. Jeong YB, Kwon KS, Kim SD, et al. Effect of discontinuation of 5alpha-reductase inhibitors on prostate volume and symptoms in men with BPH: a prospective study. Urology. 2009;73:802.
61. Kaplan SA, Walmsley K, Te AE. Tolterodine extended release attenuates lower urinary tract symptoms in men with benign prostatic hyperplasia. J Urol. 2005;174:2273.
62. Athanasopoulos A, Gyftopoulos K, Giannitsas K, et al. Combination treatment with an alpha-blocker plus an anticholinergic for bladder outlet obstruction: a prospective, randomized, controlled study. J Urol. 2003;169:2253.
63. Blake-James BT, Rashidian A, Ikeda Y, et al. The role of anticholinergics in men with lower urinary tract symptoms suggestive of benign prostatic hyperplasia: a systematic review and meta-analysis. BJU Int. 2007;99:85.
64. Kaplan S, Gonzalez R, Te A. Combination of alfuzosin and sildenafil is superior to monotherapy in treating lower urinary tract symptoms and erectile dysfunction. Eur Urol. 2007;51:1717.
65. Roehrborn CG, McVary KT, Elion-Mboussa A, et al. Tadalafil administered once daily for lower urinary tract symptoms secondary to benign prostatic hyperplasia: a dose finding study. J Urol. 2008;180:1228.
66. Stief CG, Porst H, Neuser D, et al. A randomised, placebo-controlled study to assess the efficacy of twice-daily vardenafil in the treatment of lower urinary tract symptoms secondary to benign prostatic hyperplasia. Eur Urol. 2008;53:1236.
67. Dmochowski R, Roehrborn C, Klise S, et al. Urodynamic effects of once daily tadalafil in men with lower urinary tract symptoms secondary to clinical benign prostatic hyperplasia: a randomized, placebo controlled 12-week clinical trial. J Urol. 2010;183:1092.
68. Tuncel A, Nalcacioglu V, Ener K, et al. Sildenafil citrate and tamsulosin combination is not superior to monotherapy in treating lower urinary tract symptoms and erectile dysfunction. World J Urol. 2010;28:17.
69. Chung DE, Te AE, Staskin DR, et al. Efficacy and safety of tolterodine extended release and dutasteride in male overactive bladder patients with prostates >30 grams. Urology. 2010;75:1144.

# 7 The Surgical Treatment of Benign Prostatic Hyperplasia

James C. Ulchaker

The surgical treatment options for bladder outlet obstruction (BOO) secondary to benign prostatic hyperplasia (BPH) have dramatically increased in number over the past 20 years. However, each of these new modalities continues to be measured against the gold standard treatment of transurethral resection of the prostate (TURP). Herein, we will present the current approaches to the surgical treatment for BPH. We will discuss open surgical options, as well as endoscopic and minimally invasive treatment options. Also, in 2010, the American Urological Association updated its BPH Practice Guidelines. These guidelines will be presented after each subsection in bold letters [1].

**AUA BPH Guideline Recommendation: Surgery is recommended for patients who have renal insufficiency secondary to BPH, who have recurrent UTI's, bladder stones or gross hematuria due to BPH, and those who have LUTS refractory to other therapies. The presence of a bladder diverticulum is not an absolute indication for surgery unless associated with recurrent UTI or progressive bladder dysfunction.**

**[Based on review of the data and Panel consensus.]**

J.C. Ulchaker, MD, FACS (✉)
Glickman Urologic and Kidney Institute,
Cleveland Clinic, 9500 Euclid Avenue Q10-1,
Cleveland, OH 44195, USA
e-mail: ULCHAKJ@ccf.org

## Open Simple Prostatectomy

Open simple prostatectomy continues to be an excellent treatment option for patients with very large prostates (>100 g) in size who suffer from severe lower urinary tract symptoms and/or have the complications of acute urinary retention, persistent hematuria, recurrent urinary tract infections, or bladder calculi. It can be performed via a suprapubic, retropubic, or laparoscopic approach. The suprapubic prostatectomy, also known as the transvesical prostatectomy, consists of enucleating the prostatic adenoma through an incision in the lower anterior bladder wall. This approach allows excellent visualization of the bladder neck, intravesical middle lobe, and large bladder calculi. It does, however, make the visualization of the prostatic apex more difficult, and thus, control of prostatic bleeding vessels in the prostatic capsule once the adenoma has been removed may be more difficult to control. In the retropubic approach, the anterior prostatic capsule is incised and the prostatic adenoma is removed via this capsular incision through digital dissection. This approach allows excellent visualization of the prostatic apex thus potentially decreasing the risk of urinary incontinence postoperatively. However, there is less direct access to the bladder if desired for other confounding factors. More recently, a robotic/laparoscopic approach has been developed. This approach allows direct access and visualization to both the bladder and prostate and may have the advantage

D.A. Shoskes (ed.), *Urological Men's Health: A Guide for Urologists and Primary Care Physicians*, Current Clinical Urology, DOI 10.1007/978-1-61779-900-6_7,
© Springer Science+Business Media New York 2012

of lessening the total blood loss compared to the other approaches. Historically, 3–10% of men undergoing open prostatectomy will require one or more units of blood in the perioperative period [2–4]. Thus, having proper type and screens as well as blood products available during this period is mandatory. Lastly, the risks of urinary incontinence, bladder neck contracture, as well as erectile dysfunction and ejaculatory disorders should be discussed with patients preoperatively.

Postoperatively patients are maintained on Foley catheter drainage and at times three-way catheterization with irrigation is necessary. The catheter is also maintained on traction. Early ambulation is encouraged to decrease the risk of potential deep venous thrombosis (DVT) and subsequent pulmonary embolus (PE). Bladder irrigations are weaned as tolerated. I usually maintain the catheter for a 1-week duration and pelvic drains are removed before discharge.

**AUA BPH Guideline Option: Open prostatectomy is an appropriate and effective treatment alternative for men with moderate to severe LUTS and/or who are significantly bothered by these symptoms. The choice of approach should be based on the patient's individual presentation including anatomy, the surgeon's experience, and discussion of the potential benefit and risks for complications. The panel noted that there is usually a longer hospital stay and a larger loss of blood associated with open procedures.**

**There are insufficient published data on which to base a treatment recommendation for laparoscopic or robotic prostatectomy.**

**[Based on review of the data and Panel consensus.]**

## Transurethral Resection of the Prostate

TURP is the most popular surgical treatment for benign prostatic hyperplasia and has been that way for the past 100 years. In 1986, it was estimated that 350,000 medicare patients had a TURP that year; however, these numbers have fallen to less than 200,000 per year in the medicare age patient group, but still remains the most popular surgical treatment procedure performed in the USA. The most common reason for recommending surgical intervention in men are for those men who suffer from moderate to severe lower urinary tract symptoms that significantly interfere with their quality of life. Other indications are to relieve acute urinary retention, recurrent urinary tract infections, persistent hematuria, and azotemia.

TURP is usually performed under general or spinal anesthesia. Perioperative antibiotics are administered. The traditional monopolar TURP is performed using glycine or mannitol as nonhemolytic fluids for irrigation. The monopolar surgical loop is electrically activated and prostatic tissue is resected under direct visualization using a 24–28 French resectoscope. The prostatic chips are subsequently irrigated from the bladder, hemostatis is obtained, and a Foley catheter is placed at the end of the procedure. Depending on the degree of hematuria, a two- or three-way catheter is used on moderate traction and saline irrigation may be instituted until the urine clears. These procedures usually occur on an in-patient basis with hospital stays being anywhere from 1 to 3 days. There are many potential intraoperative and postoperative complications, which can occur with TURP. These potential complications have spurred the development of TURP modification such as the introduction of bipolar technology, as well as other minimally invasive techniques, which will be discussed further in this chapter.

Intraoperative complications of TURP include blood loss requiring blood transfusions, excessive fluid absorption, and TURP syndrome. Postoperative complications include urinary incontinence, erectile dysfunction, retrograde ejaculation, urethral stricture, and bladder neck contracture to name a few.

In the AUA cooperative study [5], TUR syndrome occurred in 2% of the patients undergoing TURP. This syndrome is caused by a significant drop in the patient's serum sodium to <125 milliequivalents per deciliter (meq/dl). The risk of this syndrome development increases with both the size of the prostate and the resection time under anesthesia. Associated conditions with TURP syndrome include mental confusion, nausea, vomiting, hypertension, bradycardia, and visual disturbance. This syndrome is treated by giving the patient 3% hypertonic saline very slowly over a number of hours. Once the patient's serum sodium has reached 120–125 meq/dl of sodium, the hypertonic saline is discontinued and normal saline with the use of diuretics is initiated. It normally takes 24–48 h for serum sodium level to normalize. During that time, the initiation of other supportive care may be necessary.

Because of these complications, the standard monopolar TURP in now being challenged by the use of bipolar resection devices. These devices consist of bipolar electrical energy used to generate a plasma kinetic activity that allows the prostatic resection to be performed with the use of normal saline as its irrigant. The use of saline will thus eliminate the development of hyponatremia secondary to venous fluid absorption. Thus, this technology may be safer for patients.

In summary, TURP was introduced as a method of treatment that was less invasive than open prostatectomy. The results of TURP are listed in Table 7.1. TURP remains the gold standard treatment for obstructive BPH causing moderate to severe symptoms in lower urinary tract symptoms in men. However, because of the potential complications, numerous modifications to TURP have been developed as well as other minimally invasive treatment modalities.

**AUA BPH Guideline Option: TURP is an appropriate and effective primary alternative for surgical therapy in men with moderate to severe LUTS and/or who are significantly bothered by these symptoms. The choice of a monopolar or bipolar approach should be based on the patient's presentation, anatomy, the surgeon's experience and discussion of the potential risks and likely benefits.**

**Overall, there is insufficient evidence to recommend using 5-ARIs in the setting of a pre-TURP to reduce intraoperative bleeding or reduce the need for blood transfusions.**

**[Based on review of the data and Panel consensus.]**

## Transurethral Needle Ablation of the Prostate

Transurethral needle ablation (TUNA) of the prostate is an outpatient procedure in which low level radiofrequency energy is delivered by needles placed into the prostatic adenoma that produce localized necrotic lesions. The procedure is performed under topical anesthesia for men with symptomatic BPH and causes reproducible necrotic lesions within the prostate parenchyma. The generator produces a monopolar radiofrequency signal of 490 kHz that allows tissue heating to be created by tissue resistance to the current as it flows from the active to the passive electrode. The radiofrequency produces molecular or ionic agitation with collision of particles that relates to the frequency of the energy, and these result in a central hot core inside the prostate and away from the urethra [8]. Interestingly, radiofrequency is

**Table 7.1** Studies of transurethral needle ablation with 12-month follow-up

| | | Symptom score | | Peak urinary flow | |
|---|---|---|---|---|---|
| Study | No. patients | Preoperative | Postoperative | Preoperative | Postoperative |
| Roehrborn et al. [6] | 130 | 23.7 | 11.9 | 7.8 | 14.6 |
| Bruskewitz et al. [7] | 65 | 24.7 | 11.1 | 8.7 | 15.0 |
| Schulman et al. [8] | 36 | 21.6 | 7.8 | 9.9 | 16.8 |
| Campo et al. [9] | 72 | 20.8 | 6.2 | 8.2 | 15.9 |
| Ramon et al. [10] | 68 | 22.0 | 10.0 | 8.8 | 11.5 |
| Rosario et al. [11] | 58 | 22.0 | 10.0 | 8.8 | 11.5 |
| Steele and Sleep [12] | 41 | 22.4 | 7.0 | 6.6 | 10.2 |
| Millard et al. [13] | 20 | 19.0 | 8.2 | 3.0 | 11.4 |

*Reprinted with permission from Campbell-Walsh urology, 10th edn. Philadelphia, PA: Saunders Elseiver; 2011*

significantly affected by blood flow and has almost no effect on blood vessels larger than 3 mm in diameter [14].

This system has undergone numerous changes over the past 15 years with the most recent system being called Prostiva™. Unlike the original TUNA device, the newest version has a significantly improved optical system, and thus can be placed under direct visualization, and produce an improved angle between the catheter and needles. The newest configuration of the needles within the Teflon sheath ensures that the necrotic area is created deep within the prostatic adenoma and spares the prostatic urethra. This modification allows for increased patient comfort and an improvement in postprocedure urinary symptoms.

During the Prostiva procedure, the patient is placed in the dorsal lithotomy position and a topical anesthetic with intraurethral lidocaine jelly as well as a 1% intravesical liquid lidocaine is administered. From a personal perspective, the best result is obtained allowing these medications to sit for a period of time (15 min). For a comfort standpoint, a spinal or general anesthetic can be administered in less compliant patients. Prostatic blocks can also be applied using 1% injected lidocaine to the periprostatic nerves. Proper needle deployment is essential to ensure that the appropriate areas of prostatic anesthetic treatment occur. The number of prostatic needle placements is dependent on the size and architecture of the prostate. Variable Foley catheter times have been reported and are very subjectively dependent.

A number of studies have been reported revealing 12-month follow-up data (see Table 7.1). The average posttreatment symptom score decreased by an average of 13.1 or a 58% symptom improvement. I personally feel the best data occurs from Bruskewitz et al. [7] in which the symptom score improved 24.7 to 11.1 and the flow rate improvement improved from 8.7 to 15 $cm^3/s$. The TURP group improved significantly greater from 23.3 to 8.3 $cm^3/s$ and flow rate improved up to a maximum of 20.8 $cm^3/s$. The adverse effects profile included a urinary retention rate between 13.3% and 41.6%. This most commonly occurred within the first 24 h of catheter removal. The urinary tract infection rate was reported to be 3.1%. All other complications were noted to have a rate of 1½% or less. The reoperation rate was reported to be 14%; however, this rate was recorded at less than 2 years postprocedure.

In summary, the TUNA procedure is easy to perform with a low complication rate. Modest symptom and flow improvements have been reported. The TUNA can be performed under a topical anesthetic or local periprostatic block. A 40% urinary retention rate was noted in the first 24-h post catheter removal. The long-term efficacy of this treatment has not been clearly defined as there are no large series of patients having long-term follow-up.

**AUA BPH Guideline Option: TUNA of the prostate is an appropriate treatment alternative for bothersome moderate or severe LUTS secondary to BPH.**

[**Based on review of the data and Panel consensus.**]

## Transuretheral Microwave Therapy

Transurethral microwave therapy (TUMT) has been widely used in a variety of forms over the last two decades including both low- and high-energy devices as well as cooled and noncooled thermocatheters. TUMT is the least operator-dependent of the BPH interventions and predicting responders is difficult and inconsistent. During microwave therapy, heat is delivered to the prostatic adenoma via a specialized urethral catheter with a microwave antenna. This creates temperatures within the prostate parenchyma up to 70°C, while the specialized cooling device, if applicable, maintains the urethral temperature at about 44°C. These heat changes cause damage to sympathetic nerve endings and induction of apoptosis. In 1996, Larsen et al. reported their histologic studies showing that tissue exposed to a minimum of 45°C for about 60 min suffered significant hemorrhagic necrosis [15]. The border between viable and necrotic tissue was sharply defined. Numerous investigators have also researched the potential role that sympathetic nerve degeneration secondary to inner prostatic heating is modified by the treatment. Nerve fiber disruption is caused by this thermal damage, and a lack of nerve fiber activation in the prostatic smooth muscle layer leads to decreased tone of the urethra and potentially improved flow and urinary symptoms. Finally, heat has been implicated as the cause of prostatic apoptosis; however, no exam mechanism for this has yet been determined. It is speculated that high temperatures cause necrosis of prostatic cells, whereas lower temperatures for longer periods of time induce program cell death or apoptosis.

The literature is filled with numerous short-term studies using microwave therapy; however, the majority of these studies have been performed in high-energy cooled thermotherapy procedures. A summary of these studies revealed that TUMT is not as effective as TURP in improving urinary outflow obstruction. The symptomatic improvement that occurs with TUMT seems to be energy dose related. However, even when no objective signs of improvement are seen in comparative trials, the improvement in symptom score caused by TUMT can be considerable. TUMT is associated with a lengthy period of catheterization after treatment, thus causing increased rates of urinary tract infections and retention. The success associated with TUMT is not seen in every patient and a relatively high number of nonresponders in many series are noted. Finally, the exact place that TUMT fits in the BPH armamentarium has yet to be determined. Perhaps, the optimal place for TUMT maybe in medical nonresponders.

**AUA BPH Guideline Option: TUMT is effective in partially relieving LUTS secondary to BPH and may be considered in men with moderate or severe symptoms.**

[**Based on review of the data and Panel consensus**.]

## Laser Therapy

Laser (light amplification by the stimulated emission of radiation) has been used by the urologic community for the last quarter century. Early results were met with only poor to mild success. Over the years, four main types of lasers have been used to treat the prostate. Each of these lasers emits energy at a different wavelength and carries differing energy principals based on absorption and tissue penetration characteristics. The first laser was the neodymium:yttrium–aluminum–garnet (Nd:YAG), which emits light at a wavelength of 1,064 nanometers (nm). This light energy is poorly absorbed by both water and hemoglobin and thus penetrates deeply into human tissue. Because of these characteristics, a thermo coagulation zone is produced just under the surface of the prostatic urothelium. Hemostasis is excellent. Eventually, the coagulated tissue sloughs and, over a period of months, complete healing occurs.

The holmium:yttrium–aluminum–gartnet (Ho:YAG) laser emits light at a frequency of 2,120 nm (infrared range). This energy is emitted in a series of rapid pulses milliseconds and is highly absorbed by water but poorly absorbed by pigmented human tissue in an optical penetration depth of 0.4 mm. This laser can be used in both a cutting and a vaporization technique however; it is less hemostatic than other laser energy forms. The potassium-titanyl-phosphate (KTP) laser uses a specific KTP crystal to double the frequency of an Nd:YAG laser and produces a 532 nm wave length. This produces a wavelength, which is absorbed by both water and hemoglobin, allows for effective tissue vaporization at a lower level of tissue penetration. The diode laser is inefficient laser, thus requiring high-energy cooling devices and radiators which significantly increase the size of the machine. Diode lasers can occur at many different wavelengths and thus have varying light characteristics and physical interactions. The advantage to diode lasers is that they are significantly less expensive to build. Thus, the factors which determine whether laser coagulation or vaporization occurs are the time, power, and total amount of energy delivered to the tissue as it is applied.

A short but clear review of each of the above lasers and its clinical implications will be reviewed.

## Nd:YAG Laser

The Nd:YAG laser emitted high-energy beams (60–100 W) at a wavelength of 1,064 nm has been shown to be effective in vaporizing small amounts of tissue and produce coagulative necrosis of deeper prostatic tissue. This laser was found to be relatively ineffective, and currently is not used in the treatment of benign prostatic hyperplasia.

## Holmium:YAG Laser

The holmium:YAG laser is able to produce significant tissue vaporization and is currently used in both ablative and enucleative techniques. The current holmium laser has a maximum power of 100 W and can both resect and vaporize tissue. Holmium laser enculeation of the prostate (HoLEP) uses a 26 French continuous flow resectoscope and an end firing bare tipped fiber. The median lobe is first incised at the 5 and 7 o'clock position from the bladder neck to the verumontanum. A transverse incision is then performed just proximal to the veru to the level of the bladder neck. The median lobe is then pushed into the bladder. The lateral lobes are then enucleated by making incisions at 1 and 11 o'clock and then undermining the lobes laterally and pushing these into the bladder as well. The prostatic tissue is then morcellated into slurry and removed through the resectoscope (see Fig. 7.1). Numerous authors have published excellent results for the HoLEP technique. The procedures difficulty is that an extensive learning curve is necessary to perfect the technique and morcellation of the enucleated prostatic tissue has been reported to produce bladder perforation if not done correctly. Clinical results have revealed both excellent flow and symptom relief, similar to that of open prostatectomy; however, the risk of short-term urinary incontinence is greater than with other surgical techniques.

Holmium laser ablation of the prostate (HoLAP) uses the same 100 W holmium laser

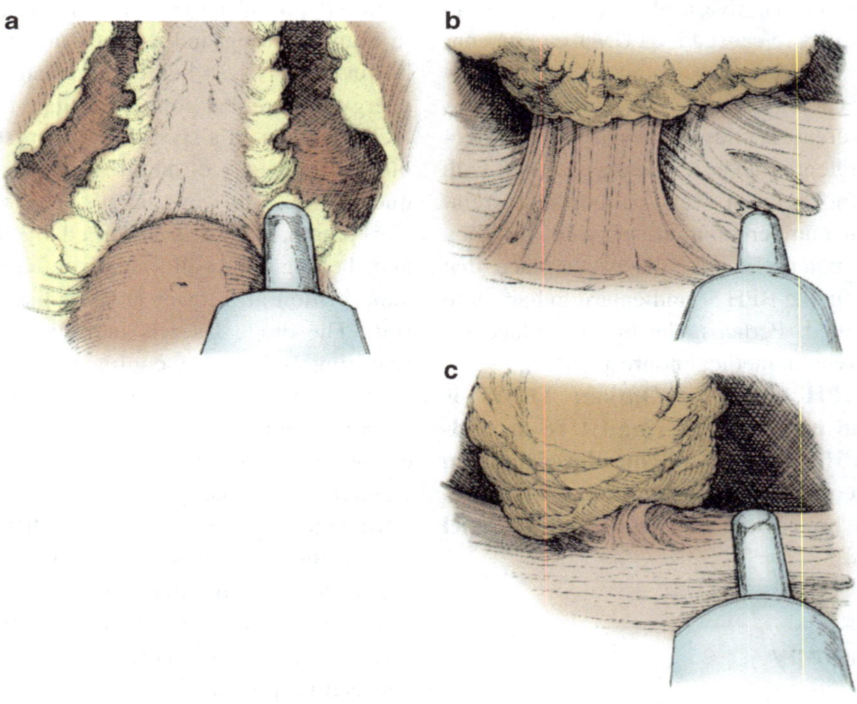

**Fig. 7.1** Holmium laser resection. (**a**) Bilateral bladder neck incisions. (**b**) Undermining the median lobe. (**c**) Releasing the median lobe. *Reprinted with permission from Campbell-Walsh urology, 10th edn. Philadelphia, PA: Saunders Elseiver; 2011*

box generator, but uses a side fire fiber to deliver its energy. The bladder neck, middle lobe, and lateral lobes are vaporized until an open prostatic channel is achieved. Short-term results have produced moderate results; however, the procedure was best served for small prostates. Hemostasis is adequate, but a significant amount of time is required to produce the desired tissue effects.

## Green Light Laser

Photo selective vaporization of the prostate (PVP) uses a KTP laser (80–180 W) of energy delivered through a 23 French continuous flow cystoscope and a 600 micron side firing glass fiber in a noncontact mode. This is usually performed under general anesthesia; however, a spinal anesthetic can be used. Once again, the end point of this procedure is a TURP like cavity. Saline is the recommended irrigant of choice. Hemostasis is excellent with this procedure as the 532 nm wavelength (in the green visible spectrum) is absorbed by hemoglobin, but not by water, thus limiting blood loss. The other acronyms for this procedure, KTP and LBO (lithium borate), identify the crystal used in the laser generator.

Both the short- and moderate-term results reported in the literature appear promising for this procedure. There has been significant improvement in flow rates, postvoid residual values, and symptom scores. Minimal complications have been reported. Improvements have been made in both wattage capability of the laser box unit as well as the fiber tip. Data on the newest version of the device, XPS generator and Moxy fiber, have yet to be published.

Diode lasers have achieved moderate clinical results in the urologic literature. The Indigo laser was an interstitial diode laser which produced multiple areas of coagulative necrosis and subsequent reabsorption of tissue. While the clinical results improved with an increase in the number of interstitial prostatic treatment zones, this laser device was eliminated from the market a few years ago. Other interstitial lasers have been used in a vaporization-type fashion. While these treatments produced moderate short-term flow and symptom score improvement, significant sloughing of prostatic tissue secondary to increase depths of penetration of this energy produced moderate-term complications and secondary procedures.

Laser technology in the use of benign prostatic hyperplasia continues to evolve. Continued improvements are recurring in each of these different laser modalities and this field continues to be an emerging technology.

**AUA BPH Guideline Option: Transurethral laser enucleation, transurethral side firing laser ablation, and photo selective vaporization are appropriate and effective treatment alternatives to transurethral resection of the prostate and open prostatectomy in men with moderate to severe LUTS and/or those who are significantly bothered by these symptoms. The choice of approach should be based on the patient's presentation, anatomy, the surgeon's level of training and experience, and a discussion of the potential benefit and risks for complications. Generally, transurethral laser approaches have been associated with shorter catheterization time and length of stay, with comparable improvements in LUTS. There is a decreased risk of the perioperative complication of transurethral resection syndrome. Information concerning certain outcomes, including retreatment and urethral strictures, is limited due to short follow-up. As with all new devices, comparison of outcomes between studies should be considered cautiously given the rapid evolution in technologies and power levels. Emerging evidence suggests a possible role of transurethral enucleation and laser vaporization as options for men with very large prostates (>100 g). There are insufficient data on which to base comments on bleeding.**

[**Based on review of the data and Panel consensus.**]

## Transurethral Incision of the Prostate

Transurethral Incision of the Prostate (TUIP) has been around for many years. Orandi [16] was the first clinician to report on a significant series of these patients. In his series younger men with high bladder necks and small prostates underwent an incision of the prostatic urethra from inside the bladder neck to lateral to the verumontanum. This incision was carried down to the prostatic capsule at the 5 and 7 o'clock positions. Orandi reported less retrograde ejaculation, a technically easy procedure to perform, and low morbidities. A 10% re-operation rate was reported by the same investigator in 1985 [17]. This procedure continues to be performed today using cold knives, hot knives, and holmium laser technology.

**AUA BPH Guideline Option: TUIP is an appropriate and effective treatment alternative in men with moderate to severe LUTS and/or who are significantly bothered by these symptoms when a prostate size is less than 30 g. The choice of approach should be based on the patient's individual presentation including anatomy, the surgeon's experience and discussion of potential benefits and risks for complications.**

**[Based on review of the data and Panel consensus.]**

## Intra-Prostatic Stents

Intra-prostatic stents were first used after stents had been reported to be beneficial in the cardiovascular literature. These were first performed in men who were unfit because of other medical conditions for surgery. Early stents were either composed of a metal alloy or woven mesh. These stents expanded the urethra to up to 42 French. Numerous complications were noted using these stents including hematuria, encrustation, migration, breakage, bacteruria, or stress urinary incontinence if these stents were not placed in the proper position. Recently, temporary or biodegradable stents have been investigated. These were developed in an effort to produce the positive findings of the permanent stents without some of the undesirable complications. Most of these stents have either been made from Nitinol (nickel–titanium) alloy or PGA. These types of stents have produced moderate success; however, patient pain and expense of the device have produced its limitations. Extensive work is currently being done with biodegradable stents. In the future, these may be used as drug delivery systems as well as treatment for obstructive voiding symptoms.

## Conclusion

The past quarter century has produced significant new technologies in the treatment of benign prostatic hyperplasia. Some of these have been beneficial, while others have produced minimal improvements. While TURP remains the "gold standard" therapy, many newer treatment modalities have been able to produce similar results with a lower complication rate. I look forward to the next quarter century and the new treatment options yet to be developed.

**AUA BPH Guideline Recommendation: Surgery is recommended for patients who have renal insufficiency secondary to BPH, who have recurrent UTI's, bladder stones or gross hematuria due to BPH, and those who have LUTS refractory to other therapies. The presence of a bladder diverticulum is not an absolute indication for surgery unless associated with recurrent UTI or progressive bladder dysfunction.**

**[Based on review of the data and Panel consensus.]**

## References


1. McVary KT, Roehrborn CG, Avins AL, et al. Update on AUA guideline on the management of benign prostatic hyperplasia. J Urol. 2011;185:1793–803.
2. Serretta V, Morgia G, Fondacaro L, et al. Open prostatectomy for benign prostatic enlargement in Southern Europe in the late 1990s: a contemporary series of 1,800 interventions. Urology. 2002;60(4):623–7.
3. Varkarakis I, Kyriakakis Z, Delis A, et al. Long-term results of open transvesical prostatectomy from a contemporary series of patients. Urology. 2004;64(2):306–10.
4. Zargooshi J. Open prostatectomy for benign prostate hyperplasia: short-term outcome in 3,000 consecutive patients. Prostate Cancer Prostatic Dis. 2007;10(4):374–7.
5. Mebust WK, Holtgrewe HL, Cockett AT, et al. Transurethral prostatectomy: immediate and

postoperative complications: a cooperative study of 13 participating institutions evaluating 3,885 patients. J Urol. 1989;141(2):243–7.

6. Roehrborn CG, Issa MM, Bruskewitz R, et al. Transurethral needle ablation (TUNA) for benign prostatic hyperplasia: 12-month results of a prospective multicenter study. Urology. 1998;51:415–21.
7. Bruskewitz R, Issa MM, Roehrborn CG, et al. A prospective, randomized, 1-year clinical trial comparing transurethral needle ablation (TUNA) to transurethral resection of the prostate for the treatment of symptomatic benign prostatic hyperplasia. J Urol. 1998;159:1588–94.
8. Schulman CC, Zlotta AR, Rasor JS, et al. Transurethral needle ablation (TUNA): safety, feasibility and tolerance of a new office procedure for the treatment of benign prostatic hyperplasia. Eur Urol. 1993;24:415–23.
9. Campo B, Bergamasghi F, Corrada P, et al. Transurethral needle ablation (TUNA) of the prostate: a clinical and urodynamic evaluation. Urology. 1997; 49:847–50.
10. Ramon J, Lynch TH, Eardley I, et al. Transurethral needle ablation of the prostate for the treatment of benign prostatic hyperplasia: a collaborative multicenter study. Br J Urol. 1997;80:128–35.
11. Rosario DJ, Woo H, Potts KL, et al. Safety and efficacy of transurethral needle ablation of the prostate for symptomatic outlet obstruction. Br J Urol. 1997;80:579–86.
12. Steele GS, Sleep DJ. Transurethral needle ablation of the prostate: a urodynamic-based study with two-year follow-up. J Urol. 1997;158:1834–8.
13. Millard RJ, Harewood LM, Tamaddon K. A study of the efficacy and safety of transurethral needle ablation (TUNA) for benign prostatic hyperplasia. Neurourol Urodyn. 1996;15:916–29.
14. Organ LW. Electrophysiological principles of radiofrequency lesion making. In: International symposium on radiofrequency lesion making procedures,Chicago, Illinois, 1976. Appl Neurophysiol. 1976;39:69–76.
15. Larson TR, Bostwick DG, Corica A. Temperature-correlated histopathologic changes following microwave thermoablation of obstructive tissue in patients with benign prostatic hyperplasia. Urology. 1996; 47:463–9.
16. Orandi A. Transurethral incision of the prostate. J Urol. 1973;110:229–31.
17. Orandi A. Transurethral incision of the prostate (TUIP): 646 cases in 15 years—a chronological appraisal. Br J Urol. 1985;57:703–7.

# Rational Herbal and Complementary Interventions for Prevention and Treatment of Urological Disorders in Men

8

Mark A. Moyad

## Introduction

Arguably, almost every area of urology is impacted by complementary medicine [1–5]. Some of these interventions have potential profound impacts independently or in combination with conventional therapy, others have no impact, and some could negatively impact treatment and overall health. Few specialties have arguably invested more energy and financial effort in determining whether certain dietary supplements impact a variety of medical conditions compared to urology [6, 7]. Therefore, a rapid review of potentially effective and noneffective complementary medicine interventions is timely. Keep in mind that heart health has been generally tantamount to urologic health when deciding which complementary interventions to recommend or discourage [8].

## BPH/LUTS

Benign Prostatic Hyperplasia (BPH) or Lower Urinary Tract Symptoms (LUTS) has a consistent history of being positively impacted by heart healthy lifestyle changes. Again, reminding patients that almost anything heart healthy is beneficial for prostate health is an easy to construe and memorable mantra [9–11]. Thus, it is also empirical that heart unhealthy changes appear to increase the risk of exacerbation of BPH such as minimal to no aerobic exercise, obesity, poor mental health, dyslipidemia, coronary heart disease, hypertension, diabetes, tobacco use… all tend to have a potential dramatic negative impact via multiple mechanisms including increased sympathetic tone, cholesterol, oxidative stress, etc. [12–19].

### Beta-Sitosterol Supplements and Cholesterol Reducing Mechanisms

Phytosterols are found in diverse plants and plant oils, are somewhat similar in structure to cholesterol except for a minor difference that allows for a unique benefit [20]. They are not synthesized in humans and poorly absorbed, rapidly excreted from the liver compared to cholesterol, and rarely found in large concentrations in human tissues. The primary phytosterols found in diet are sitosterol, stigmasterol, and campesterol. Beta-sitosterol is the phytosterol arguably found in higher quantities in the diet. Phytosterols inhibit the absorption of exogenous cholesterol from dietary and bile sources in the intestinal tract. LDL cholesterol reduction occurs when phytosterols are consumed, but HDL and triglycerides

M.A. Moyad, MD, MPH (✉)
Jenkins/Pokempner Director of Preventative and Alternative Medicine, Department of Urology, University of Michigan Medical Center, 1500 East Medical Center Drive, Ann Arbor, MI 48109, USA
e-mail: moyad@umich.edu

D.A. Shoskes (ed.), *Urological Men's Health: A Guide for Urologists and Primary Care Physicians*, Current Clinical Urology, DOI 10.1007/978-1-61779-900-6_8,
© Springer Science+Business Media New York 2012

are not affected. The inhibition of cholesterol absorption may produce a relative cholesterol resource pool reduction that is followed by upregulation of cholesterol synthesis and LDL receptors, which can increase LDL removal from the circulation. This is essentially a similar mechanism whereby several healthy dietary fats found in many healthy foods such as almonds or pistachios may also reduce LDL and improve some specific urologic outcomes [21, 22].

Approximately, more than 40 clinical trials of phytosterols have been conducted that have ranged from 1 month to 1 year in duration [20, 23, 24]. Plant sterols have been added to multiple diverse foods such as margarine, mayonnaise, milk, orange juice, olive oil, and yogurt with a reduction in LDL by approximately 10–15% when approximately 2,000 mg per day is consumed. In general, 1,600–3,000 mg of plant sterol supplemental or tablet consumption can also reduce LDL approximately 4–15%. Plant sterols have the ability to inhibit the absorption of some fat-soluble vitamins, so there has been some debate as to whether multivitamin consumption should occur with the use of these products. Perhaps, in the author's opinion, a children's multivitamin should be consumed by an adult utilizing plant sterol supplements because of some concerns over the excessive exposure of nutrients such as folic acid from some high-dose adult multivitamins [8].

The primary mechanism of action of the plant sterols appears to occur through dietary cholesterol uptake inhibition and a minor anti-inflammatory response, which arguably suggests that they are weaker or somewhat inferior mimics of the drug ezetimibe (Zetia®), which can reduce LDL by approximately 20% with 10 mg standard recommended dosage [25, 26].

Basic science research has recently demonstrated the ability of ezetimibe to favorably impact prostate tissue and inhibit BPH [27]. Interestingly, ezetimibe is commonly added to statin therapy or other lipid- lowering agents to achieve synergistically further reduce LDL [25, 26]. Thus, it is logical to conclude that beta-sitosterol by itself or with other cholesterol-lowering medications could favorably impact BPH. Despite some data to suggest minimal clinical impact of statins on established BPH over a short period of time [28, 29], other new epidemiologic and past basic science investigations suggest potentially favorable impacts on BPH prevention and progression with cholesterol-lowering prescribed medications [30–32].

Several past meta-analysis and one recent clinical guidelines summary have suggested that beta-sitosterol supplements could provide some benefit for men with BPH/LUTS [33–35]. Beta-sitosterol in some studies is an extract that contains a variety of phytosterols, which were usually extracted from South African star grass (Hypoxis rooperi). Researchers reported a mean positive difference versus placebo for IPSS of –4.9 points, peak urinary flow rate was 3.91 ml/sec, and residual volume was –28.62 ml. Beta-sitosterol had no short-term impact on prostate size, which is of interest because there is some preliminary evidence that it could partially inhibit 5-alpha-reductase [36]. The approximately 8% withdrawal rates was similar to placebo. Most common adverse events with beta-sitosterol were gastrointestinal in 1.6% and erectile dysfunction in 0.5%. These analyses were conducted from four trials with 519 men [34].

Why not just utilize or recommend beta-sitosterol, a heart-healthy ingredient, with or without medications for BPH? The dosage range the trials have been from 0.30 mg of beta-sitosterol-beta-D-glucoside to approximately 200 mg per day. Yet, the dosage recommended in national cholesterol treatment guidelines is 2,000–3,000 mg a day to reduce LDL by 6–15%, and the National Cholesterol Education Panel (NCEP) recommendations the following: "Plant stanol/sterol esters (2 g/day) are a therapeutic option to enhance LDL cholesterol lowering" [37]. It should be of interest that no recent studies of beta-sitosterol have been published, but if patients are going to use a cost-effective product for cholesterol reduction, it is theoretically possible that a secondary benefit may be the prevention or reduction of some aspect of BPH/LUTS.

A total of 18 Pygeum africanum clinical trials were reviewed in a meta-analysis from 2002, which suggested a potential benefit with this supplement [38]. This product is an extract of the African prune tree. The mean duration time of clinical trials was only 64 days, but men were more than two times as likely to report an improvement in overall symptoms with this product. Nocturia decreased by 19%, residual volume by 24%, and peak urine flow increased by 23%. The withdrawal rate of 12% was similar to placebo. Adverse effects were also similar to placebo, but the most commonly reported adverse effects were gastrointestinal. In general, studies utilized a standardized extract effective at approximately 100–200 mg per day. It is also of interest that one of the main components of Pygeum africanum and even saw palmetto is phytosterols that include beta-sitosterol [39, 40]. However, a serious issue with Pygeum exists and that is the demand compared to precious supply because the bark is derived from an endangered tree [41]. Despite previous suggestions of the need for a major clinical trial to support past positive clinical and mechanistic benefits such as the inhibition of growth factor influenced pathways [42], the future supply of true Pygeum similar to what was utilized in past studies will probably somewhat limit the design of any future trial.

Saw palmetto has some similar and different issues compared to pygeum and beta-sitosterol. There appears to be few limitations to the supply of this herbal compound, and it has arguably a diverse number of heart healthy compounds apart from beta-sitosterol including the primary monounsaturated fat found in olive oil known as oleic acid, and a variety of other potentially healthy dietary fats that may have the ability to increase HDL and lower cardiovascular events [43–46]. Although recent low dose (320 mg/day) and even dose-escalation (up to 960 mg/day), major clinical trials of approximately 1–1.5 years on this intervention have failed to find a benefit for saw palmetto [47, 48]. Adverse events were similar to a placebo at even the highest dosages, which is why it still may be a safe option for mild symptoms, and one cannot ignore that other major trials outside of the USA have been positive [49, 50], and in one case equaled or even surpassed in subgroups the benefits observed with an alpha-blocker [50]. How do clinicians resolve this strange clinical conundrum? Saw palmetto was not subject to placebo control in many of these positive studies, yet neither was the drug option. It is also possible that some of the European and other saw palmetto options have greater concentrations of isolated single drug-like compounds compared to what was utilized in the USA. [51]. Saw palmetto is cost-effective and arguably could be considered a first-line safe product for mild symptoms that could then be discarded after a several months if proven ineffective [52], or when combined with beta-sitosterol and pygeum. More severe symptoms should arguably not be handled by a dietary supplement. And, regardless of pharmacologic and/or dietary supplement usage, never underestimate the importance of strongly encouraging heart healthy lifestyle changes to the patient.

## Chronic Nonbacterial Prostatitis/ Chronic Pelvic Pain Syndrome/ Interstitial Cystitis

Complementary medicine for chronic nonbacterial prostatitis and interstitial cystitis (IC) should be well known and at least they have a history of being heart healthy and some even reduce blood pressure in prehypertensive patients [53–57]. Doses of 1,000 mg per day of a quercetin complex have provided significant pain relief and improved quality of life in 1 month or less for many individuals. Interestingly, positive preliminary clinical studies began to publish over a decade ago with these complexes. The reader is encouraged to review the latest information on quercetin complex agents for nonbacterial prostatitis for example from experts that have conducted past and ongoing clinical studies with these agents [58].

Cernitin or a pollen extract also continues to receive positive results but recommending specific dosages is not as easy based on the difficulty in standardizing the specific ingredients used in these supplements in clinical trials [54, 55]. Regardless, pollen extract is an option for nonbacterial chronic prostatitis that has the potential to reduce pain and improve quality of life.

Heart healthy lifestyle changes that have also displayed some preliminary profound effects in this area of urologic health appear less publicized.

A lifestyle clinical study from Florence, Italy was double-blind, randomized and found encouraging results because the participants failed conventional treatments [59]. Participants (mean age of 36–38 years, BMI of 22, mean symptom duration 5.5–6 months) experienced pain in the pelvic region for 3 or more months continuously and scored a minimum of 15 points on NIH-CPSI with at least six or more points on the pain subscale. A total of 52 individuals were placed in the exercise group and 51 were assigned to the placebo/stretching group. The outcome measures were the NIH-CPSI, Beck Depression Inventory, State Anxiety Inventory-Y (SAI-Y), and a pain visual analog scale (VAS). These evaluations were determined at baseline, 6 and 18 weeks. The exercise group participated in vigorous walking three times per week for 40 min each session to achieve 70/80% of the predicted age-based maximum heart rate. The placebo/stretching group performed several stretching exercises, but had to maintain their heart rate under 110 beats per minute for the entire session. Approximately, 25% of the participants dropped out of the study by 18 weeks. Significant differences between the two groups favored the exercise group for total NIH-CPSI ($p=0.006$), pain ($p=0.0009$), quality of life subscales ($p=0.02$), and VAS ($p=0.003$). No difference was observed for other parameters. Responders were considered those that experienced a decrease of six or more points in total NIH-CPSI (58% exercise vs. 43% placebo), 25–49% (39% vs. 35%), and 50% (19% vs. 5%) or more decrease from baseline in total NIH-CPSI. A 25% placebo response of this magnitude is expected from other clinical trials. It is of interest that pain is the symptom that is arguably the most influential variable and quality of life predictor and should be one of the primary targets of any therapy or combination treatment. Exercise induces release of endogenous opioids and reduces sympathetic activity to prostate and surrounding tissues [60–62].

## Bladder/Kidney/Prostate Cancers

Smoking is not just correlated with only lung cancer risk, but also bladder cancer [63–65]. Additionally, smoking after bladder or prostate cancer treatment may also increase the risk of cancer recurrence and cardiovascular disease. Interestingly, obesity is associated with a higher risk of several cancers but kidney cancer (renal cell) has arguably the strongest correlation [66–70]. Hypertension, lack of exercise, smoking, and perhaps dyslipidemia may also be associated with increased risks of kidney cancer. Most heart healthy behaviors are simply correlated with a potential lower risk of kidney and prostate cancer [2, 3, 8].

There is evidence to suggest that mega-doses of most dietary supplements or antioxidants do not appear to provide benefit and may even encourage tumor growth in multiple situations [6, 71–84]. Similar to the evidence that existed in terms of cardiovascular risk increases with larger intakes of dietary supplements [72, 75, 81].

How does this relate to bladder cancer? In a preliminary randomized study from the 1990s, there was a suggestion that mega-doses of a supplement as opposed to a recommended daily allowance (RDA) pill may reduce the risk of non-muscle invasive bladder cancer recurrence after BCG therapy [85]. However, a larger follow-up study was needed to confirm these preliminary findings, which was recently published [86]. Participants who were BCG naïve with carcinoma in situ, Ta or T1 bladder cancer were randomized to receive intravesical BCG or BCG+interferon alpha-2b, and then further randomized to receive an RDA (minimal intake) or mega-dose supplement. Each RDA pill of vitamins contained 25% of the recommended daily dose and participants ingested two tablets twice daily of either the RDA, or the mega-dose supplement. Each mega-dose tablet contained 9,000 IU of vitamin A, 25 mg of B6, 500 mg of vitamin C, 400 IU of vitamin D3, 400 mcg of folate, 100 IU of vitamin E, and 7.6 mg of zinc. Induction BCG was given weekly for 6 weeks, and then at 4, 7, 13, 19, 25, and 37 months. The primary endpoint was biopsy confirmed recurrence or cytology that was positive. A total of 670 patients were randomized and at 24-month median follow-up there were no significant differences between the RDA and mega-dose supplements groups. The following recurrence-free survival numbers were: BCG+RDA 63%, BCG+mega-dose supplement 59%, BCG+Interferon+RDA 55%, and BCG+Interferon+mega-dose supplement 61%. Mega-dose supplements, and/or interferon alpha-2b added to BCG did not impact time to recurrence in the subjects with nonmuscle invasive bladder cancer. There was a minimal nonsignificant increased risk of recurrence with BCG and the mega-dose supplement.

When the initial bladder cancer and mega-dose study published in the 1990s in the Journal of Urology, it was clearly a unique, bold and wonderful contribution in the field of complementary medicine [85], and these mega-dose vitamins probably did reduce the risk of recurrence in my opinion in that older publication. Why? Researchers arguably recruited a population of individuals that had deficiencies in a variety of vitamins and minerals. Fast-forward almost two decades and participants in these trials are no longer deficient, but they appear to be oversupplemented with antioxidants from foods, beverages, and a multitude of dietary supplements [8, 87]. This provides an almost insurmountable barrier to conduct a large clinical trial of a truly deficient healthy population over a long period of time, despite some authors calling for the need for such studies [88]. When nutritional clinical trials are designed, these deficiencies are more prevalent, but by the time the trial commences they may no longer exist [6, 8, 71, 87].

The more recent bladder cancer trial utilizing the mega-dose supplement itself had added folic acid and vitamin D to it versus the original formulation from the preliminary successful study [85, 86]. Why was the formula altered from what was potentially successful in the preliminary study, because of some minimal or even moderate laboratory and population data? Would this be allowed in a definitive phase three pharmaceutical studies, where the phase 1 or 2 had a successful outcome and safety with a specific dose and formulation, and it was simply changed in the phase 3 trial? Arguably these nutrients, especially folic acid, also have data to suggest that they could also increase recurrence of certain cancers or other abnormalities when given at these higher doses [77–80]. In reality, lower doses of these supplements may be providing the benefits needed without adding the significant increased risks or overall concerns for most individuals [89, 90]. Of more interest to the reader, over the past 20 years multiple randomized trials and some observational studies suggest that a potentially heart and digestive healthy probiotic (Lactobacillus casei) found in some types of yogurt, and available as potential dietary supplement at 3 g per day may reduce the risk of bladder cancer or recurrence after conventional treatment [91–96]. Why isn't this supplement being utilized for specific bladder cancer patients along with lifestyle changes?

An additional note concerning the future of urologic cancer prevention including prostate, kidney, or bladder cancer may be that the only dietary supplement that may look promising in the future in this capacity is one that produces a heart healthy outcome. For example, the increasing interest and accumulating positive overall data concerning cholesterol lowering to potentially reduce the risk of aggressive prostate cancer or perhaps slow the progression of this disease has become fascinating [97]. However, it has been difficult for over a decade for this author to get the attention of some researchers and companies in order to make such a clinical trial occur. Therefore, red yeast rice extract, a dietary supplement with a natural amount of a statin mimic in it is going to be tested in active surveillance patients in a clinical trial [98]. This study represents a major step forward in not only the mind set of how to potentially prevent urologic cancer, but to potentially at the very least attempt to also reduce the risk of the number one cause of death in men [99]. Other supplements right now for cancer prevention tend to receive more hyperbole, such as vitamin D, but the overall general health data using larger quantities of this supplement is not only misrepresented [100–102], but recent evidence suggests a potential increased risk of prostate cancer with higher blood levels of this vitamin [103].

## Infertility

Heart unhealthy behaviors or lifestyle changes also negatively impact male fertility [104]. Obesity, high cholesterol and blood pressure, lack of exercise, improper diet, stress, depression and multiple other heart disease risk factors that increase oxidative stress all have some minor or major impact on fertility and should be addressed immediately to change patients lives and improving overall health [105–107].

Of enormous additional interest is that some recent authoritative and influential medical reviews appear to be recommending antioxidant supplements for some male fertility issues [108, 109]. For example, a recent Cochrane review is one of the most extensive published in male fertility and dietary supplements, because it reviewed and analyzed 34 clinical trials with 2,876 couples [109]. The authors concluded that numerous diverse antioxidant supplements appears to have a significant positive role in improving the outcomes of live birth and pregnancy rates in couples participating in Assisted Reproduction Techniques (ART). The P-value for live births was 0.0008 and for pregnancy rates it was $p<0.00001$. Critics of this analysis on "live births" will likely point toward the small number of such events ($n=20$) that occurred from a total of 214 couples in only three trials that was used in this part of the analysis, or the "pregnancy rates," which were derived from 96 pregnancies in 15 trials that included 964 couples. However, this should not change the relevance of these positive findings with supplements because they have to remain a viable option for some men given the low cost of most "antioxidants" utilized in these clinical trials. Furthermore, adverse events were similar to a placebo with no serious side events reported in any trial.

Thus, which specific dietary supplements, what dosage and frequency should be recommended for male fertility issues? This extensive review could not identify one or several ideal individual antioxidants or combination products from these trials [109], so clinicians and patients appeared to be left with unanswered clinical inquires. However, perhaps it is not as difficult to recommend several supplements for infertility. Complementary medicines that have a past overall safety record that may be heart healthy should be the only ones recommended for fertility from this past review [109], especially if there is equivalent efficacy among all the positive trials. For example, CoQ10 at 200–300 mg/day [110], L-carnitine at 2,000–3,000 mg/day [111–115], omega-3 fatty acids (fish oil) [116–118], and vitamin C [119–121], but not high-dose supplements that have a potential heart or overall male unhealthy profile [8, 87], such as folic acid [77, 78], selenium and vitamin E [71, 73], or even mega-doses of zinc [84].

## Sexual Dysfunction

Arguably, one of the most prime examples of how heart healthy lifestyle changes positively impact urologic health has to be in the area of male and female sexual dysfunction [122–127]. These changes can also improve the efficacy of prescription erectile dysfunction medications [128]. Several compounds also deserve attention as an over-the-counter first-line safe option for erectile dysfunction (ED) of psychogenic or mixed etiology. For example, Korean Red Ginseng at a dosage of 1,800–3,000 mg a day or even at half these doses when advanced concentration methods have been used have begun to receive adequate support and recommendations from recent state-of-the-art clinical recommendations [129]. This would appear to represent the first safe dietary supplement to achieve such a status in urology. The problem is that quality control with ginseng has been an issue, so that the clinician and patient should seek reputable companies that standardize the ginsenosides (active ingredients) in the Korean ginseng [130]. Another dietary supplement that is a combination of pycnogenol (approximately 80 mg) and arginine (approximately 3 g) is also achieving a considerable and impressive amount of clinical data and should also be considered as an option even for those with potentially impaired nitric oxide levels as represented by comorbidities [131, 132]. Whether or not either of these supplements can be combined with standard prescription ED medications is not known at this time, but arginine has the potential to reduce blood pressure whereby ginseng does not consistently have this ability. It is even plausible that these two dietary supplements may be ideal for different types of men with ED. Regardless, both of these supplements are hopefully changing the perception that this author has witnessed for over a decade, because the reality is that several over-the-counter options for ED may now be potential options in the clinical setting. And, another important point is that the cost of the over the counters is generally affordable and their side effect profile is manageable for most men and this is not necessarily the case with ED prescription pills for some men [132–135].

## Stones and Urinary Tract Infections

Heart healthy recommendations also appear to be options for those at an increased risk for kidney stones [136–139]. Recent data also suggests that individuals at risk for nephrolithiasis may also be at risk for cardiovascular disease [140]. Peyronie's disease has had several potential supplements discussed and even recommended with mixed results [141–143], but preliminary novel data on coenzyme Q10 at 300 mg a day appears to be promising [144]. CoQ10 may also slightly lower blood pressure in prehypertensive patients and may reduce some statin side effects, but further research on interactions with warfarin is needed [145].

Increasing global antibiotic resistance to multiple pathogens is concerning [146]. Other nonantibiotic options are needed as potential alternatives to prevalent conditions including recurrent urinary tract infections (UTIs). Cranberry drink and supplements have garnered some interest as a potential viable option for recurrent UTIs but the beverage has had compliance and high withdrawal rate issues [147]. A recent clinical trial with cranberry supplementation may not have been as effective compared to antibiotics over a 1-year period but still the safety and efficacy should be of interest to the clinician [148]. This was a double-blind trial of 221 premenopausal women who were randomized to 12-month prophylaxis utilization of TMP-SMX 480 mg once daily, or 500 mg twice daily of cranberry capsules. Mean number of symptomatic UTIs over 12 months, percentage of patients with at least 1 symptomatic UTI, median time to first UTI, and the development of antibiotic resistance (indigenous *Escherichia coli*) were all primary endpoints. After approximately 1 year, the mean number of participants with at least 1 symptomatic UTI was significantly ($p=0.02$) lower in the TMP-SMX group (1.8 vs 4.0) and the percentage of women with at least 1 symptomatic UTI was higher in the cranberry group (78 vs 71%). Median time to first UTI was 8 months on the antibiotic compared to 4 months with cranberry. Approximately 91% of the asymptomatic bacteriuria *E coli* isolates were TMP-SMX resistant after 1 month compared to 28% with cranberry. Antibiotic resistance was not increased in the cranberry arm of the study. Thus, TMP-SMX at 480 mg per day was more effective than 500 mg bid cranberry capsules to prevent recurrent UTIs in premenopausal women, but at the limitation of causing antibiotic resistance. It was also concerning that the antibiotic resistance was so high in such a short period of time (1 month), and a "simultaneous increase" in resistance to fluoroquinolones and amoxicillin also occurred. There is little doubt that antibiotics are more effective than a dietary supplement but when examining the risk versus benefit ratio some clinicians will be more eager to try cranberry supplements for some patients, such as those that are worried about drug-resistance with long-term use. A final note about cranberry supplements is that the issue of a high oxalate concentration in some products may be concerning. Cranberry supplements should report their oxalate content in my opinion based on a past wonderful study that should receive more attention [149].

## Conclusion

Heart healthy appears to be equivalent to urologic health. In fact, large and diverse (American Cancer Society, American Heart Association, and the American Diabetes Association) health care preventive organizations are becoming unified in this belief [150], because life-altering lifestyle recommendations for patients are not mutually exclusive, and neither are dietary supplements [8]. They impact multiple clinical endpoints and have the highest overall probability of impacting all-cause morbidity and mortality. This is critical in my opinion, because again the forest has to take precedence over the tree in order to improve the overall state of urologic health. Again, Heart health = Urologic health should be the unified mantra for urologic practitioners because it is also easy to construe for patients, simple and rapid for the clinician to recommend and arguably has the best chance of immediately improving the lives of your patients.

## References


1. Moyad MA. Calcium oxalate kidney stones: another reason to encourage moderate calcium intakes and other dietary changes. Urol Nurs. 2003;23:310–3.
2. Moyad MA. Step-by-step lifestyle changes that can improve urologic health in men, part I: what do I tell my patients? Prim Care. 2006;33:139–63.
3. Moyad MA. Step-by-step lifestyle changes that can improve urologic health in men, part II: what do I tell my patients? Prim Care. 2006;33:165–85.
4. Moyad MA, Roach 3rd M. Promoting wellness for patients on androgen deprivation therapy: why using numerous drugs for drug side effects should not be first-line treatment. Urol Clin North Am. 2011;38:303–12.
5. Kane CJ, Raheem OA, Bent S, Avins AL. What do I tell patients about saw palmetto for benign prostatic hyperplasia. Urol Clin North Am. 2011;38:261–77.
6. Lippman SM, Klein EA, Goodman PJ, et al. Effect of selenium and vitamin E on risk of prostate and other cancers: the Selenium and Vitamin E Cancer Prevention Trial (SELECT). JAMA. 2009;301:39–51.
7. Lee J, Andriole G, Avins A, et al. Redesigning a large-scale clinical trial in response to negative external trial results: the CAMUS study of phytotherapy for benign prostatic hyperplasia. Clin Trials. 2009;6:628–36.
8. Moyad MA. Promoting wellness for patients with prostate cancer, 3rd edn. Ann Arbor: Ann Arbor Media Publishing; 2011.
9. Moyad MA. Lifestyle changes to prevent BPH: heart healthy=prostate healthy. Urol Nurs. 2003;23:439–41.
10. Sea J, Poon KS, McVary KT. Review of exercise and the risk of benign prostatic hyperplasia. Phys Sportsmed. 2009;37:75–83.
11. Parsons JK, Im R. Alcohol consumption is associated with a decreased risk of benign prostatic hyperplasia. J Urol. 2009;182:1463–8.
12. Parsons JK. Benign prostatic hyperplasia and male lower urinary tract symptoms: epidemiology and risk factors. Curr Bladder Dysfunct Rep. 2010;5:212–8.
13. Moyad MA, Lowe FC. Educating patients about lifestyle modifications for prostate health. Am J Med. 2008;121(8 Suppl 2):S34–42.
14. Parsons JK. Lifestyle factors, bengin prostatic hyperplasia, and lower urinary tract symptoms. Curr Opin Urol. 2011;21:1–4.
15. Zhang X, Zhang J, Chen J, et al. Prevalence and risk factors of nocturia and nocturia-related quality of life in the Chinese population. Urol Int. 2011;86:173–8.
16. Wong SY, Woo J, Leung JC, Leung PC. Depressive symptoms and lifestyle factors as risk factors of lower urinary tract symptoms in Southern Chinese men: a prospective study. Aging Male. 2010;13:113–9.
17. Mongiu AK, McVary KT. Lower urinary tract symptoms, bengin prostatic hyperplasia, and obesity. Curr Urol Rep. 2009;10:247–53.
18. Parsons JK, Bergstrom J, Barrett-Connor E. Lipids, lipoproteins and the risk of benign prostatic hyperplasia in community-dwelling men. BJU Int. 2008;101:313–8.
19. Parsons JK. Modifiable risk factors for benign prostatic hyperplasia and lower urinary tract symptoms: new approaches to old problems. J Urol. 2007;178:395–401.
20. Jones PJ, AbuMweis SS. Phytosterols as functional food ingredients: linkages to cardiovascular disease and cancer. Curr Opin Clin Nutr Metab Care. 2009;12:147–51.
21. Berryman CE, Preston AG, Karmally W, Deckelbaum RJ, Kris-Etherton PM. Effects of almond consumption on the reduction of LDL-cholesterol: a discussion of potential mechanisms and future research directions. Nutr Rev. 2011;69:171–85.
22. Aldemir M, Okulu E, Neselioglu S, Erel O, Kayigil O. Pistachio diet improves erectile function parameters and serum lipid profiles in patients with erectile dysfunction. Int J Impot Res. 2011;23:32–8.
23. Guardamagna O, Abello F, Baracco V, et al. Primary hyperlipidemias in children: effect of plant sterol supplementation on plasma lipids and markers of cholesterol synthesis and absorption. Acta Diabetol. 2011;48(2):127–33.
24. Malinkowski JM, Gehret MM. Phytosterols for dyslipidemia. Am J Health Syst Pharm. 2010;67:1165–73.
25. Hamilton P. Role of ezetimibe in the management of patients with atherosclerosis. Coron Artery Dis. 2009;20:169–74.
26. Dujovne CA, Suresh R, McCrary Sisk C, et al. Safety and efficacy of ezetimibe monotherapy in 1624 primary hypercholesterolaemic patients for up to 2 years. Int J Clin Pract. 2008;62:1332–6.
27. Pelton K, Di Vizio D, Insabato L, et al. Ezetimibe reduces enlarged prostate in an animal model of benign prostatic hyperplasia. J Urol. 2010;184:1555–9.
28. Mills IW, Crossland A, Patel A, Ramonas H. Atorvastatin treatment for men with lower urinary tract symptoms and benign prostatic enlargement. Eur Urol. 2007;52:503–9.
29. Stamatiou KN, Zaglavira P, Skolarikos A, Sofras F. The effects of lovastatin on conventional medical treatment of lower urinary tract symptoms with finasteride. Int Braz J Urol. 2008;34:555–61.

30. Hall SA, Chiu GR, Link CL, et al. Are statin medications associated with lower urinary tract symptoms in men and women? Results from the Boston Area Community Health (BACH) Survey. Ann Epidemiol. 2011;21:149–55.
31. St Sauver JL, Jacobsen SJ, Jacobson DJ, et al. Statin use and decreased risk of benign prostatic enlargement and lower urinary tract symptoms. BJU Int. 2011;107:443–50.
32. Padayatty SJ, Marcelli M, Shao TC, Cunningham GR. Lovastatin-induced apoptosis in prostate stromal cells. J Clin Endocrinol Metab. 1997;82:1434–9.
33. Wilt TJ, MacDonald R, Ishani A. Beta-sitosterol for the treatment of benign prostatic hyperplasia: a systematic review. BJU Int. 1999;83:976–83.
34. Wilt T, Ishani A, MacDonald R, et al. Beta-sitosterols for benign prostatic hyperplasia. Cochrane Database Syst Rev. 2000;(2):CD001043.
35. McNicholas T, Kirby R. Benign prostatic hyperplasia and male lower urinary tract symptoms (LUTS). Clin Evid (online). 2011.
36. Cabeza M, Bratoeff E, Heuze I, et al. Effect of beta-sitosterol as inhibitor of 5-alpha-reductase in hamster prostate. Proc West Pharmacol Soc. 2003;46:153–5.
37. National Cholesterol Education Porgram (NCEP) Expert Panel on Detection, Evaluation, and Treatment of High Blood Cholesterol in Adults (Adult Treatment Panel III). Third Report of the National Cholesterol Education Program (NCEP) Expert Panel on Detection, Evaluation, and Treatment of High Blood Cholesterol in Adults (Adult Treatment Panel III) final report. Circulation. 2002;106:3143–421.
38. Wilt T, Ishani A, Mac Donald R, Rutks I, Stark G. Pygeum africanum for bengin prostatic hyperplasia. Cochrane Database Syst Rev. 2002;(1):CD001044.
39. McQueen CE, Bryant PJ. Pygeum. Am J Health Syst Pharm. 2001;58:120–3.
40. Suzuki M, Ito Y, Fujino T, et al. Pharmacological effects of saw palmetto extract in the lower urinary tract. Acta Pharmacol Sin. 2009;30:227–81.
41. Stewart KM. The African cherry (*Prunus africana*): can lessons be learned from an over-exploited tree. J Ethnopharmacol. 2003;89:3–13.
42. Edgar AD, Levin R, Constantinou CE, Denis L. A critical review of the pharmacology of the plant extract of Pygeum africanum in the treatment in the treatment of the LUTS. Neurourol Urodyn. 2007;26:458–63.
43. Lopez-Miranda J, Perez-Jimenez F, Ros E, et al. Olive oil and health: summary of the II international conference on olive oil and health consensus report, Jaen and Cordoba (Spain) 2008. Nutr Metab Cardiovasc Dis. 2010;20:284–94.
44. Mensink RP, Zock PL, Kester AD, Katan MB. Effects of dietary fatty acids and carbohydrates on the ratio of serum total to HDL cholesterol and on serum lipids and apolipoproteins: a meta-analysis of 60 controlled trials. Am J Clin Nutr. 2003;77:1146–55.
45. Kochikuzhyil BM, Devi K, Fattepur SR. Effect of saturated fatty acid-rich dietary vegetable oils on lipid profile, antioxidant enzymes and glucose tolerance in diabetic rats. Indian J Pharmacol. 2010;42:142–5.
46. Yamagishi K, Iso H, Yatsuya H, et al. for the JACC Study Group. Dietary intake of saturated fatty acids and mortality from cardiovascular disease in Japanese: the Japan Collaborative Cohort Study for Evaluation of Cancer Risk. Am J Clin Nutr. 2010;92:759–65.
47. Bent S, Kane C, Shinohara K, et al. Saw palmetto for benign prostatic hyperplasia. N Engl J Med. 2006;354:557–66.
48. Barry MJ, Meleth S, Lee JY, et al. for the Complementary and Alternative Medicine for Urological Symptoms (CAMUS) Study Group. Effect of increasing doses of saw palmetto extract on lower urinary tract symptoms: a randomized trial. JAMA. 2011;306:1344–51.
49. Sinescu I, Geavlete P, Multescu R, et al. Long-term efficacy of Serenoa repens treatment in patients with mild and moderate symptomatic benign prostatic hyperplasia. Urol Int. 2011;86:284–9.
50. Debruyne F, Boyle P, Calais Da Silva F, et al. Evaluation of the clinical benefit of permixon and tamsulosin in severe BPH patients-PERMAL study subset analysis. Eur Urol. 2004;45:773–9.
51. Carballido J, Ruiz-Cerda JL, Unda M, et al. Economic evaluation of medical treatment of benign prostatic hyperplasia (BPH) in the specialized care setting in Spain. Application to the cost-effectiveness of two drugs frequently used in its treatment. Actas Urol Esp. 2008;32:916–25.
52. Geavlete P, Multescu R, Geavlete B. Serenoa repens extract in the treatment of benign prostatic hyperplasia. Ther Adv Urol. 2011;3:193–8.
53. Shoskes DA, Zeitlin SI, Shahed A, Raffer J. Quercetin in men with category III chronic prostatitis: a preliminary prospective, double-blind, placebo-controlled trial. Urology. 1999;54:960–3.
54. Wagenlehner FM, Schneider H, Ludwig M, et al. A pollen extract (Cernilton) in patients with inflammatory chronic prostatitis-chronic pelvic pain syndrome: a multicentre, randomized, prospective, double-blind, placebo-controlled phase 3 study. Eur Urol. 2009;56: 544–51.
55. Asakawa K, Nandachi N, satoh S, et al. Effects of cernitin pollen extract (Cernilton) on inflammatory cytokines in sex-hormone-induced nonbacterial prostatitis rats [in Japanese]. Hinyokika Kiyo. 2001;47: 459–65.
56. Katske F, Shoskes DA, Sender M, Poliakin R, Gagliano K, Rajfer J. Treatment of interstitial cystitis with a quercetin supplement. Tech Urol. 2001;7(1):44–6.
57. Boots AW, Haenen GRMM, Bast A. Health effects of quercetin: from antioxidant to nutraceutical. Eur J Pharmacol. 2008;585:325–37.
58. Shoskes DA, Nickel JC. Quercetin for chronic prostatitis/chronic pelvic pain syndrome. Urol Clin North Am. 2011;38:279–84.
59. Giubilei G, Mondaini N, Minervini A, Saieva C, Lapini A, Serni S, Bartoletti R, Carini M. Physical

activity of men with chronic prostatitis/chronic pelvic pain syndrome not satisfied with conventional treatments-could it represent a valid option? The physical activity and male pelvic pain trial: a double-blind, randomized study. J Urol. 2007;177:159–65.
60. Pool JL. Role of sympathetic nervous system in hypertension and benign prostatic hyperplasia. Br J Clin Pract Suppl. 1994;74:13–7.
61. Esch T, Stefano GB. The neurobiology of stress management. Neuro Endocrinol Lett. 2010;31:19–39.
62. McVary KT, Rademaker A, Lloyd GL, Gann P. Autonomic nervous system overactivity in men with lower urinary tract symptoms secondary to benign prostatic hyperplasia. J Urol. 2005;174(4 Pt 1): 1327–433.
63. Grossman HB, Stenzl A, Moyad MA, Droller MJ. Bladder cancer: chemoprevention, complementary approaches and budgetary considerations. Scand J Urol Nephrol Suppl. 2008;218:213–33.
64. Vilensky D, Lawrentschuk N, Hersey K, Fleshner NE. A smoking cessation program as a resource for bladder cancer patients. Can Urol Assoc J. 2011; May 1:1–7, epub ahead of print.
65. Joshu CE, Mondul AM, Meinhold CL, et al. Cigarette smoking and prostate cancer recurrence after prostatectomy. J Natl Cancer Inst. 2011;103(10):835–8.
66. Moyad MA. Obesity, interrelated mechanisms, and exposures and kidney cancer. Semin Urol Oncol. 2001;19:270–9.
67. Khurana V, Caldito G, Ankem M. Statins might reduce risk of renal cell carcinoma in humans: case–control study of 500,000 veterans. Urology. 2008;71:118–22.
68. Lipworth L, Tarone RE, McLaughlin JK. Renal cell cancer among African Americans: an epidemiologic review. BMC Cancer. 2011;11:133.
69. Chow WH, Dong LM, Devesa SS. Epidemiology and risk factors for kidney cancer. Nat Rev Urol. 2010;7:245–57.
70. Ljungberg B, Campbell SC, Cho HY, et al. The epidemiology of renal cell carcinoma. Eur Urol. 2011;60: 615–21.
71. Klein EA, Thompson Jr IM, Tangen CM, et al. Vitamin E and the risk of prostate cancer: the Selenium and Vitamin E Cancer Prevention Trial (SELECT). JAMA. 2011;306:1549–56.
72. Miller 3rd ER, Pastor-Barriuso R, Dalal D, et al. Meta-analysis: high-dosage vitamin E supplementation may increase all-cause mortality. Ann Intern Med. 2005;142:37–46.
73. Duffield-Lillico AJ, Slate EH, Reid ME, et al. for the Nutritional Prevention of Cancer Study Group. Selenium supplementation and secondary prevention of nonmelanoma skin cancer in a randomized trial. J Natl Cancer Inst. 2003;95:1477–81.
74. Stranges S, Marshall JR, Natarajan R, et al. Effects of long-term selenium supplementation on the incidence of type 2 diabetes: a randomized trial. Ann Intern Med. 2007;147:217–23.
75. Sesso HD, Buring JE, Christen WG, et al. Vitamins E and C in the prevention of cardiovascular disease in men: the Physicians' Health Study II randomized controlled trial. JAMA. 2008;300:2123–33.
76. Moyad MA. Selenium and vitamin E supplements for prostate cancer: evidence or embellishment? Urology. 2002;59(4 Suppl 1):9–19.
77. Figueriredo JC, Grau MV, Haile RW, et al. Folic acid and risk of prostate cancer: results from a randomized clinical trial. J Natl Cancer Inst. 2009;101:432–5.
78. Cole BF, Baron JA, Sandler RS, et al. for Polyp Prevention Study Group. Folic acid for the prevention of colorectal adenomas: a randomized clinical trial. JAMA. 2007;297:2351–59.
79. Collin SM, Metcalfe C, REfsum H, et al. Circulating folate, vitamin B12, homocysteine, vitamin B12 transport proteins, and risk of prostate cancer: a case–control study, systematic review, and meta-analysis. Cancer Epidemiol Biomarkers Prev. 2010;19: 1632–42.
80. Bailey RL, Mills JL, Yetley EA, et al. Unmetabolized serum folic acid and its relation to folic acid intake from diet and supplements in a nationally representative sample of adults aged>or =60 y in the United States. Am J Clin Nutr. 2010;92:383–9.
81. Clarke R, Halsey J, Lewington S, et al. for the B-vitamin Treatment Trialists' Collaboration. Effects of lowering homocysteine levels with B vitamins on cardiovascular disease, cancer, and cause-specific mortality. Meta-analysis of 8 randomized trials involving 37,485 individuals. Arch Intern Med. 2010;170:1622–31.
82. Giovannucci E, Chan AT. Role of vitamin and mineral supplementation and aspirin use in cancer survivors. J Clin Oncol. 2010;28:4081–5.
83. Lawson KA, Wright ME, Subar A, et al. Multivitamin use and risk of prostate cancer in the National Institutes of Health-AARP Diet and Health Study. J Natl Cancer Inst. 2007;99:754–64.
84. Moyad MA. Zinc for prostate disease and other conditions: a little evidence, a lot of hype, and a significant potential problem. Urol Nurs. 2004;24: 49–52.
85. Lamm DL, Riggs DR, Shriver JS, et al. Megadose vitamins in bladder cancer: a double-blind clinical trial. J Urol. 1994;151:21–6.
86. Nepple KG, Lightfoot AJ, Rosevear HM, et al. Bacillus Calmette-Guerin with or without interferon alpha-2b and megadose versus recommended daily allowance vitamins during induction and maintenance intravesical treatment of nonmuscle invasive bladder cancer. J Urol. 2010;184:1915–9.
87. Moyad MA. Dr. Moyad's no bogus science health advice. Ann Arbor: Ann Arbor Media Group; 2009.
88. Morris MC, Tangney CC. A potential design flaw of randomized trials of vitamin supplements. JAMA. 2011;305:1348–9.
89. Tighe P, Ward M, McNulty H, et al. A dose-finding trial of the effect of long-term folic acid intervention: implications for food fortification policy. Am J Clin Nutr. 2011;93:11–8.
90. Hercberg S, Galan P, Preziosi P, et al. The SU.VI. MAX study: a randomized, placebo-controlled trial

of the health effects of antioxidant vitamins and minerals. Arch Intern Med. 2004;164:2335–42.
91. Aso Y, Akazan H. Prophylactic effect of a Lactobacillus preparation on the recurrence of superficial bladder cancer. BLP Study Group. Uro Int. 1992;49:125–9.
92. Aso Y, Akaza H, Kotake T, et al. for the BLP Study Group. Preventive effect of a *Lactobacillus casei* preparation on the recurrence of superficial bladder cancer in a double-blind trial. Eur Urol. 1995;27:104–9.
93. Naito S, Koga H, Yamaguchi A, et al. for the Kyushu University Urological Oncology Group. Prevention of recurrence with epirubicin and lactobacillus casei after transurethral resection of the bladder. J Urol 2008;179:485–90.
94. Ohashi Y, Nakai S, Tsukamoto T, et al. Habitual intake of lactic acid bacteria and risk reduction of bladder cancer. Urol Int. 2002;68:273–80.
95. Larsson SC, Andersson SO, Johansson JE, Wolk A. Cultured milk, yogurt, and dairy intake in relation to bladder cancer risk in a prospective study of Swedish women and men. Am J Clin Nutr. 2008;88: 1083–7.
96. di Giuseppe R, Di Castelnuovo A, Melegari C, et al. on behalf of the Moli-sani Project Investigators. Nutr Metab Cardiovasc Dis. 2010;22:347–54.
97. Solomon KR, Freeman MR. The complex interplay between cholesterol and prostate malignancy. Urol Clin North Am. 2011;38:243–59.
98. Moyad MA, Klotz LH. Statin clinical trial (REALITY) for prostate cancer: an over 15-year wait is finally over thanks to a dietary supplement. Urol Clin N Am. 2011;38:325–31.
99. Moyad MA. Heart healthy equals prostate healthy equals statins: the next cancer chemoprevention trial. Part I. Curr Opin Urol. 2005;15:1–6.
100. Glendenning P, Zhu K, Inderjeeth C, et al. Effects of three monthly oral 150,000 IU cholecalciferol supplementation on falls, mobility and muscle strength in older postmenopausal women: a randomized controlled trial. J Bone Miner Res. 2011; Sept 28, epub ahead of print.
101. Sanders KM, Stuart AL, Williamson EJ, et al. Annual high-dose oral vitamin D and falls and fractures in older women: a randomized controlled trial. JAMA. 2010;303:1815–22.
102. Shapses SA, Manson JE. Vitamin D and prevention of cardiovascular disease disease and diabetes: why the evidence falls short. JAMA. 2011;305:2565–66.
103. Albanes D, Mondul AM, Yu K. Serum 25-hydroxy vitamin d and prostate cancer risk in a large nested case–control study. Cancer Epidemiol Biomarkers Prev. 2011;20:1850–60.
104. Cabler S, Agarwal A, Flint M, du Plessis SS. Obesity: modern man's fertility nemesis. Asian J Androl. 2010;12:480–9.
105. Kasturi SS, Tannir J, Brannigan RE. The metabolic syndrome and male infertility. J Androl. 2008;29:251–9.
106. Brannian JD. Obesity and fertility. S D Med. 2011;64:251–4.
107. Campagne DM. Should fertilization treatment start with reducing stress? Hum Reprod. 2006;21: 1651–8.
108. Agarwal A, Sekhon LH. The role of antioxidant therapy in the treatment of male infertility. Hum Fertil (Camb). 2010;13:217–25.
109. Showell MG, Brown J, Yazdani A, Stankiewicz MT, Hart RJ. Antioxidants for male subfertility. Cochrane Database Syst Rev. 2011;(1):CD007411.
110. Littarru GP, Tiano L. Clinical aspects of coenzyme Q10: an update. Nutrition. 2010;26:250–4.
111. Balercia G, Regoli F, Armeni T, et al. Placebo-controlled double-blind randomized trial on the use of L-carnitine, L-acetylcarnitine, or combined L-carnitine and L-acetylcarnitine in men with idiopathic asthenozoospermia. Fertil Steril. 2005;84:662–71.
112. Lenzi A, Lombardo F, Sgro P, et al. Use of carnitine therapy in selected cases of male factor infertility: a double-blind crossover trial. Fertil Steril. 2003;79: 292–300.
113. Li Z, Chen GW, Shang XJ, et al. A controlled randomized trial of the use of combined L-carnitine and acetyl-L-carnitine treatment in men with oligoasthenozoospermia. Zhong Hua Nan Ke Xue. 2005;11: 761–4.
114. Peivandi S, Abasali K, Narges M. Effects of L-carnitine on infertile men's spermogram: a randomized clinical trial. J Reprod Infertil. 2010;10:331.
115. Lombardo F, Gandini L, Agarwal A, et al. A prospective double blind placebo controlled cross over trial of carnitine therapy in selected cases of male infertility. Fertil Steril. 2002;78 Suppl 1:68–9.
116. Marchioli R, Barzi F, Bomba E, et al. Early protection against sudden cardiac death by n-3 polyunsaturated fatty acids after myocardial infarction: time-course analysis of the results of the Gruppo Italiano per lo Studio della Sopravvivenza nell'Infarto Miocardico (GISSI)-Prevenzione. Circulation. 2002;105:1897–903.
117. Matsuzaki M, Yokoyama M, Saito Y, et al. for the JELIS investigators. Incremental effects of eicosapentaenoic acid on cardiovascular events in statin-treated patients with coronary artery disease. Circ J. 2009;73:1283–90.
118. Conquer JA, Martin JB, Tummon I, Watson L, Tekpetey F. Effect of DHA supplementation on DHA status and sperm motility in asthenozoospermic males. Lipids. 2000;35:149–54.
119. Colagar AH, Marzony ET. Ascorbic acid in human seminal plasma: determination and its relationship to sperm quality. J Clin Biochem Nutr. 2009;45: 144–9.
120. Vitamin C content in foods. http://www.vitamincfoundation.org/usda.html. Accessed 20 Mar 2011.
121. Moyad MA, Combs MA, Baisley JE, Evans M. Vitamin C with metabolites: additional analysis suggests favorable changes in oxalate. Urol Nurs. 2009;29:383–5.
122. Esposito K, Giugliano F, Di Palo C, et al. Effect of lifestyle changes on erectile dysfunction in obese men. JAMA. 2004;291(24):2978–84.

123. Giugliano D, Giugliano F, Esposito K. Sexual dysfunction and the Mediterranean diet. Public Health Nutr. 2006;9:1118–20.
124. Hannan JL, Maio MT, Komolova M, Adams MA. Beneficial impact of exercise and obesity interventions on erectile function and its risk factors. J Sex Med. 2009;6 Suppl 3:254–61.
125. Horasanli K, Boylu U, Kendirci M, Miroglu C. Do lifestyle changes work for improving erectile function? Asian J Androl. 2008;10:28–35.
126. Esposito K, Maiorino MI, Bellastella G, et al. Determinants of female sexual dysfunction in type 2 diabetes. Int J Impot Res. 2010;22:179–84.
127. Esposito K, Giugliano D. Lifestyle/dietary recommendations for erectile dysfunction and female sexual dysfunction. Urol Clin North Am. 2011;38:293–301.
128. Maio G, Saraeb S, Marchiori A. Physical activity and PDE5 inhibitors in the treatment of erectile dysfunction: results of a randomized controlled study. J Sex Med. 2010;7:2201–8.
129. Khera M, Goldstein I. Erectile Dysfunction. Clinical Evidence (online); 2011.
130. Kiefer D, Pantuso T. Panax ginseng. Am Fam Phys. 2003;68:1539–42.
131. Meldrum DR, Gambone JC, Morris MA, et al. The link between erectile and cardiovascular health: the canary in the coal mine. Am J Cardiol. 2011;108:599–606.
132. Ledda A, Belcaro G, Cesarone MR, Dugall M, Schonlau F. Investigation of a complex plant extract for mild to moderate erectile dysfunction in a randomized, double-blind, placebo-controlled, parallel-arm study. BJU Int. 2010;106:1030–3.
133. Tsertsvadze A, Yazdl F, Fink H, et al. Oral sildenafil citrate (Viagra) for erectile dysfunction: a systematic review and meta-analysis of harms. Urology. 2009;74:831–6.
134. Mulhall JP, McLaughlin TP, Hartnett JP, et al. Medication utilization behavior in patients receiving phosphodiesterase type 5 inhibitors for erectile dysfunction. J Sex Med. 2005;2:848–55.
135. Lee DJ, Cheetham P, Badani KK. Penile rehabilitation protocol after robot-assisted radical prostatectomy: assessment of compliance with phosphodiesterase type 5 inhibitor therapy and effect on early potency. BJU Intl. 2009;105:382–8.
136. Meschi T, Nouvenne A, Borghi L. Lifestyle recommendations to reduce the risk of kidney stones. Urol Clin North Am. 2011;38:313–20.
137. Siener R, Jansen B, Watzer B, Hesse A. Effect of n-3 fatty acid supplementation on urinary risk factors for calcium oxalate stone formation. J Urol. 2011; 185: 719–24.
138. Taylor EN, Stampfer MJ, Mount DB, Curhan GC. DASH-style diet and 24-hour urine composition. Clin J Am Soc Nephrol. 2010;5:2315–22.
139. Taylor EN, Fung TT, Curhan GC. DASH-style diet associates with reduced risk for kidney stones. J Am Soc Nephrol. 2009;20:2253–9.
140. Reiner AP, Kahn A, Eisner BH, et al. Kidney stones and subclinical atherosclerosis in young adults: the CARDIA Study. J Urol. 2011;185:920–5.
141. Gur S, Limin M, Hellstrom WJ. Current status and new developments in Peyronie's disease: medical, minimally invasive and surgical treatment options. Expert Opin Pharmacother. 2011;12:931–44.
142. Safarinejad MR, Hosseini SY, Kolahi AA. Comparison of vitamin E and propionyl-L-carnitine, separately or in combination, in patients with early chronic Peyronie's disease: a double-blind, placebo controlled, randomized study. J Urol. 2007;178(4 Pt 1):1398–403.
143. Cavallini G, Biagiotti G, Koverech A, Vitali G. Oral propionyl-l-carnitine and intraplaque verapamil in the therapy of advanced and resistant Peyronie's disease. BJU Int. 2002;89:895–900.
144. Safarinejad MR. Safety and efficacy of coenzyme Q10 supplementation in early chronic Peyronie's disease: a double-blind, placebo-controlled randomized study. Int J Impot Res. 2010;22:298–309.
145. Wyman M, Leonard M, Morledge T. Coenzyme Q10: a therapy for hypertension and statin-induced myalgia? Cleve Clin J Med. 2010;77:435–42.
146. Miyakis S, Pefanis A, Tsakris A. The challenge of antimicrobial drug resistance in Greece. Clin Infect Dis. 2011;53:177–84.
147. Jepson RG, Craig JC. Cranberries for preventing urinary tract infections. Cochrane Database Syst Rev. 2008;(1):CD001321.
148. Beerepoot MJ, Riet GT, Nys S, et al. Cranberries vs antibiotics to prevent urinary tract infections. Arch Intern Med. 2011;171:1270–8.
149. Terris MK, Issa MM, Tacker JR. Dietary supplementation with cranberry concentrate tablets may increase the risk of nephrolithiasis. Urology. 2001; 57:26–9.
150. Eyre H, Kahn R, Robertson RM, et al. for the ACS/ADA/AHA Collaborative Writing Committee Members. Preventing cancer, cardiovascular disease, and diabetes: a common agenda for the American Cancer Society, the American Diabetes Association, and the American Heart Association. Circulation. 2004;109:3244–55.

# Androgen Decline in the Aging Male: Making Sense of the "Male Menopause"

9

Daniel A. Shoskes

## Introduction

As men age, there is commonly a change in the function and efficiency of testosterone production along the hypothalamic–pituitary–testicular axis, resulting in declining measured serum testosterone. Many of the clinical changes associated with low testosterone are nonspecific and often associated with aging alone (e.g., low energy level, erectile dysfunction). Testosterone replacement therapy (TRT) will usually increase testosterone levels, but may have a variable effect on these symptoms. The clinical challenge is to accurately diagnose clinically meaningful low testosterone levels and institute therapy that can improve symptoms and quality of life (Fig. 9.1).

Given these difficulties, it is not surprising that nomenclature is not standardized. While common in the popular press, "male menopause" is probably the least helpful term, since there are few correlates with the better defined female menopause. Testosterone deficiency syndrome is a commonly used term, but does imply a set constellation of symptoms. Androgen Decline in the Aging Male (ADAM) is both descriptive and helps differentiate young men, with their separate concerns such as fertility and does not presuppose any set of symptoms.

D.A. Shoskes, MD, MSc, FRCS(C) (✉)
Department of Urology, The Glickman Urologic and Kidney Institute, Cleveland Clinic, Cleveland, OH 44195, USA
e-mail: dshoskes@mac.com

## Epidemiology

On a population basis, serum testosterone levels begin to decline in men in their mid-40s, and this decline continues for the rest of life [1]. The Massachusetts Male Aging Study measured testosterone serially in a "well" cohort of men not seeking medical attention for other reasons. They found an initial incidence of low testosterone of 6% which doubled to 12% on subsequent measures [2]. Serial measures are important, as one natural history study did show return to normal testosterone on subsequent measures in up to 50% of men [3]. In a European cross-sectional study, 11.8% of men had low testosterone associated with low-normal or normal leutenizing hormone (LH) [4].

Low testosterone is associated with a number of other comorbid conditions. It is important to emphasize that these associations do not equate with causality and that testosterone replacement may therefore not improve the associated illnesses. Having a testosterone measurement in a physician's office "for cause" raises the incidence of TDS from the cross-sectional studies to as high as 39% [5]. Conditions that increase the risk of TDS include metabolic syndrome, obesity, type II diabetes [6], osteoporosis, renal failure, and treatment with

D.A. Shoskes (ed.), *Urological Men's Health: A Guide for Urologists and Primary Care Physicians*, Current Clinical Urology, DOI 10.1007/978-1-61779-900-6_9,
© Springer Science+Business Media New York 2012

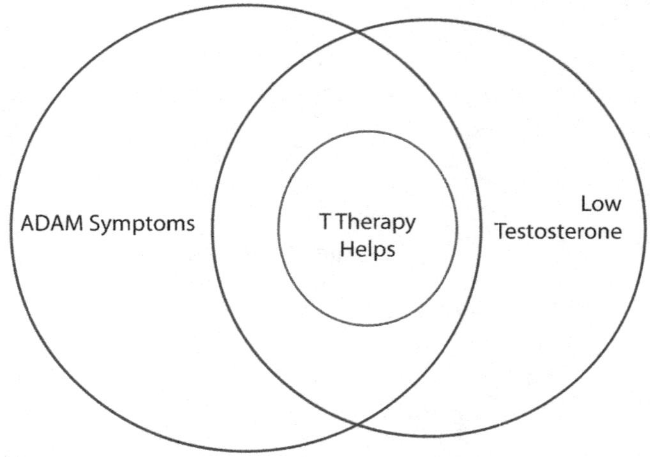


**Fig. 9.1** Clinical challenge in managing low testosterone: both the symptoms of adrogen decline in the aging male and low testosterone are common, the challenge is identifying patients with a causal relationship who will benefit from testosterone replacement therapy

steroids or opioids [7]. Indeed, 77% of men with end-stage renal disease had low testosterone [8].

Low testosterone is also associated with decreased survival, although given the tight linkage with advancing age and comorbidities, a cause and effect relationship is difficult to prove. In a key study, Shores et al. examined a database of male patients older than 40 from the Veteran's Administration. Including those with at least two testosterone measures and excluding men with a diagnosis of prostate cancer, they found consistent low testosterone in 53% [9]. Risk for all-cause mortality was 20% in men with normal testosterone and 35% in men with low testosterone. Increased mortality with low testosterone persisted in a multivariable analysis of other comorbidities and even when mortality in the first year was excluded. In men with renal failure, low testosterone independently predicted all-cause and cardiac mortality [10]. In Europe, a prospective health study in Pomerania found that low testosterone independently increased risk of death from cardiovascular disease and cancer [11]. A recent meta-analysis confirms this association [12].

## Clinical Presentation and Diagnosis

A biochemical diagnosis of low testosterone is greatly dependent on accurate measurement. Testosterone release is diurnal with the highest levels in the early morning, and week-to-week variability is common. Therefore, it is important to collect blood in the morning (before 11 a.m.) and to confirm a diagnosis of low testosterone with at least two measurements several days apart. With either the first or second testosterone measurement, it is important to measure pituitary hormones LH and prolactin. Significant elevations could point to a pituitary adenoma, and medical therapy for hyperprolactinemia (e.g., in renal failure) can improve serum testosterone [13]. Testosterone binds in the bloodstream to Sex Hormone Binding Globulin (SHBG) and this bound form is biologically inactive. Both free testosterone and testosterone bound to albumin is active and the two together form "bioavailable testosterone." Most labs will offer a free testosterone, which is a calculated value based on the SHBG [14]. In general, values for total testosterone >360 ng/dl (12 nmol/L) are "normal," those below 250 ng/dl (9 nmol/L) are "abnormal," and between these two values are "borderline." In general, "borderline" values in the face of clinical symptoms of ADAM should be treated as "abnormal." The typical equivalent clinical breakpoints for free testosterone are >60 ng/dl and <40 ng/dl. For patients who are about to start testosterone replacement therapy, it is also necessary to measure hemoglobin and PSA (if age is >39).

Declining testosterone values seldom if ever should be treated without corresponding clinical manifestations. Symptoms associated with age-related declines in testosterone that also are amenable to improvement with testosterone replacement include low libido [15], erectile dysfunction, low energy [16], depressed mood [17], low muscle mass, osteoporosis, and hot flashes. Screening questionnaires have been developed for the symptoms of low testosterone and all have some correlation with biochemical testosterone values. The ADAM questionnaire has ten yes/no questions that are not quantitative and have some ambiguity (e.g., "are you falling asleep after dinner?"; well, eventually yes) [18]. It can be used as a screening test for low testosterone but not to monitor response to therapy. The Aging Male Survey (AMS) questionnaire has 17 questions, each on a 5-point scale of none to extremely severe that are grouped into psychologic (e.g., anxiety), somatovegetative (e.g., sleep problems, decreased strength) and sexual. It can be used to screen for low testosterone and also as an outcome measure [19]. A recent European multicenter study looked for associations between symptoms of ADAM and low testosterone in 3,369 men between age 40 and 79 and concluded that minimal criteria for ADAM should be the presence of at least three sexual symptoms (low sexual desire, poor morning erections, erectile dysfunction) with a total testosterone <320 ng/dl and a free testosterone <64 pg/dl [15].

The history for a patient evaluated for ADAM should include the sexual and constitutional symptoms described above. In addition, a history of anatomic, medical or surgical events that could affect testosterone production should be sought including cryptorchidism, scrotal and inguinal surgery, pituitary surgery or radiation, prior fertility, development of secondary sexual characteristics, history or renal or hepatic failure, chemotherapy (for cancer or autoimmune diseases), and prior use of anabolic steroids (prescribed or illicit). Components of the complete physical exam should include observation of bodily hair and habitus, gynecomastia, and genital exam to include size, position, and number of testes and size and consistency of the prostate.

## Testosterone Replacement Therapy

The true indications, benefits, and risks of TRT are still controversial. Data is limited by lack of long-term follow-up, biochemical target values and ability to tell clinical associations apart from clinical causality. In particular, it is difficult to make a compelling case to treat low testosterone as an isolated biochemical finding in the absence of any clinical changes or complaints. Nevertheless, few aging (or indeed young) men will deny the presence of any possible symptoms (e.g., decreased sexual performance, fatigue). Therefore, it is reasonable to treat a man with symptoms attributable to ADAM and low or borderline testosterone values (total $T<350$ ng/ml, free $T<60$ pg/ml) for at least 3 months, confirm that treatment improves the testosterone levels and assess the impact on symptoms.

There are several contradictions to TRT. Elevation of PSA and/or a prostate nodule should prompt prostate biopsy; however, the role of TRT in prostate cancer patients is controversial and evolving (see below). Breast cancer, uncontrolled congestive heart failure, and polycythemia remain strong contraindications. Men seeking fertility should not be offered TRT, as this therapy will lower sperm count. Instead, short-term therapy with clomiphene or similar agents is indicated [20].

There are multiple effective forms of testosterone that can be used for TRT (Table 9.1). Oral agents are not unfortunately on that list. Testosterone in pill form is associated with liver toxicity and is not available in the USA. A buccal form is available but inconvenient, often irritating and offers no benefit over other forms. The most common TRT modalities are parenteral and transdermal.

Parenteral TRT can be given intramuscularly (im) or subcutaneously. In the USA, the only im form available is testosterone cypionate, which must be given every 2–4 weeks. It is often the least expensive form of TRT but suffers from the need of frequent administration (as an office visit or self-administered by the patient) and wide swings of testosterone levels ranging from supraphysiologic for a few days after administration to hypogonadal prior to the next injection. A longer acting form, testosterone undecanoate is available outside the USA and is given every 3 months once stable levels are reached. The other parenteral choice is subcutaneous slow release pellets, sold in the USA as Testopel. The pellets have

**Table 9.1** Summary of common forms of testosterone therapy in the USA

| Route | Type | Commerical name | Typical dose | Advantages | Disadvantages |
|---|---|---|---|---|---|
| Intramuscular | Testosterone cypionate | Depot testosterone | 200–400 mg q2–4 weeks | Inexpensive | Pain, inconvenience, wide swings in levels |
| Subcutaneous | Testosterone pellets | Testopel | 10–15 pellets q3–6 months | Convenient, no transmission risk, high compliance | Unable to remove if side effects |
| Transdermal | Patch | Androderm | 1–5 mg patch daily | Minimal transmission risk | Skin irritation common |
| | Liquid | Axiron | 2–4 pumps (30–90 mg) to axillae daily | Fast drying, axilla relatively protected | Application has a learning curve |
| | Gel | Testim | 1–2 tubes (5–10 mg) daily to shoulders | Individual tubes convenient for travel | Odor |
| | | Androgel (1% or 1.62%) | 5–10 mg daily to shoulders/chest (1–8 pumps depending on concentration) | New concentrated form reduces volume needed | Messy |
| | | Fortesta | 40–70 mg per day (4–7 pumps) to thighs | Fast drying | Applied near genitals |

75 mg of testosterone and typically 10–15 pellets are placed subcutaneously in the buttock area, which will provide adequate coverage for 3–6 months [21]. In our experience, the insertion procedure is simple with a short learning curve and has a low incidence of wound infection or pellet extrusion. Advantages are simple compliance and no risk of transdermal transmission of drug to others.

Transdermal preparations include patches, liquids, and gels. Patches, such as Androderm, are applied daily and are rotated to different sites; however, the primary limitation is skin irritation. Patches do minimize the risk for skin transmission to others. There are three gel formulations currently available in the USA: Androgel (1% or 1.62%), which is applied to the chest or shoulders, Testim 1% which applied to the shoulders, and Fortesta which is applied to the thigh. A liquid preparation, Axiron, is applied to the underarms. Secondary transfer to women and children is possible, and it is important after application to thoroughly wash the hands and cover the treated skin with clothing. In 3–4 h once all the medication is absorbed, the area should ideally be washed before making direct skin contact with others.

## Monitoring of Patients on TRT

Patients starting TRT require clinical and biochemical monitoring, both for response to therapy and for side effects/complications. The first set of labs should be done 6–12 weeks after therapy starts and monitored quarterly for the first year, twice in the second year and then annually if no problems develop. We typically include total testosterone, PSA, and hemoglobin (to monitor for polycythemia). For men on daily therapy (patch, gel, liquid), testosterone should be drawn about 2 h after application. The appropriate target testosterone value on therapy is unknown and guidelines suggest a "mid or low normal range" [22], which we interpret to be a total testosterone between 450 and 600 ng/dl. A rise in PSA of up to 20% would be expected as a response in a benign prostate gland, but a higher increase should prompt consideration of prostate biopsy [23]. Similarly, hemoglobin and hematocrit typically rise [24], but a hematocrit >55% should prompt dose reduction or cessation. Since elevation of liver function tests is only seen with the unavailable oral forms, they do not need monitoring during parenteral or transdermal therapy.

Clinically, patients should be assessed for improvement in their index ADAM symptoms, realizing that an initial placebo effect is possible. Libido should improve by 3 months; however, other symptoms may take 6 months or more to improve. Lack of any improvement at 6 months suggests that the symptoms were unrelated to low testosterone. It is important to document that testosterone was actually increased to the normal range in men without clinical improvement. Potential clinical side effects that should prompt dose reduction or discontinuation are irritability, gynecomastia, worsening of lower urinary tract symptoms from an enlarged prostate and new or worsening sleep apnea, although the data linking sleep apnea and TRT is weak [25].

## Clinical Benefits of TRT

While long-term studies are lacking, there is considerable evidence that TRT can be of benefit to men with many clinical and biologic effects of ADAM, both urologic and systemic. In a 2-year prospective randomized trial in men with metabolic syndrome, TRT improved waist circumference, fasting glucose, BMI and biochemical surrogate markers of atherosclerosis [26]. In a randomized controlled trial of men with type II diabetes, TRT reduced insulin resistance and improved glycemic control [27]. In a meta-analysis of studies looking at ADAM and cardiovascular risk, men with low testosterone had increased risk of cardiovascular risk and mortality and TRT in this population improved surrogate markers such as treadmill test duration [28].

Specific benefits are seen in men suffering from erectile dysfunction with ADAM and TRT, although due to the often multifactorial nature of the erectile dysfunction, TRT alone may not be sufficient. In a registry of men receiving Testim for at least 1 year, there was improvement in sexual function in all subgroups, including those taking PDE5 inhibitors, and this improvement correlated best with testosterone increase after 6 months of therapy [29]. In a recent study of men who did not respond to PDE5i therapy alone, addition of testosterone gel to taldalafil improved sexual function if the starting testosterone was <300 ng/ml [30]. Most men will begin to see improvement in sexual functioning on TRT by 3 months [31].

Despite these benefits, it must be emphasized that TRT should be used with specific target symptoms related to ADAM and that the general health benefits and safety of TRT in any man with a low measured testosterone alone is not proven. In a recent study of 209 elderly men with low testosterone and limited mobility associated with other chronic illnesses, there was a significantly higher incidence of cardiac events in the TRT group vs. placebo [32].

## Testosterone Replacement Therapy and Prostate Cancer

The relationship between prostate cancer growth and testosterone is well established and androgen ablation remains the cornerstone of treatment for metastatic disease. It has always been assumed that if no testosterone is bad for prostate cancer that more testosterone must be "good" and TRT continues to carry warnings about increased risk of development and spread of prostate cancer. Recent data, although not conclusive, is challenging this dogma. Accumulating data would support the hypothesis that while prostate cancer does require testosterone to grow, a "saturation" level is reached at relatively low serum levels and increases above this level (as one would find with TRT in a man with ADAM) does not increase risk for development or growth of cancer [33].

Pathologic studies suggest a higher Gleason grade of tumor is associated with low serum testosterone [34], although another study only found this association with testosterone <100 ng/dl [35]. In men with erectile dysfunction after successful treatment for prostate cancer, TRT appears safe whether after radical prostatectomy [36] or brachytherapy [37]. Most provocatively, a recent small study of 13 men with known prostate cancer on active surveillance showed that TRT did not lead to local progression or metastatic disease in any of the patients [38].

While these data are provocative, it should still be the standard of care that prostate cancer screening be done in age-appropriate men with ADAM. Hypogonadal men with a history of prostate cancer, whether treated with surgery, radiation or active surveillance, should only be treated with testosterone in conjunction with careful monitoring and a complete disclosure of risks and limitations of the data as it evolves.

## References

1. Simon D, Preziosi P, Barrett-Connor E, et al. The influence of aging on plasma sex hormones in men: the Telecom Study. Am J Epidemiol. 1992;135:783–91.
2. Araujo AB, O'Donnell AB, Brambilla DJ, et al. Prevalence and incidence of androgen deficiency in middle-aged and older men: estimates from the Massachusetts Male Aging Study. J Clin Endocrinol Metab. 2004;89:5920–6.
3. Travison TG, Shackelton R, Araujo AB, et al. The natural history of symptomatic androgen deficiency in men: onset, progression, and spontaneous remission. J Am Geriatr Soc. 2008;56:831–9.
4. Tajar A, Forti G, O'Neill TW, et al. Characteristics of secondary, primary, and compensated hypogonadism in aging men: evidence from the European Male Ageing Study. J Clin Endocrinol Metab. 2010;95:1810–8.
5. Mulligan T, Frick MF, Zuraw QC, Stemhagen A, McWhirter C. Prevalence of hypogonadism in males aged at least 45 years: the HIM study. Int J Clin Pract. 2006;60:762–9.
6. Dhindsa S, Miller MG, McWhirter CL, et al. Testosterone concentrations in diabetic and nondiabetic obese men. Diabetes Care. 2010;33:1186–92.
7. Haring R, Ittermann T, Volzke H, et al. Prevalence, incidence and risk factors of testosterone deficiency in a population-based cohort of men: results from the study of health in Pomerania. Aging Male. 2010;13: 247–57.
8. Carrero JJ, Qureshi AR, Nakashima A, et al. Prevalence and clinical implications of testosterone deficiency in men with end-stage renal disease. Nephrol Dial Transplant. 2011;26(1):184–90.
9. Shores MM, Matsumoto AM, Sloan KL, Kivlahan DR. Low serum testosterone and mortality in male veterans. Arch Intern Med. 2006;166:1660–5.
10. Carrero JJ, Qureshi AR, Parini P, et al. Low serum testosterone increases mortality risk among male dialysis patients. J Am Soc Nephrol. 2009;20:613–20.
11. Haring R, Volzke H, Steveling A, et al. Low serum testosterone levels are associated with increased risk of mortality in a population-based cohort of men aged 20–79. Eur Heart J. 2010;31:1494–501.
12. Araujo AB, Dixon JM, Suarez EA, Murad MH, Guey LT, Wittert GA. Clinical review: endogenous testosterone and mortality in men: a systematic review and meta-analysis. J Clin Endocrinol Metab. 2011; 96(10):3007–19.
13. Saha MT, Saha HH, Niskanen LK, Salmela KT, Pasternack AI. Time course of serum prolactin and sex hormones following successful renal transplantation. Nephron. 2002;92:735–7.
14. Ly LP, Sartorius G, Hull L, et al. Accuracy of calculated free testosterone formulae in men. Clin Endocrinol (Oxf). 2010;73:382–8.
15. Wu FC, Tajar A, Beynon JM, et al. Identification of late-onset hypogonadism in middle-aged and elderly men. N Engl J Med. 2010;363:123–35.
16. Kelleher S, Conway AJ, Handelsman DJ. Blood testosterone threshold for androgen deficiency symptoms. J Clin Endocrinol Metab. 2004;89:3813–7.
17. Joshi D, van Schoor NM, de Ronde W, et al. Low free testosterone levels are associated with prevalence and incidence of depressive symptoms in older men. Clin Endocrinol (Oxf). 2010;72:232–40.
18. Morley JE, Charlton E, Patrick P, et al. Validation of a screening questionnaire for androgen deficiency in aging males. Metabolism. 2000;49:1239–42.
19. Moore C, Huebler D, Zimmermann T, Heinemann LA, Saad F, Thai DM. The Aging Males' Symptoms scale (AMS) as outcome measure for treatment of androgen deficiency. Eur Urol. 2004;46:80–7.
20. Taylor F, Levine L. Clomiphene citrate and testosterone gel replacement therapy for male hypogonadism: efficacy and treatment cost. J Sex Med. 2010;7: 269–76.
21. Cavender RK, Fairall M. Subcutaneous testosterone pellet implant (Testopel) therapy for men with testosterone deficiency syndrome: a single-site retrospective safety analysis. J Sex Med. 2009;6: 3177–92.
22. Wang C, Nieschlag E, Swerdloff R, et al. Investigation, treatment, and monitoring of late-onset hypogonadism in males: ISA, ISSAM, EAU, EAA, and ASA recommendations. Eur Urol. 2009;55:121–30.
23. Gerstenbluth RE, Maniam PN, Corty EW, Seftel AD. Prostate-specific antigen changes in hypogonadal men treated with testosterone replacement. J Androl. 2002;23:922–6.
24. Fernandez-Balsells MM, Murad MH, Lane M, et al. Clinical review 1: adverse effects of testosterone therapy in adult men: a systematic review and meta-analysis. J Clin Endocrinol Metab. 2010;95: 2560–75.
25. Hanafy HM. Testosterone therapy and obstructive sleep apnea: is there a real connection? J Sex Med. 2007;4:1241–6.
26. Aversa A, Bruzziches R, Francomano D, et al. Effects of testosterone undecanoate on cardiovascular risk factors and atherosclerosis in middle-aged men with late-onset hypogonadism and metabolic syndrome: results from a 24-month, randomized, double-blind, placebo-controlled study. J Sex Med. 2010;7:3495–503.

27. Kapoor D, Goodwin E, Channer KS, Jones TH. Testosterone replacement therapy improves insulin resistance, glycaemic control, visceral adiposity and hypercholesterolaemia in hypogonadal men with type 2 diabetes. Eur J Endocrinol. 2006;154:899–906.
28. Corona G, Rastrelli G, Monami M, et al. Hypogonadism as a risk factor for cardiovascular mortality in men: a meta-analytic study. Eur J Endocrinol. 2011; 165(5):687–701.
29. Khera M, Bhattacharya RK, Blick G, Kushner H, Nguyen D, Miner MM. Improved sexual function with testosterone replacement therapy in hypogonadal men: real-world data from the Testim Registry in the United States (TRiUS). J Sex Med. 2011;8(11):3204–13.
30. Buvat J, Montorsi F, Maggi M, et al. Hypogonadal men nonresponders to the PDE5 inhibitor tadalafil benefit from normalization of testosterone levels with a 1% hydroalcoholic testosterone gel in the treatment of erectile dysfunction (TADTEST study). J Sex Med. 2011;8:284–93.
31. Rhoden EL, Morgentaler A. Symptomatic response rates to testosterone therapy and the likelihood of completing 12 months of therapy in clinical practice. J Sex Med. 2010;7:277–83.
32. Basaria S, Coviello AD, Travison TG, et al. Adverse events associated with testosterone administration. N Engl J Med. 2010;363:109–22.
33. Morgentaler A, Traish AM. Shifting the paradigm of testosterone and prostate cancer: the saturation model and the limits of androgen-dependent growth. Eur Urol. 2009;55:310–20.
34. Botto H, Neuzillet Y, Lebret T, Camparo P, Molinie V, Raynaud JP. High incidence of predominant gleason pattern 4 localized prostate cancer is associated with low serum testosterone. J Urol. 2011;186:1400–5.
35. Salonia A, Gallina A, Briganti A, et al. Preoperative hypogonadism is not an independent predictor of high-risk disease in patients undergoing radical prostatectomy. Cancer. 2011;117:3953–62.
36. Khera M. Androgens and erectile function: a case for early androgen use in postprostatectomy hypogonadal men. J Sex Med. 2009;6 Suppl 3:234–8.
37. Sarosdy MF. Testosterone replacement for hypogonadism after treatment of early prostate cancer with brachytherapy. Cancer. 2007;109:536–41.
38. Morgentaler A, Lipshultz LI, Bennett R, Sweeney M, Avila DJ, Khera M. Testosterone therapy in men with untreated prostate cancer. J Urol. 2011;185:1256–60.

# 10 Evaluation and Treatment of Peyronie's Disease

Lawrence S. Hakim

While erectile dysfunction (ED) affects more than 50% of men over the age of 40, Peyronie's disease (PD) is an important potency-threatening condition of male sexual dysfunction, occurring in 3–8% of men [1]. The clinical presentation of Peyronie's disease may be immediately obvious: a curved or bent penis, a palpable penile scar or plaque, complaints of decreased penile length, diminished penile stretch, less rigidity, penile numbness, and erectile dysfunction, as illustrated in Fig. 10.1. This is different than "congenital" curvature of the penis as seen in children and young adults. Peyronie's disease is known to be associated with Dupuytren's disease. In a recent study from the Netherlands, 22% of men with PD in their series also had evidence of Dupuytren's contractures [2]. While the etiology of Peyronie's disease can vary and is not always known in every case, it is often thought to be a result of solitary or repeated injury during sexual activity. Studies have demonstrated that erectile dysfunction and coital trauma constituted the only two independent risk factors for Peyronie's disease [3]. MRI studies obtained during coitus, illustrating the forces on the erect penis in or against the vagina during intercourse, tend to support this theory [4].

Peyronie's disease is often associated with diminished erectile function. The penis may become firm up to the point of the plaque and remain soft beyond that point. In some instances, the patient may see a narrowed "bottleneck" or an "hourglass" shape of the penis as well. The plaque can also inhibit the normal veno-occlusive function of the corpora and prevent the penis from storing blood during erection. As a result of this, the patient may be unable to have intercourse because of a soft and curved penis. In addition, the penile curvature may be uncomfortable or painful during intercourse for one's sexual partner.

To achieve the ultimate goal of therapy, the restoration of a less curved, stable, more pliable, and rigid erection, which allows comfortable penetration for both the patient and his partner, a number of effective procedures have been used, including intralesional injection therapy, vacuum or stretching devices, surgical plication, or plaque incision or excision and grafting. For patients who have poor erectile function, insertion of a penile implant with subsequent repair of any residual curvature is an excellent treatment option enabling restoration of both normal sexual function with a straightened erection [5].

Because no single treatment is appropriate for everyone, it is critical to make an accurate diagnosis prior to treatment, and such factors as plaque size, stability and location, penile curvature, stretch and baseline erectile function, should be determined prior to instituting any form of intervention. This is most effectively done using a directed approach, which provides for compre-

L.S. Hakim, MD, FACS (✉)
Department of Urology, Cleveland Clinic Florida, 2950 Cleveland Clinic Blvd., Weston, FL 33331, USA
e-mail: hakiml@ccf.org

D.A. Shoskes (ed.), *Urological Men's Health: A Guide for Urologists and Primary Care Physicians*, Current Clinical Urology, DOI 10.1007/978-1-61779-900-6_10,
© Springer Science+Business Media New York 2012

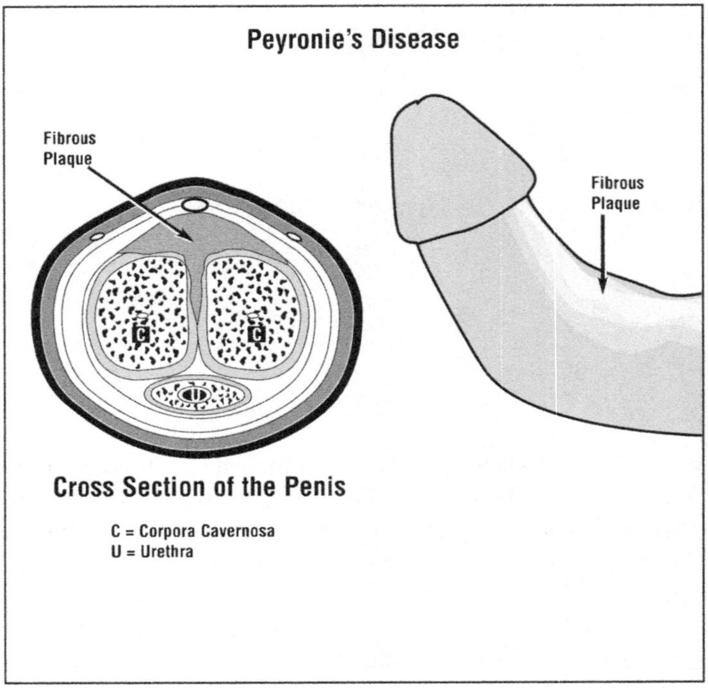


**Fig. 10.1** Anatomy of Peyronie's disease

hensive evaluation of both the patient and his partner as sexual dysfunction is a couple's disease. Penile curvature and poor erectile function can directly affect both patient and partner (i.e., dyspareunia). Both patient and partner sexual issues need to be addressed as part of any couples sexual function evaluation to assure the greatest chance of success [6].

In addition, setting realistic goals is essential prior to the initiation of any form of therapy for Peyronie's disease in order to assure maximal patient and partner satisfaction. Numbness and loss of length do not always improve or resolve despite any type of therapeutic intervention. In addition, since many patients with Peyronie's disease do not require any form of intervention, evaluation of the plaque's impact on the couple's sexual function should also be considered when discussing the role of therapy, if needed.

## Diagnostic Evaluation

As in any form of sexual dysfunction, the initial evaluation of the male with Peyronie's disease begins with a sexual, psychosocial, and medical history. The presence of associated risk factors, such as penile injury or trauma, as well as systemic vascular disease should be assessed. An important part of the history involves the length of time that the plaque has been present. Is it stable? Has the plaque been present for greater than 1 year? Is it getting larger? Is it getting smaller? Has the plaque changed location or orientation? All of these factors are important parts of the diagnostic evaluation and history, as men often delay seeking help for any sexually related condition and they have a direct impact as to the role and form of intervention that will be offered [7].

Other associated forms of sexual dysfunction, including poor libido and ejaculatory dysfunction, should be evaluated and treated appropriately. Patient and partner education with regard to various intercourse positions and noncoital sexual activities is often an important part of the management of this disease.

Once a complete history has been obtained, a thorough physical examination and routine laboratory tests are in order. Specifically, assessment of the penile plaque, if present, is of foremost importance. In most cases, a clearly palpable penile plaque will be identified on physical examination, and in fact may be the reason for the patient's concern (i.e., cancer scare). Factors including the plaque location, size, and consistency, as well as the presence of any pain or tenderness, are useful during the decision-making process.

Another penile lesion, which may be confused with Peyronie's disease or plaque, during the diagnostic evaluation is "sclerosing lymphangitis," a superficial ropelike lesion, usually located at the coronal sulcus. It is most commonly seen in men who engage in extremely vigorous sex and is thought to be due to repeated penile trauma during intercourse. A thrombosed vein is felt on physical examination, which usually resolves spontaneously after a period of abstinence.

In some situations, Peyronie's disease may present with decreased penile stretch or deformity with no specific, palpable plaque. Evaluation of penile length, stretch, and sensation are an important part of the directed genital examination to make the diagnosis of Peyronie's disease.

In addition to a directed history and physical examination, a variety of further specific diagnostic examinations such as vascular, neurologic, hormonal, and psychologic testing may be used to further corroborate the findings.

Office-based hemodynamic testing is typically utilized to objectively measure the degree of penile curvature. Evaluation of the penile curvature or deformity in the erect state is critical, as a baseline prior to any type of intervention for Peyronie's curvature. This is usually assessed following intracorporal injection of vasoactive agents, such as prostaglandin, phentolamine, papaverine, or some mixture of these drugs (i.e., Trimix). Redosing of vasoactive drugs may be necessary to achieve maximal corporal smooth muscle relaxation and realize the best-quality erection in order to demonstrate the actual penile deformity. Specifically, when assessing the Peyronie's plaque in the erect state, factors including the size, degree of penile curvature, direction of curvature (dorsal, ventral, lateral, or some combination), extent and location are critical when deciding on intervention.

One mechanism of Peyronie's disease associated erectile dysfunction is secondary to hemodynamic changes in the corpora cavernosa. PD is a clinically and sonographically heterogeneous condition and the addition of high-resolution color duplex Doppler ultrasonography rapidly and objectively characterizes both the penile hemodynamics and the anatomy of the lesion with a simple, safe, low-cost, noninvasive office-based test [8]. Erectile function can be evaluated by assessing penile blood flow and storage capacity dynamically. Decreased compliance of the penile fibroelastic frame induced by Peyronie's plaques may result in an inability to expand the trabeculae against the tunica albuginea and compress the subtunical venules. The clinical consequence of such hemodynamic alterations in the "trapping" mechanism is excessive outflow of lacunar blood through the subtunical venules, leading to decreased penile rigidity and a diminished ability to sustain an erection. This modality allows for objective understanding of the disease, both for the patient and his partner, as well as the physician. In addition, this diagnostic test allows the clinician to establish a baseline prior to intervention and tailor the best treatment strategy by offering an objective means of monitoring improvement following the initiation of therapy and throughout the course of management.

Additional noninvasive erectile function tests may include penile biothesiometry to evaluate sensation preoperatively. Anatomic changes other than curvature seen with Peyronie's disease, such as an "hourglass-deformity" should be documented in the erect state, as well. The severity of the deformity, as well as the associated erectile function and storage ability are critical factors when determining the appropriate therapeutic intervention.

More invasive diagnostic tests, such as dynamic infusion pharmaco-cavernosometry and cavernosography may be utilized to better understand these changes in the individual patient. Pharmacocavernosography in the erect state in men with Peyronie's disease typically demonstrates penile deformity and a focal, site-specific pattern of abnormal venous drainage.

Objective evaluation of penile hemodynamics and storage ability is critical during the preoperative evaluation, as any therapeutic intervention for

Peyronie's disease may have some adverse impact upon erectile function. Hence, documentation of the baseline erectile function is imperative, from both medical and medico-legal perspectives.

## Goals of Therapy

Among men with Peyronie's disease, there is a very high prevalence of emotional and relationship problems often as a result of the loss of penile length and inability to have intercourse. Medical and surgical therapies may enhance quality of life through their ability to improve sexual function. Further research will characterize the ways in which individual symptoms affect emotional and psychological well-being [9].

Setting realistic goals is essential prior to instituting any form of therapy, especially for Peyronie's disease and erectile dysfunction. The "goal of therapy" for Peyronie's disease is to achieve a degree of penile straightening or improved pliability, combined with adequate erectile function (with or without the need for medication or surgery) to enable comfortable intercourse and sexual activity for both the patient and his partner. Penile numbness and loss of length do not always improve or resolve despite any type of therapeutic intervention. Patients with Peyronie's disease must understand all the advantages and disadvantages of the various therapeutic options, including active surveillance or no therapy, prior to treatment. Although excellent treatment options are available, each person needs to be diagnosed and evaluated individually by a doctor who is an expert in this area because no one treatment is appropriate for everyone. However, based on our experience, the majority of men with Peyronie's disease with or without erectile dysfunction can be helped, often without the need for surgical intervention.

## Treatment Options

After an appropriate diagnosis is made and vascular testing performed, the physician will prescribe treatment tailored to the individual. For specific patients, active surveillance may be an appropriate option. In rare cases, the disease and resultant curvature may resolve spontaneously. In many cases, the plaque typically runs its course and often stabilizes after 6–12 months. It is for this reason that early treatment should typically be conservative, consisting of nonsurgical management, especially in cases where erectile function is normal and the patient is able to achieve successful intercourse with minimal or no discomfort. However, once the plaque is stable or calcified, conservative therapy tends to be less successful, and more invasive treatments may be needed, especially if severe curvature or ED prevents satisfactory intercourse [10].

Various therapeutic options are available for patients who have Peyronie's disease, including medical and surgical intervention [11]. Conservative medical treatments, including antioxidants such as Vitamin E, Pentoxifylline, Potaba and Colchicine, an anti-gout medicine that has been shown to improve inflammation, have been suggested [12]. It has been suggested that these medicines taken during the initial, acute phase of the disease process, may play some role in improving the outcome, although clear objective data demonstrating their usefulness is minimal. It is more likely, however, that time alone is the critical factor in those rare cases where spontaneous resolution is observed.

Studies have suggested that phosphodiesterase type-5 inhibitors (PDE5I), such as sildenafil, vardenafil, or tadalafil, may have a role in the management of Peyronie's disease through their antifibrotic action and their potential for penile scar remodeling. While early science is encouraging, further research is necessary in order to establish the usefulness of this strategy [13, 14].

An association between Peyronie's disease and low levels of serum testosterone levels has been suggested. In a recent study from Cavallini and associates, plaque area and penile curvature were found to be more severe in hypogonadal PD men compared to PD men with normal testosterone levels. In addition, men with PD were found to have a lower serum ratio of bioavailable testosterone to free testosterone than healthy controls.

In those patients with PD, supplementation with testosterone was also demonstrated to improve the efficacy of intralesional verapamil therapy [15].

A number of studies have demonstrated the efficacy of intralesional therapy, or injecting medication directly into the plaque [16]. This is done in an attempt to reduce, soften, or eliminate the plaque and its resultant curvature.

Although minimal success was initially reported using steroids or collagenase injections, placebo-controlled clinical trials have clearly demonstrated that the use of intralesional interferon and intralesional verapamil can help to improve the penile curvature condition with minimal side effects [17]. In fact, up to 80% of men undergoing a 3- to 6-month course of intralesional therapy with Interferon (Intron A) or verapamil noted significant decrease in plaque size, improvement in penile curvature, as well as patient and partner comfort and ease of intercourse [18]. The advantage of this form of therapy is that in addition to being safe and effective, it allows many men to improve their Peyronie's condition and to have comfortable sexual intercourse without the need for surgery. Currently, phase III trials evaluating a new formulation of intralesional collagenase to reduce penile curvature is underway. Intralesional injections should only be performed by a physician who is very experienced in this form of therapy, in order to maximize success and reduce the chance of damage to the neurovascular bundle and erectile tissue.

The use of topical medications, such as verapamil, applied to the penis, directly over the plaque, in an attempt to decrease plaque size and improve curvature, have also been suggested. While anecdotal reports abound regarding the efficacy of topical therapy, clear objective data is lacking. The use of iontophoresis to improve penetration of the chemical has also been suggested as a means to improve penetration into the plaque and may prove to be beneficial [19].

The use of external beam radiation and directed lithotripsy (shock wave energy) treatments for Peyronie's disease have been suggested and reported in the medical literature [20]. However, it is believed that these treatments may damage the underlying corporal (erectile) tissue and neurovascular structures and may, in fact, worsen the overall erectile function of the penis. Further large-scale trials need to be performed in order to determine the safety and efficacy of these treatment modalities in Peyronie's disease [21].

As there is no known reliable nonsurgical treatment for PD, the principle of modeling the tunica albuginea, which has been shown to be useful prior to penile implant surgery, has been applied to the treatment of PD. Specifically, the use of vacuum therapy and external penile traction to mechanically straighten the penile curvature of Peyronie's disease has been suggested as an alternative conservative therapy. Preliminary studies have demonstrated statistically significant improvement in penile length, angle of curvature, and pain after 12 weeks of using the vacuum pump [22]. The studies suggest that vacuum therapy and external penile traction therapy may improve or stabilize the curvature of PD, is safe to use, and might reduce the number of patients going on to surgery [23].

## Surgical Treatment Options

Surgical intervention for Peyronie's disease is usually not considered until the condition has stabilized, usually after 12 months, and medical therapy has not been effective. At that point if there is still significant penile curvature and/or sexual dysfunction, surgical options may be considered. It is recommended that only a surgeon very experienced in these types of procedures perform this surgery. Depending on the location, extent and degree of curvature, in addition to the degree of erectile dysfunction, the most appropriate procedure will be determined [24].

In patients with normal erectile function, a number of effective "straightening" procedures may be used, including plication surgery, or various plaque incision and grafting procedures [25–27]. In cases of an extensive dorsal plaque, often with involvement of the neurovascular bundle, use of a ventral Nesbit-type plication may be appropriate in order to minimize the risk of penile numbness and resultant erectile dysfunction.

A) DIAGNOSIS:

Patient and Partner History:
- Medical, Sexual and Psychosocial History
- History of Penile Trauma and Pain
- Length of Time of Plaque/Deformity/Curvature
- Stability of Plaque/Deformity/Curvature
- Prior Therapies (including Herbals/Vitamins)
- Rule out: Ejaculatory or orgasmic dysfunction
- Endocrinologic and Laboratory Evaluation

Physical Examination:
- Complete Genitourinary Examination
- Palpable Penile Plaque (Location, Size, Severity)
- Penile stretch, length, sensation, pain

Vascular Evaluation in the Erect State:
- Abnormal penile curvature (Location, Size, Severity)
- Hourglass deformity (Location, Size, Severity)
- Office intracavernosal injection test
- Penile duplex Doppler ultrasonography
- Dynamic Infusion Pharmacocavernosography and cavernosography

Neurologic Evaluation: (performed in selected patients)
- Biothesiometry
- Vibration perception sensitivity testing

B) THERAPEUTIC ALTERNATIVES:

1) Normal erectile function and minimal curvature or deformity
   a. Consider Active Surveillance, if curvature not bothersome to patient or partner
   b. Consider conservative therapy if needed (i.e. stretching device, VED, Intralesional tx)
2) Normal erectile function and significant curvature or deformity
   a. Consider first line conservative medical therapy (i.e. Intralesional therapy, with or w/o stretching device or VED)
   b. Consider surgical intervention if medical therapy ineffective or not desired by patient (i.e. plication, plaque incision/excision and grafting)
   c. Consider need for PDE5I tx
3) Poor erectile function (not responsive to PDE5I) with significant curvature or deformity.
   a. Consider first line conservative medical therapy (i.e. Intralesional therapy, with or w/o stretching device or VED) to achieve maximal improvement in curvature or deformity prior to surgery
   b. Consider implantation of inflatable penile prosthesis with repair of residual curvature or deformity (via molding, plaque incision/excision, possible grafting)

**Fig. 10.2** Peyronie's disease: management algorithm

For patients who have moderate to severe erectile dysfunction in addition to penile plaque and curvature, insertion of an inflatable penile prosthesis (IPP) with repair of any residual curvature is an excellent treatment option for restoring both normal sexual function and a straight erection [28]. Men with PD undergoing IPP placement should be counseled regarding potential penile length loss and residual curvature, neither of which typically interfere with coitus but may reduce satisfaction [29].

## Summary

While the overall incidence of Peyronie's disease in the general population is <10%, it is a devastating process that affects both the unfortunate man and his partner. Numerous advances have been made in understanding the underlying physiologic mechanisms causing Peyronie's disease. Improved clinical techniques for the diagnosis and treatment of Peyronie's disease have allowed us to enter a new and exciting era in the field of sexual medicine. While the evaluation process should be individualized for each patient, a simple, algorithm for the evaluation and management of patients with Peyronie's disease is described below in Fig. 10.2.

## References


1. Serefoglu EC, Hellstrom WJ. Treatment of Peyronie's disease: 2012 update. Curr Urol Rep. 2011;12(6):444–52. http://dx.doi.org/10.1007/s11934-011-0212-2. Accessed 5 Aug 2011.
2. Nugteren HM, Nijman JM, de Jong IJ, van Driel MF. The association between Peyronie's and Dupuytren's disease. Int J Impot Res. 2011;23(4):142–5.
3. Casabé A, Bechara A, Cheliz G, De Bonis W, Rey H. Risk factors of Peyronie's disease. What does our clinical experience show? J Sex Med. 2011;8(2):518–23.
4. Faix A, Lapray JF, Callede O, Maubon A, Lanfrey K. Magnetic resonance imaging (MRI) of sexual intercourse: second experience in missionary position and initial experience in posterior position. J Sex Marital Ther. 2002;28 Suppl 1:63–76.
5. Hellstrom WJ, Bivalacqua TJ. Peyronie's disease: etiology, medical, and surgical therapy. J Androl. 2000; 21(3):347–54.
6. Hakim LS, Platt M. The couple's disease: finding a cure for your 'lost' love life. NY: DHP Publishers; 2002.
7. Mulhall JP, Alex B, Choi JM. Predicting delay in presentation in men with Peyronie's disease. J Sex Med. 2010;7(6):2226–30.
8. Smith JF, Brant WO, Fradet V, Shindel AW, et al. Penile sonographic and clinical characteristics in men with Peyronie's disease. J Sex Med. 2009;6(10): 2858–67.
9. Smith JF, Walsh TJ, Conti SL, Turek P, Lue T. Risk factors for emotional and relationship problems in Peyronie's disease. J Sex Med. 2008;5(9):2179–84.
10. Ralph D, Gonzalez-Cadavid N, Mirone V, Perovic S, Sohn M, Usta M, Levine L. The management of Peyronie's disease: evidence-based 2010 guidelines. J Sex Med. 2010;7(7):2359–74.
11. Gur S, Limin M, Hellstrom WJ. Current status and new developments in Peyronie's disease: medical, minimally invasive and surgical treatment options. Expert Opin Pharmacother. 2011;12(6):931–44.
12. Safarinejad MR, Asgari MA, Hosseini SY, Dadkhah F. A double-blind placebo-controlled study of the efficacy and safety of pentoxifylline in early chronic Peyronie's disease. BJU Int. 2010;106(2):240–8.
13. Gonzalez-Cadavid NF, Rajfer J. Treatment of Peyronie's disease with PDE5 inhibitors: an antifibrotic strategy. Nat Rev Urol. 2010;7(4): 215–21.
14. Chung E, Deyoung L, Brock GB. The role of PDE5 inhibitors in penile septal scar remodeling: assessment of clinical and radiological outcomes. J Sex Med. 2011;8(5):1472–7.
15. Cavallini G, Biagiotti G, Lo Giudice C. Association between Peyronie's disease and low serum testosterone levels: detection and therapeutic considerations. J Androl. 2011. http://www.andrologyjournal.org/cgi/rapidpdf/jandrol.111.012948v1. Accessed 5 Aug 2011.
16. Greenfield JM, Shah SJ, Levine LA. Verapamil versus saline in electromotive drug administration for Peyronie's disease: a double-blind, placebo controlled trial. J Urol. 2007;177(3):972–5.
17. Hellstrom WJ, Kendirci M, Matern R, Cockerham Y, et al. Single-blind, multicenter, placebo controlled, parallel study to assess the safety and efficacy of intralesional interferon alpha-2B for minimally invasive treatment for Peyronie's disease. J Urol. 2006;176(1):394–8.
18. Kendirci M, Usta MF, Matern RV, Nowfar S, et al. The impact of intralesional interferon alpha-2b injection therapy on penile hemodynamics in men with Peyronie's disease. J Sex Med. 2005;2(5):709–15.
19. Vardi Y, Levine LA, Chen J, Hatzimouratidis K, Sohn M. Is there a place for conservative treatment in Peyronie's disease? J Sex Med. 2009;6(4):903–9.
20. De Berardinis E, Busetto GM, Antonini G, Giovannone R, Gentile V. Extracorporeal shock wave therapy in the treatment of Peyronie's disease: long-term results. Arch Ital Urol Androl. 2010;82(2):128–33.
21. Chitale S, Morsey M, Swift L, Sethia K. Limited shock wave therapy vs. sham treatment in men with Peyronie's disease: results of a prospective randomized controlled double-blind trial. BJU Int. 2010;106(9):1352–6.
22. Rahim AA, Giraffe G, Rahim TA, Dixon M, et al. The role of vacuum pump therapy to mechanically straighten the penis in Peyronie's disease. BJU Int. 2010;106(8):1178–80.
23. Levine LA, Newell M, Taylor FL. Penile traction therapy for treatment of Peyronie's disease: a single-center pilot study. J Sex Med. 2008;5(6):1468–73.
24. Mulhall J, Anderson M, Parker M. A surgical algorithm for men with combined Peyronie's disease and erectile dysfunction: functional and satisfaction outcomes. J Sex Med. 2005;2(1):132–8.
25. Richardson B, Pinsk MR, Hellstrom WJ. Incision and grafting for severe Peyronie's disease. J Sex Med. 2009;6(8):2084–7.
26. Lentz AC, Carson 3rd CC. Peyronie's surgery: graft choices and outcomes. Curr Urol Rep. 2009;10(6): 460–7.
27. Chung E, Clendenin E, Lesser L, Brock G. Five-year follow-up of Peyronie's graft surgery: outcomes and patient satisfaction. J Sex Med. 2011;8(2):594–600.
28. Levine LA, Demetrious RJ. A surgical algorithm for penile prosthesis placement in men with erectile failure and Peyronie's disease. Int J Impot Res. 2000; 12(3):147–51.
29. Levine LA, Benso J, Hoover C. Inflatable penile prosthesis placement in men with Peyronie's disease and drug-resistant erectile dysfunction: a single-center study. J Sex Med. 2010;7(11):3775–83.

# Primary Care Evaluation and Treatment of Erectile Dysfunction

11

Martin Miner and Jacob Rajfer

Primary care for adults is provided by a variety of clinicians including nurse practitioners, physicians' assistants, family physicians, internists, and gynecologists. The values and roles of individual clinicians are complex because they may depend on the individual's value system and practice model [1]. Most primary care clinicians will routinely address problems with high morbidity and mortality, disabling conditions, conditions for which there are clear standards of care, and perhaps those with well-established management guidelines. The demands of their patient and the personal interest of the clinician will also affect the choice of issues that the clinician addresses.

Issues that involve quality of life commonly fall into a lower priority category. Patients may not feel that they are important or clinicians do not recognize "improving quality of life" as being a high priority. This is especially true when the quality-of-life issue involves very personal issues and more difficult language. Addressing quality-of-life issues around sexual dysfunction is even more difficult; partly because there are complex psychosocial issues involved and treatments are not well standardized (except for erectile dysfunction). Social taboos about discussing sex or considering sex a legitimate personal need also hinder communication about sexual dysfunction.

M. Miner, MD (✉)
Department of Family Medicine and Urology, Warren Albert School of Medicine, Brown University, Men's Health Center, The Miriam Hospital, 164 Summit Avenue, Providence, RI 02906, USA
e-mail: Martin_Miner@brown.edu

J. Rajfer, MD
Department of Urology, UCLA School of Medicine, Los Angeles, CA, USA

Harbor-UCLA Medical Center, Torrance, CA, USA
e-mail: JRajfer@ucla.edu

## Trends in Primary Care Involvement in Sexual Health

Many factors have recently changed the work of primary care clinicians. Trends in population demographics, the aging of patients, managed care, and medical technology have altered demand and actual primary care activity. The mean age of patients visiting primary care clinicians has increased and patients have become more ethnically and racially diverse [2]. The duration of visits to the doctor is decreasing with a recent study of the length of ambulatory visits to primary care clinicians having a mean of 16.3 min [3], possibly associated with the availability of nonphysician support personnel and with the issues around health maintenance organizations as payers. These and other changes, such as an increase in single-specialty and multispecialty group practice, computerization of the office, more complex reimbursement methods, and an increasingly educated patient population have occupied some of the energy that would better be turned toward patient care and prevention of disease.

D.A. Shoskes (ed.), *Urological Men's Health: A Guide for Urologists and Primary Care Physicians*, Current Clinical Urology, DOI 10.1007/978-1-61779-900-6_11,
© Springer Science+Business Media New York 2012

Health-care clinicians have been ambivalent about sexuality for a long time. Most early research was done by nonphysician social scientists [4]. Medical school instruction related to sex is limited to (1) some anatomy and physiology, (2) information about AIDS and sexually transmitted diseases, and (3) lectures on "alternative" lifestyles such as homosexuality. There is a conspicuous absence of courses on sex in general. Clinicians avoid discussing sexual concerns even when a problem is suspected, citing lack of knowledge and skills as a common reason [5]. Clinicians are often concerned that a sexual dysfunction like erectile dysfunction (ED) will become a complex, time-consuming condition that cannot be managed properly under pressures of current reimbursement methods [6]. However, pioneering primary care clinicians, including both physician and nonphysician clinicians reviewed the impact of sexual problems on health and psychosocial issues and reviewed possible management strategies [7, 8].

The motivation for primary care clinicians to help patients with sexual dysfunction should be high [9]. Unfortunately, while general sexual dissatisfaction is very high among men, reported at a rate of 75% noting at least one problem with dissatisfaction, avoidance, infrequency, or noncommunication [10], 70% of men with ED go untreated [11]. Specific sexual dysfunction is prevalent, reported in approximately one-third of men over age 18, with premature ejaculation as the most common sexual dysfunction reported by men followed by ED [10, 12]. Yet, men continue not to seek treatment, mistakenly believing that ED is a normal part of aging, or embarrassed to discuss the condition with their clinicians.

Experiencing a sexual dysfunction is highly associated with a number of unsatisfying personal experiences and relationships. Men with ED experience a diminished quality of life when measured as low physical satisfaction, low emotional satisfaction, and low general happiness [13]. Reports of low self-esteem and relationship difficulties indicate the effect of ED on function and satisfaction with daily life activities. There are also some preliminary reports that sexual dysfunction can contribute to initiating clinical anxiety and depression syndromes. If "morbidity" is defined as the consequences resulting from an abnormally functioning, diseased organ or body system, then ED clearly has a recognizable morbidity.

## Inquiry and Management of ED Is a Primary Care Priority

Several factors make primary care the ideal place for discussions about sexual issues [14]. First, longitudinal and personal relationships with patients is an asset in discussing and resolving sexual problems, second, the multifactorial issues around ED are appropriately evaluated by the patient's clinician, and third, the long-term follow-up to be certain that a sexual dysfunction is resolved is well suited to primary care.

Recently, ED has been found to be more relevant than simply a quality-of-life issue with psychosocial morbidity. The comorbidities most often presenting with ED are those frequently seen in primary care practices. Diabetes, dyslipidemias, hypertension, coronary artery disease, cigarette smoking and smoking-related illness, lower urinary tract symptoms (LUTS) associated with benign prostatic hyperplasia (BPH), depression, acute or chronic anxiety and stress and obesity all represent risk factors for the presence of ED [15–18]. Organic ED is likely to be a reliable signal for systemic vascular disease and possibly for vascular endothelial function and may even be the first recognized evidence of the presence of yet-undiscovered vascular risk factors such as hypertension, hyperlipidemia, or diabetes [19]. In a study of men seeking medical advice for ED, many were newly diagnosed with a comorbid condition following seeking attention for the ED complaint. These included a new diagnosis of hypertension (18%), diabetes (16%), benign prostatic hypertrophy (15%), ischemic heart disease (5%), prostate cancer (4%), and depression (1%) [20]. Up to 15% of previously healthy men presenting with ED have abnormal blood glucose levels [21]. Abnormal cholesterol profiles were discovered in 60% of men complaining of ED without a prior history of cardiac disease [22]. In a study of 200 men with ED who underwent lipid profiling (that had not been previously performed), 75% of these men with ED had dyslipidemia [23].

In a study involving patients receiving care in Canadian primary care clinicians' offices, a significant relationship was noted between ED and hyperglycemia, diabetes mellitus, and metabolic syndrome [24]. Another large self-reporting survey study noted that traditional modifiable risk factors for cardiovascular disease (CVD) were independently associated with ED, including diabetes mellitus (DM) (OR, 2.69), obesity (OR, 1.60), current smoking (OR, 1.74), and hypertension (OR, 1.56). These authors implied that mitigation of these risk factors might not only ameliorate ED but also improve health outcomes [25].

Recent studies support the relationship between ED and actual CVD. The first study using stress myocardial perfusion computed tomography found that men with ED exhibited more severe coronary heart disease (CHD) and left ventricular dysfunction than those without ED [26]. A prospective analysis of men randomly assigned to the placebo arm of the Prostate Cancer Prevention Trial (PCPT) revealed that men with ED are at significantly greater risk ($p<0.001$) of having a cardiovascular event—angina, myocardial infarction (MI), or stroke—than those without ED. Furthermore, the findings indicate that the relationship between incident ED (the first report of ED of any grade) and CVD is comparable to that associated with current smoking, family history of MI, or hyperlipidemia [27]. A subsequent study of almost 300 men with coronary artery disease symptoms reported that these men experienced ED symptoms first, on average 3 years beforehand [28].

Once it is recognized that ED is more than simply a quality-of-life issue, it is a simple step to acknowledge that ED is a very common and important problem among patients seen in a primary care office [29]. If ED is truly a signal of endothelial dysfunction and both CVD risk and actual disease, then identifying ED, especially vasculogenic ED, becomes a priority [30]. "A flagging penis should raise the red flag of warning to evaluate the patient for arterial disease elsewhere" [31]. "By monitoring a patient's sexual well-being, added insight into the progression of his CVD can be obtained and his treatment adjusted accordingly [32].

Clinicians are accustomed to asking patients about exercise "tolerance" or "capacity" in order to evaluate cardiovascular function and reserve. With the recognition of the relation between ED and CVD, it would not be difficult for clinicians to add a brief question about erectile "tolerance" or "capacity" with the understanding of potentially identifying CVD risk factors or actual disease among men who report ED. Some epidemiologic experts have noted the higher death rate and likely lower health status among middle-aged men in the USA compared with England probably caused by the increased prevalence of hypertension, diabetes, and nonhypertension CVD [33]. Although the death rate evens out as the men get beyond middle age, the increased rate of vascular risk factors in the USA puts even more obligation on American clinicians to inquire about erectile function among middle-aged men. If clinicians more thoroughly screened ED patients for CVD in particular for hypertension, risk reduction might offset the development or progression of CVD [34].

We are also learning that being part of a good relationship is not only just a quality-of-life issue, but also can promote good health. A popular idea in the lay press, that loving, supportive relationships can make you healthier, has support in clinical studies. The breakdown of a significant personal relationship is one of the most stressful life events and impacts on general health and quality of life [35]. Although sex is not essential for supportive, healthy relationships, the amount of sexual intimacy in loving relationships has been correlated with relationship satisfaction [36]. ED negatively affects relationships with one survey of ED sufferers noting that 80% of respondents indicating some form of relationship difficulty because of their ED and 12% saying that the condition prevented them from forming relationships [14].

## Talking to Patients and Partners

Patients may either present with symptoms of erectile dysfunction or have risk factors that prompt screening. Since the yield of screening is related to the frequency of ED in the population, men who should be screened include: those over 40 years of age, those with a predisposing comorbidity such as a CVD including hypertension, diabetes, or depression, or anyone else who the clinician feels may be having difficulty with physical intimacy.

Patients with sexual concerns report feeling most comfortable discussing these issues with their family clinician and expect to receive advice and treatment [12]. Introduction of sexual activity as a legitimate topic for conversation with patients can be done passively or actively. Examples of passive approaches to engaging the patient would be to leave pamphlets about sex-related topics or self-evaluation material such as the Sexual Health Inventory for Men (SHIM) in the waiting room or to hang educational posters in patient care areas. Inclusion of one or more questions about sexual activity in a printed history form completed by the patient requires more active patient participation.

Clinicians initiate more of the verbal interaction than do patients and control the content, pace, and length of the interview. A truly active approach for initiating discussions about sexual activity is probably the most efficient discussion-initiating technique (Table 11.1). Clinicians should develop ease with one of these more active approaches and incorporate it into discussions with patients. Questions about sexual matters are appropriate either during the initial formal history, during the review of systems, during a follow-up visit, or during appropriate stages of the physical examination. These questions need to be sensitive to cultural, religious, and educational differences. Using terminology, that is, clear, simple, and respectful of the patient's feelings can facilitate communication as can the use of synonyms that will increase the likelihood that language common to the patient will be used. Gender difference between a female clinician and a male patient may initially cause some discomfort, but many men report feeling more comfortable discussing sexual issues with female clinicians [37]. Being polite and respectful, yet displaying an appropriate level of interest in the patient's personal life is the best overall approach to encouraging conversation about sexual activity.

**Table 11.1** Discussing sexual matters

| |
|---|
| *Your approach sets the tone* |
| – Take the initiative |
| – Use language that is simple and direct |
| – Maintain a sense of privacy and confidentiality |
| – Keep your attitude nonjudgmental, caring, and respectful |
| – Provide explanations and allow for questions |
| – Acknowledge and explore patient's responses |
| – Promote optimistic attitude |
| *Taking a sexual history* |
| – Routinely ask all patients about their sexual history |
| – Add sexual health questions on patient history forms |
| – Use a screening test (e.g., SHIM) to uncover ED when performing a comprehensive evaluation |
| – Give patients the opportunity to discuss sexual problems they now have or may develop in the future |
| – Discuss sexually transmitted disease prevention |
| *Ask questions to clarify the problem more precisely* |
| – How severe is the problem? |
| – What caused the problem? |
| – How long has the problem existed? |

Initially using "open-ended" questions such as "Tell me a little about your sexual activities?" "Have you been sexually active with a partner in the past 6 months?" or simply "How's your sex life?" encourages the patient to speak more openly. In men with chronic illnesses or risk factors for ED, asking: "How has your illness affected your sex life?" This question may be preceded with a brief statement about the importance of sexual activity to an individual's health. "In order to protect your health, I need to ask you some questions about your sexual life. Are you romantically or sexually involved with anyone?" Occasionally, a question about "concerns" is useful because it is both open ended and problem oriented [18]. "Do you or your partner have any sexual concerns?" Offering some specific examples might also be useful. "Do you or your partner have any sexual difficulties or concerns such as with your interest level, erections, ejaculation?" Questions should be used that cannot be answered by a simple "yes" or "no" since these will close off discussion [18].

Another technique is to use a permission-giving question that tells the patient that you will not be surprised if he reports a problem, demonstrates respect and sensitivity to the patient. An example of this would be to say to a patient with diabetes "Many of my male patients with diabetes report some difficulty having an erection. Have you noticed any problems?" This allows the patient to answer openly without anticipating that the physician would be surprised or shocked by their answer. Using synonyms such as "getting hard," or "coming" may help the patient understand the question better. Encouraging a patient's response with "facilitating" gestures such as good eye contact, nodding affirmatively, summing up what the patient has told you and expressing optimism that the problem can be resolved improves communication.

If the primary care clinician plans to further manage sexual disorders, it is helpful to obtain further information about the characteristics of the specific problem. The first characteristic is to determine whether the problem is *psychogenic or organic*. An organic etiology refers to the ED being caused by either a vascular, neurogenic, or hormonal issue or any combination of the three. To distinguish most psychogenic ED disorders from potentially organically induced disorders, ask some combination of three questions: (1) "Do you ever wake up with an erection before having to urinate?" (2) "If you touch yourself, can you get an erection?" (3) "Can you get an erection at any time of night or day, during any form of sexual activity, with any partner?" A positive response to these questions indicates stress or anxiety as the trigger of the ED, rather than a physical cause or a medication adverse effect.

The second characteristic is to determine whether the problem is *lifelong or acquired*. Dysfunctions that are more recently acquired are more amenable to briefer treatments while those that are lifelong often require further psychotherapy or clinical investigation. The third characteristic is *generalized or situational*. Situational problems hint at difficulties with specific partners or in specific situations that implies a psychogenic etiology.

Asking sexual partners about each other's sexual function is often very useful. Women ranked "partner sexual difficulties" as a common sexual concern [38]. If both members of a couple are in the office, it becomes easy to introduce the topic by asking "How are you two doing together? ... How are you doing with sex?" If only one member of a couple is available, questions can still be asked both about the present patient and the partner. When a sexual dysfunction is identified, talking to the partner can reveal a different picture that may substantially affect management, and can also have a therapeutic effect [39, 40]. Relationships have a profound effect on sexual health and often need to be explored to amplify the likelihood of successful resolution of the problem.

More often, if the patient or partner is not asked about sexual issues, they will bring up problems at the end of the visit. Although this may seem like an afterthought, for many it may be one of the major (if not the major) reasons for the visit. An initial impression that their problem is being dismissed can considerably delay or prevent them from seeking further help [41]. If inadequate time exists to discuss the issue at that time, recognition should be made of the patient's problem or concern and another time should be scheduled to discuss it further. Just spending time clarifying the nature of the problem can lead to more effective treatment and may, in itself, be therapeutic [41]. Alternatively, the patient can be given a referral to another clinician if the primary care clinician is uncomfortable, but even a proper referral requires some further exploration.

Knowing about a patient's sexuality is important to the clinician who is truly interested in the patient's health and happiness. "Do you have sex with men, women, or both?" is a common way of demonstrating an acceptance of varying sexual orientations. Using the term "partner" rather than "spouse" or "wife" conveys the fact that the clinician is not making any assumptions regarding sexual orientation. Gay men are more likely to confide important information and to follow a provider's advice if they feel accepted and understood.

From a practical point of view, the majority of cases of ED that present to the physician's office today is due to a vascular problem. More specifically, it is not an issue with getting blood into the penis, but it is due to the inability of the corporal tissue to trap the blood within the penis. This inability to store the incoming blood in the corpora or what is euphemistically called venous leakage is due to a dysfunction of the corporal smooth muscle, which can be caused by a variety of diseases, e.g., diabetes, hypogonadism, aging, etc. as a result of their impact, directly or indirectly, on the corporal smooth muscle. Venous leakage can be found in between two-thirds to three-quarters of all men who present with ED. In fact, the first inkling by a patient of a problem with this muscle is the increase in the refractory period that men experience as they age. In clinical terms, when this increase in refractory period progresses, patients begin to develop what they express as "difficulty maintaining my erection."

## The Next Step After Identifying ED

The primary care clinician who identifies the patient with ED has accomplished a lot. This information can be used to (1) initiate evaluation for psychologic and organic comorbid conditions including risk factors for neurovascular disease, (2) refer the patient to an appropriate clinician, (3) open up further discussion to confirm whether or not ED is the primary sexual problem or whether it is secondary to a difficulty with some other phase of the male sexual cycle such as libido or ejaculation, and/or (4) work with the patient on a management plan.

## Basic Sex Counseling

Basic sex therapy can be offered by the primary care clinician [42]. Sex therapy involves teaching improvements in sexual technique and helping the patient to concentrate on pleasure rather than simply the achievement of an erection. This may be achieved by providing to the man or, ideally, to both partners in a relationship, information including factual information about sexual concerns, sexual practices, and sexual response individualized to the specific patient or couple, and by attempting to reduce performance anxiety. Encourage partners to discuss what they enjoy about sex. More specific suggestions can be offered as the next level of sex therapy encouraging couples to renew intimacy and sensuality in the relationship and to extend foreplay for each other. The use of topical lubricants or estrogen replacement therapy for the woman may be essential, especially if increased sexual activity is anticipated. The clinician needs to have some specific knowledge about sexual performance and response to provide this level of counseling. The most detailed level of therapy often requires the assistance of a sex therapist and should be considered when the patient has been unable to understand or implement any of the more basic hints or when the counseling interventions have not worked.

## ED Management Promotes Good Health in Men

Men tend to underuse health services for medical problems or for health promotion and disease prevention. Identified factors that impact upon a man's decision to present to a physician include (1) support, (2) help seeking, and (3) barriers [43]. Barriers in the way of men presenting to the physician include a sense of immortality and invulnerability, difficulty giving up control, a belief that seeking help is unacceptable, and a lower concern about disease prevention. Other barriers include time and access, and having to state a reason for the visit [44]. Men receive fewer services, less health information, and are less likely to receive advice about how changes in behavior can improve health [45]. Emphasis is on common cardiovascular risk diseases including hypertension, coronary and non-CHD, and diabetes mellitus while ignoring conditions that determine the patient's quality of life [46]. When men's health issues are considered, it usually is limited to detection of prostate cancer. Specific approaches may work better in encouraging men to follow-up on medical issues.

Sexuality is a most vital part of one's health [46]. Sexual activity and good health appear to be related. Laumann noted that among men and women in his study who had no sexual partners in the past 12 months, 6% perceived that they were in "poor health" compared with 2% of the entire study population [47]. Sexual activity and happiness were also correlated in this group. The impact of ED on comorbid conditions is beginning to be studied. Patients with diabetes who also have ED showed higher levels of frustration and discouragement and a lower acceptance of diabetes. These observations were related to worse metabolic control and higher levels of depressive symptoms [48].

The epidemiology of ED demonstrates several modifiable risk factors associated with increased incidence of ED. Identification of ED helps the physician encourage healthier lifestyle activities in patients that may impact on cardiovascular risk. Men are often slow to adopt healthy lifestyles even when a full explanation is offered about cardiovascular risk. Associating healthier lifestyles with preservation or a possible improvement of impaired erectile function may motivate men to work harder to make healthier lifestyle decisions. The impact of general lifestyle changes to limit progression of ED has been reviewed noting varied results [49]. Regular moderate physical activity seemed to reduce the risk for ED [50] and possibly even improve symptoms of ED in some populations [49, 51]. This is not surprising since the positive impacts of exercise on claudication, a common lower extremity symptom in patients with peripheral vascular disease, have been well documented [52]. Exercise improvement of claudicating symptoms may be explained by mechanisms that may also impact on penile artery flow including measurable improvements in endothelial vasodilator function, muscle metabolism, blood viscosity, and inflammatory response [52].

The risk of ED may be a smoking deterrent in younger men because of its immediacy when compared with heart disease and cancer [18, 53]. Older men may also be motivated to quit smoking because of the link between smoking and ED [54].

## Evaluating the Man with ED

A targeted evaluation will often find likely etiologic factors for ED [55]. The evaluation of ED follows the same pattern as evaluation of any medical disorder. This includes a pertinent history, physical examination, and laboratory tests (Table 11.2). This history, however, must include a sexual history. It is best not to accept the

**Table 11.2** Initial evaluation of erectile dysfunction (*adapted with modification from Mikhail N. Management of erectile dysfunction by the primary care physician. Cleve Cl J Med 2005;72:293–311*)

| |
|---|
| History<br>Libido<br>Ejaculatory issues (to confirm diagnosis)<br>Understanding of sexual function<br>Hypertension<br>Diabetes<br>Hyperlipidemia<br>Smoking<br>Alcohol, substance abuse |
| Drugs (most commonly diuretics, beta-blockers, digoxin, spironolactone, antidepressants) |
| Depression ,anxiety |
| Hypogonadism |
| Thyroid dysfunction |
| Uremia |
| Pelvic surgery or trauma |
| Partner issues |
| Nocturnal or other spontaneous erections |
| Physical exam |
| Blood pressure |
| Cardiac, peripheral pulses, thyroid, testicular, prostate examination |
| Penile anatomic abnormalities |
| Gynecomastia |
| Laboratory tests |
| Fasting glucose and lipid profile |
| Blood chemistries including FBS and renal function |
| Hemoglobin; Hematocrit |
| Serum testosterone as appropriate[a] |
| Cardiac evaluation with ECG and/or exercise testing as appropriate |

[a]Although most urologic and endocrine guidelines for the evaluation of erectile dysfunction include testosterone measurement, the usefulness of this test among all men initially presenting with erectile dysfunction remains unclear

patient's label for a disorder without first questioning and getting a clear picture of the complaint. Often less educated patients misuse medical or technical terminology. Because, for example, some men confuse ED with premature ejaculation, asking if the erection is lost before or after ejaculation can clarify the problem. Learning about the patient's past sexual history and relationship history can also be very revealing [56].

Questions generally review the phases of male sexual response and focus on problems of desire, arousal/erection, orgasm/ejaculation, and sexual pain. Offering the patient several phrases that describe the same phenomenon in different ways can make the communication clearer.

For desire phase disorder—"Do you still feel in the mood, feel desire, have sexual thoughts or fantasies?" ED preceded by loss of desire can signal hormonal problems, relationship difficulties, medication adverse effects, and depression.

For arousal/erection difficulties—"Do you have trouble getting or keeping an erection, getting or keeping hard? Or both?"

Orgasm/ejaculatory phase problems can be reviewed by asking—"Do you feel you ejaculate, 'come' too quickly" (or "too slowly", or "not at all?)?" ED is common in men who, for any reason, became increasingly anxious about quick ejaculations, delayed ejaculation or perceived absence of ejaculation, as can occur with retrograde emission.

To reveal Peyronie disease or pain disorders ask about "a bend to the penis" or pain during or after sexual activity.

The medical history should include review of risk factors, and screening for psychological difficulties. A medication review, including over-the-counter preparations, may reveal the source of the problem because medications have been implicated in up to 25% of cases of ED [57]. Medications have adverse effects on all phases of sexual functioning making clarification of the patient's complaint a priority before ascribing symptoms to specific medication side effects [58]. Brief screening for depression such as "Do you sometimes feel blue, down in the dumps?" may elicit more honest responses than "Are you depressed?" Other psychiatric conditions such as anxiety may also be responsible for ED. The social history looking for stress surrounding a relationship or substance abuse including alcohol and cigarettes is critical. Finally, a review of daily activity and review of cardiovascular status is important to determine the potential risk of enhancing ED in patients who may have a sedentary lifestyle and who may be at risk (usually minimal) for an adverse cardiac event when sexual activity potential is increased [59].

The physical examination should be targeted with emphasis on several areas [60, 61]. Immature secondary sex characteristics, including hair distribution, and penile and testicular development, may represent testosterone deficiency. Keep in mind that it is good practice to offer the presence of a chaperone to patients having a genital exam. Many will say that it is not necessary, but the offer will allow the more anxious patient to have the comfort of an appropriate additional person in the exam room. Some men prefer to be examined by a clinician of their own sex. Also consider any cultural differences and explore them when necessary prior to initiating the genital exam.

Laboratory tests useful in evaluating ED look for the risk entities already discussed [62]. Prostate specific antigen should be considered for men over age 50 years, and at 40 years for high-risk patients, to evaluate prostate size and tumor presence, especially if testosterone treatment is a possibility. If there is any evidence of hypogonadism or the ED is particularly consistent at a young age, then further hormone evaluation becomes a higher priority.

The advanced diagnostic evaluation for ED includes tests like nocturnal penile tumescence studies, vascular evaluation with sonography, biothesiometry, and other tests that can be performed by the urologic subspecialist. These tests are somewhat subjective and rarely provide useful information except in cases of trauma or other major vascular injury.

If treatment is being considered for a man who has been sexually inactive for a prolonged period, a cardiac evaluation determining cardiac risk needs to be done to determine the safety of the patient's resuming an actual sex life. Although sexual activity requires only a slight increase in energy expenditure for most men in most circumstances, there is a small absolute increase in risk of an adverse cardiac event occurring during sex or within 2 h of sexual activity [59]. The Princeton Guidelines help to evaluate a man's risk for an adverse cardiac event during or shortly after sexual activity [63]. These guidelines tell us that some men with active cardiac risk factors and/or disease fall into a high or intermediate risk category for adverse cardiovascular events and require further cardiac evaluation. The vast majority of men, however, fall into the low risk category for adverse cardiovascular events with increased sexual activity and can safely be treated for erectile dysfunction [64].

## Evaluating Men with ED for Future CVD Risk

Erectile dysfunction can serve as a valuable signal of the need for cardiovascular assessment, especially in men with more established coronary risk factors [63]. Early recommendations are suggesting that men with ED should be screened for both heart disease risk and depression [65–67]. Depression is a known risk factor for CVD [68–70]. This process could lead to early diagnosis and management. The US Preventive Services Task Force has found insufficient evidence to screen low risk or patients at increased risk for the presence of CVD using resting electrocardiography, exercise treadmill testing, or electron beam computerized tomography [71]. However, clinicians should investigate men with ED for comorbid CVD-risk conditions that might then be treated at an earlier date, and these patients should be assessed for CHD risk according to recommended guidelines and algorithms [71].

Many strategies have been suggested that include office-friendly measurements of endothelial dysfunction along with more traditional risk assessment to clarify those men with ED are at increased risk for CVD [19]. A reasonable approach would be to use the Framingham equation, although this equation does not yet include ED as a potential predictor of CAD [72]. The assessment of cardiac risk after a complaint of erectile problems can potentially reduce subsequent morbidity and mortality. We need to determine whether measures of vascular endothelial function can compete with other risk factors such as age, systolic blood pressure, serum lipid fraction levels, glucose, and insulin resistance. Some experts have suggested that men with ED are probably candidates for aggressive treatment to improve endothelial function with treatments such as statins, or angiotensin-converting enzyme inhibitors, or angiotensin receptor blockers [73].

## Treatment of ED

Treatment plans need to be goal oriented, ideally aimed at satisfying the needs of both the man and his partner and maximizing the chance of achieving patient satisfaction. Based on the desired outcome, treatment can be simply pharmacologic, or may require further comprehensive psychosocial and relationship counseling. In many cases, the partner can be brought in to participate in the discussion about the goal of treatment improving the chance of success.

### Educational and Psychosocial Interventions

In most cases, regardless of etiology, the treatment options of the physiologic impairment of ED are the same. Education is the first step in treatment and is personalized to the needs of the specific patient. The normal physiological changes associated with aging are often misunderstood by patients and lead to problems. Myths and misunderstandings about sexual activity can directly cause sexual difficulties as well as generate anxiety, guilt and worry that negatively impact on sexual response and erectile ability [18, 74]. Helping men to have realistic expectations and to better understand healthy function and honest, constructive communication with partners can encourage more satisfactory sexual interaction and a healthier sense of sexual nature. Research has demonstrated that the amount of sexual intimacy correlates with relationship satisfaction [75, 76].

The easily obtained erection begins to disappear in older men, especially those with chronic illness, such as diabetes, hypertension, or renal disease. Direct tactile stimulation of the penis may be needed to obtain and maintain an erection. The man becomes increasingly anxious thereby causing further erectile difficulties. Information from the physician about these changes of aging can be extremely reassuring.

Partner issues vary widely. Issues around partner choice, partner participation in sexual activity, and partner physiology may influence erectile function. When vaginal dryness, or vaginal atrophy leads to loss of lubrication and pain, women often lose interest in continued sexual activity.

## Lifestyle and Medication Changes

Making healthy lifestyle changes may reduce the symptoms of ED and improve general physical health [77]. Patients need to understand that what is bad for the heart is bad for the penis. Elimination of smoking tobacco is probably helpful in reducing incident erectile dysfunction [77]. Dietary issues including reduced cholesterol and trans-fats, eliminating hyperglycemia when present, and decreasing salt intake when salt-sensitive hypertension is noted, all help to diminish vascular insufficiency progression. Exercise will increase cardiac output and improve peripheral circulation. A recent study of obese men with ED without diabetes, hypertension, or dyslipidemia found that reducing caloric intake and increasing physical activity was associated with improved sexual function in about one-third of obese men. These positive changes were associated with significant improvements in erectile function, which were highly correlated with both amount of weight loss and increased activity levels [51]. Exercise training improves endothelial function in the coronary [78] and peripheral circulation [79]. Endurance programs clearly have a positive effect on vasculature probably by moving endothelial function related to an increase in NO production and decreased oxidative stress, which leads to an increase in NO availability [80]. These recommendations will help men be healthier and, hopefully, happier, although their effect on erectile functioning may not be instantly apparent.

Changing medication regimens to remove causative agents can be tried when clinically possible. Examples of this might be discontinuing a thiazide diuretic and substituting and alpha-adrenergic blocker, or weaning the patient from digoxin if the medication is not necessary. Treatment of antidepressant-induced sexual dysfunction can sometimes be managed by reducing drug dosages, altering timing of drug dosages, taking drug holidays, adding an adjunctive drug, and switching to an alternative antidepressant [81]. These substitutions and eliminations may meet with some success, but need to be individualized depending on clinical circumstances.

## Direct Pharmacologic and Surgical Treatment

Specific treatment regimens for ED include oral medications, transurethral suppositories, intracavernosal injection, vacuum devices, and surgery first-line therapies include oral medications and vacuum constriction devices. The FDA approved oral treatments include (1) sildenafil (Viagra), tadalafil (Cialis), and vardenafil (Levitra) [82]. Primary care clinicians are writing about 80–85% of all the prescriptions for PDE5 inhibitors in the USA [83].

Other pharmacologic treatments being used primarily by the urologist and much less often by primary care clinicians include intraurethral or intracavernosal injections of vasodilating medications, apomorphine, a dopamine agonist that causes central initiation of an erection through specific action in the brain, is available in Europe but not in the USA. Vacuum devices are a reasonable choice for many men who are in a stable relationship and their partners are willing to accept the inconvenience [84].

Testosterone augmentation, available as patches, gels, buccal patch injection, or insertion of subcutaneous pellets is best reserved for patients with documented hypogonadism based on the morning free-serum testosterone level. Generally, testosterone augmentation is associated with enhanced libido. This may improve erectile status by restoring interest and perhaps through other neurohormonal mechanisms, but relying solely on testosterone to restore erectile function in the dysfunctional male is inappropriate [85]. Testosterone treatment for testosterone deficiency requires thorough evaluation and monitoring for prostate cancer.

The most common surgical treatment for ED is penile implant surgery, which is primarily performed by urologists. This is a successful therapy in the properly identified patient and should be reserved for those patients who have considered or at least tried several other treatments. The surgery should be considered irreversible since the normal function of the corpora cavernosa is obliterated with this procedure. There are two types of implants—the inflatable and noninflatable or semi-rigid. These implants are essentially mechanical devices and as such can suffer from mechanical failures, which require another surgical procedure to fix the "failure."

Some clinicians have advised that ED can be managed naturally, although no controlled trials exist. A dietary program rich in whole foods including vegetables, fruits, whole grains, and legumes has been suggested with key nutrients including zinc, essential fatty acids, vitamin A, vitamin B-6, L-arginine, and vitamin E being recommended. Herbal supplements such as ginseng, gotu kola, and saw palmetto have also been discussed. Spices reported to increase sexual desire include nutmeg, saffron, parsley, vanilla, avocado, carrot oil, and celery.

## Optimizing Treatment with PDE5Is

Phosphodiesterase type 5 inhibitors (PDEIs) have been available for the treatment of erectile dysfunction since 1998. The rationale for their use is based on the fact that the NO-cGMP pathway [86] is the primary mechanism by which relaxation of the corporal smooth muscle as well as the muscle of the penile vessels occurs. Of the three available PDEIs today, both sildenafil and vardenafil have comparable pharmacokinetics, i.e., peak levels in the blood occur about 1 h after oral ingestion and the serum half-life is about 6–8 h. Both agents require an empty stomach for optimum reabsorption. On the other hand, tadalafil reaches a peak level in the blood stream about 2–3 h after ingestion while its half-life is more extended to about 17–18 h. The absorption of this agent from the gut is not negatively impacted by food.

The PDE5i all have common side effects usually referable to vasomotor function. These include headache, flushing, lightheadedness, etc. Sildenafil is associated at times with visual changes, e.g., seeing blue tint while tadalafil has been associated with back discomfort and muscle aches. All of the aforementioned side effects are dose dependent and reversible. Extremely rare but troubling side effects include nonarteretic ischemic optical neuropathy (NAION) and hearing loss both of which do not seem to be dose related.

The success rates for these PDEIs in rigorous scientific studies range from 60% to 80% in most populations and early expectations of similar success among the general population were similarly high. Unfortunately, in real life a certain percentage of men with erectile dysfunction do not seem to be achieving their desired or expected goal with these agents. The discontinuation rate for PDE5I use among men diagnosed as having erectile dysfunction by their physicians appears to be high even among those who initially responded to the medication, reaching up to 57% in 3-year follow-up [87, 88].

Discussions about appropriate expectations are keys to optimize PDE5I therapy outcomes (Table 11.3). Myths and misunderstandings about sexual activity can directly cause sexual difficulties as well as generate anxiety, guilt and

**Table 11.3** Treatment failure

| |
|---|
| a. Re-educate about appropriate goals, medication use, dose titration |
| b. Consider more detailed psychosocial problems and/ or interventions |
| c. Adjunctive pharmacotherapy |
| d. Alternative pharmacotherapy |
| e. Referral to a specialist |

worry that negatively impact on sexual response and erectile ability [18, 74]. Helping men to have realistic expectations and to understand healthy function, and honest, constructive communication with their partners can encourage more satisfactory sexual interaction and a healthier sexual life in a nonpharmacologic means. Men need to be told that although the medication is likely to have a positive and significant effect on erectile function in men with ED, the degree of effect can vary based on a variety of physiologic and psychosocial factors. The PDE5I biochemical effect does not promise 100% success in all men, and appears to be decreased in men with diabetes or who have had a radical prostatectomy [89, 90].

An algorithm meant to deal with oral treatment ED failures includes reevaluation and adjustment of therapy with (1) hypogonadism treatment if present, (2) dose titration, and (3) patient instruction on optimal use of medication. If the man is still not satisfied, this algorithm suggests considering alternative oral or local therapy with additional education and counseling followed by referral to a specialist if needed [91].

Our goal as physicians for men with ED is to (1) help improve sexual function and regain self-esteem, (2) improve the man's sense of well-being, and (3) improve relationships [92]. We know that improving physiologic erectile function in men with ED is an important part, but only one part of the desired outcome. Many other issues can influence the likelihood of achieving the desired outcomes including (1) the man's psychosocial milieu, (2) the presence of other sexual issues or risk factors for physical sexual dysfunction, (3) the availability and receptivity of a partner, and (4) partner interaction. A trusting physician–patient partnership enhances the likelihood of a successful therapeutic outcome. Optimism is an essential management tool for clinicians to use in responding to sexual issues.

## Follow-Up of Treatment for ED

Follow-up is an essential part of management of erectile dysfunction. Patients should be seen 1 month after initiation of treatment to evaluate progress. Comparison to baseline can be done by verbal exchange or by using the standardized questionnaire measuring erectile function (SHIM). Reviewing the success or lack of success of treatment, any adverse effects, and considering dose or treatment alterations is more likely to achieve the patient's goal. Further education and/or basic sex counseling can be provided to the patient with or without his partner.

## Consultation

Consultation with subspecialists may be appropriate at varying intervals when managing a man with erectile dysfunction. The major factor is the primary care clinician's comfort in discussing and managing treatment options. The obligation of the primary care clinician is to recognize ED and make the patient feel comfortable about seeking help. Initial workup and treatment can be planned by the primary care clinician who has good communication skills about sexual activity and who is knowledgeable about first-line treatments. Common indications for referral to an appropriate specialist include (1) significant penile anatomic disease, (2) a younger patient with a history of pelvic or perineal trauma, (3) cases requiring vascular or neurosurgical intervention, (4) complicated endocrinopathies, (5) complicated psychiatric or psychosocial problems, or (6) patient or physician desire for further evaluation [6]. Urologists can be helpful in difficult or complex erectile dysfunction situations or when the patient presents with an anatomical problem such as Peyronie's disease. An endocrinologist may be consulted to assist in managing men with difficult to control diabetes, hypogonadism, or evidence of pituitary dysfunction.

Sex therapists are practitioners in the medical or mental health field who, in addition to their basic clinical education, have had additional training in sex therapy including evaluation and treatment options. Sex therapists have more time to talk with the patient, to work with couples suggesting enhancement techniques, and to educate couples that there are many ways of having pleasurable sexual relations without a firm erection. These could be physicians, ministers, and mental health professionals. The American Association of Sex Therapists and Counselors can provide a directory for your state of trained, certified sex therapists (www.aasect.org/Home/). Most major teaching hospitals have such a trained individual on their staffs.

## References


1. Lamberts H, Hofmans-Okkes I. Values and roles in primary care. J Fam Pract. 1996;42:178–80.
2. Stafford RS, Saglam D, Causino N, et al. Trends in adult visits to primary care physicians in the United States. Arch Fam Med. 1999;8:26–32.
3. Blumenthal D, Causino N, Chang YC, et al. The duration of ambulatory visits to physicians. J Fam Pract. 1999;48:264–71.
4. Bullough VL. American physicians and sex research and expertise 1900–1990. J Hist Med. 1997;52: 236–53.
5. Broekman CPM, Van Der Werf T, Bosch JJ, Slob AK. An investigation into the management of patients with erection problems in general practice. Int J Impot Res. 1994;6:67–72.
6. Becker BL. Streamlined office management. Article consultant: Baum N, Patient Care Supplement Spring 1999; 17–21.
7. Herrick P. Problems in human sexuality encountered in primary care. PA J. 1976;6(1):3–10.
8. Stine CC, Collins M. Male sexual dysfunction. Prim Care. 1989;16:1031–56.
9. Hakim J, Subit M, Maroon M. Screening for erectile dysfunction in the primary care practice: results of a survey. W V Med J. 2005;101:67–70.
10. Laumann EO, Paik A, Rosen RC. Sexual dysfunction in the United States: prevalence and predictors. JAMA. 1999;281:537–44.
11. Kubin M, Wagner G, Fugl-Meyer AR. Epidemiology of erectile dysfunction. Int J Impot Res. 2003;15: 63–71.
12. Dunn KM, Croft PR, Hackett GI. Sexual problems: a study of prevalence and need for healthcare in the general population. Fam Pract. 1998;15:519–24.
13. Jonler M, Moon T, Branaan W, et al. The effect of age, ethnicity and geographical location on impotence and quality of life. Br J Urol. 1995;75:651–5.
14. Dunn KM, Croft PR, Hackett GI. Association of sexual problems with social, psychological, and physical problems in men and women: a cross-sectional population survey. J Epidemiol Community Health. 1999; 53:144–8.
15. Anderson MA, Mulhall JP. Epidemiology of erectile dysfunction. In: Mulcahy JJ, editor. Male sexual function. New York: Igaku-shoin; 2001. First Edition.
16. McVary KT, Carrier S, Wessells H. Smoking and erectile dysfunction. J Urol. 2001;166:1624–32.
17. Seftel A, Rosen R, Kuritzky L. Physician perceptions of sexual dysfunction related to benign prostatic hyperplasia (BPH) symptoms and sexual side effects related to BPH medications. Int J Impot Res. 2007; 19(4):386–92.
18. Weeks GR, Gambescia N. Erectile dysfunction: integrating couples therapy, sex therapy, and medical treatment. New York: WW Norton and Co; 2000. p. 43–4.
19. Sadovsky R, Miner M. Erectile dysfunction is a signal of risk for cardiovascular disease: a primary care view. Prim Care Clin Office Pract. 2005;32: 977–93.
20. Curkendall SM, Jones JK, Glasser D, et al. Incidence of medically detected erectile dysfunction and related diseases before and after Viagra (sildenafil citrate). Eur Urol. 1998;37 Suppl 2:81.
21. DeWire DM. Evaluation and treatment of ED. Am Fam Phys. 1996;53:2102–7.
22. Billups K, Fiedrich S. Assessment of fasting lipid panels and Doppler ultrasound testing in men presenting with erectile dysfunction and no other medical problems. J Urol. 2000;163:147.
23. Roumeguere T, Wespes E, Carpentier Y, et al. Erectile dysfunction is associated with a high prevalence of hyperlipidemia and coronary heart disease risk. Eur Urol. 2003;44:355–9.
24. Grover SA, Lowensteyn I, Kaouache M, et al. The prevalence of erectile dysfunction in the primary care setting. Arch Intern Med. 2006;166:213–9.
25. Gaigal CS, Wessels H, Pace J, et al. Predictors and prevalence of erectile dysfunction ion in men referred for nuclear stress testing. Arch Intern Med. 2006; 166:201–6.
26. Min JK, Williams KA, Okwuosa TM, et al. Prediction of coronary heart disease by erectile dysfunction in men referred for nuclear stress testing. Arch Intern Med. 2006;166:201–6.
27. Thompson IM, Tangen CM, Goodman PJ, et al. Erectile dysfunction and subsequent cardiovascular disease. JAMA. 2005;294(23):2996–3002.
28. Montorsi P, Ravagnani PM, Galli S, et al. Association between erectile dysfunction and coronary artery disease. Role of coronary clinical presentation and extent of coronary vessels involvement: the COBRA trial. Eur Heart J. 2006;27(22):2632–9.
29. Sadovsky R, Mulhall J. The potential value of ED inquiry and management. IJCP. 2003;57:601–8.
30. Billups KL, Bank AJ, Padma-Nathan H, et al. Erectile dysfunction is a marker for cardiovascular disease: results of the minority health institute expert advisory panel. J Sex Med. 2005;2:40–52.
31. Richardson D, Vinik A. Etiology and treatment of erectile failure in diabetes mellitus. Curr Diab Rep. 2002;2:501–9.
32. Halcox JP, Schenjke WH, Zalos G, et al. Prognostic value of coronary vascular endothelial dysfunction. Circulation. 2002;106:653–8.

33. Banks J, Marmot M, Oldfield Z, Simith JP. Disease and disadvantage in the United States and England. JAMA. 2006;295:2037–45.
34. Young SE, Mainous AG, Diaz VA, Everett C. Practice patterns in sildenafil prescribing. Fam Med. 2006;38(2):110–5.
35. Holmes TH, Rahe RH. Social adjustment rating scale. J Psychosom Res. 1967;11:213–8.
36. Birchler GR, Webb LJ. Discriminating interactive behavior in happy and unhappy marriages. J Consult Clin Psychol. 1977;45:494–5.
37. Gott M, Galena E, Hinchiff S, Elford M. "Opening a can of worms": GP and practice nurse barriers to talking about sexual health in primary care. Fam Pract. 2004;21:528–36.
38. Nusbaum MR, Gamble G, Heiman J. The high prevalence of sexual concerns among women seeking routine gynecological care. J Fam Pract. 2000;49:229–32.
39. Ackerman MD, Carey MP. Psychology's role in the assessment of sexual dysfunction: historical precedents, current knowledge, and methods. J Consult Clin Psychol. 1995;63:862–76.
40. Dunn MR. Restoration of couple's intimacy and relationship visits to reestablishing erectile function. JAOA. 2004;104 Suppl 4:S6–10.
41. Gregoire A. Assessing and managing male sexual problems. West J Med. 2000;172:49–50.
42. Sadovsky R. The role of the primary care clinician in the management of erectile dysfunction. Rev Urol. 2002;4 Suppl 3:S54–63.
43. Tudiver F, Talbot Y. Why don't men seek help? Family physicians' perspectives on help-seeking behavior in men. J Fam Pract. 1999;48:47–52.
44. Courtenay WH. Constructions of masculinity and their influence on men's well being: a theory of gender and health. Soc Sci Med. 2000;50:1385–401.
45. Penson D, Kreiger JN. Men's health. Are we missing the big picture? JGIM. 2001;16:717–8.
46. Nusbaum MRH. Sexual Health. AAFP home study assessment program 2001. Monograph 267:9.
47. Laumann E. The social organization of sexuality: sexual practices in the United States 1994. Chicago: University of Chicago Press; 1994.
48. DeBerardis G, Franciosi M, Belfigilio M, et al. Erectile dysfunction and quality of life in type 2 diabetic patients. Diabetes Care. 2002;25:284–91.
49. Derby CA, Mohr BA, Goldstein I, et al. Modifiable risk factors and erectile dysfunction: can lifestyle changes modify risk? Urology. 2000;56:302–6.
50. Pinnock CB, Stapleton AMF, Marshal VR. Erectile dysfunction in the community: a prevalence study. Med J Aust. 1999;171:353–7.
51. Esposito K, Giugliano R, DiPalo C, et al. Effect of lifestyle changes on erectile dysfunction in obese men. JAMA. 2004;291:2978–84.
52. Stewart KJ, Hiatt WR, Regensteiner JG, Hirsch AT. Exercise training for claudication. N Engl J Med. 2002;347:1941–51.
53. Latshcer F. The human costs of tobacco use. (editorial). N Engl J Med. 1994;331:618.
54. Jeremy JY, Mikhailidis DP. Cigarette smoking and erectile dysfucntion. J R Soc Health. 1998;118: 151–5.
55. Kuritzky L. Counseling the patient with erectile dysfunction: a primary care physician perspective. JAOA. 2002;102 Suppl 4:S7–11.
56. Halvorson JG. The clinical evaluation of common sexual concerns. CNS Spectrum. 2003;8(3):217–24.
57. Slag MF, Morley JE, Elson MK, et al. Impotence in medical clinic outpatients. JAMA. 1983;249: 1736–40.
58. Finfer WW, Lung M, Stagle MA. Medications that may contribute to sexual disorders. J Fam Pract. 1997;44:33–43.
59. Muller JE, Mittleman MA, Maclure M, et al. Triggering myocardial infarction by sexual activity. JAMA. 1996;275:1405–9.
60. Lue TF. Impotence: patient's goal-directed approach to treatment. World J Urol. 1990;8:67–74.
61. Althof SE, Seftel AD. The evaluation and management of erectile dysfunction. Psychiatr Clin North Am. 1995;18:171–92.
62. McLaughlin SP, Carson CC. Laboratory evaluation of the patient with erectile dysfunction. Endocrine. 2004;23:113–7.
63. Barrett-Connor E. Cardiovascular risk stratification and cardiovascular risk factors associated with erectile dysfunction. Clin Card. 2004;27 Suppl 4:8–13.
64. Kostis JB, Jackson G, Rosen R, et al. Sexual dysfunction and cardiac risk (the Second Princeton Consensus Conference). Am J Cardiol. 2005;96:85–93.
65. Sadovsky R. Erectile dysfunction is a signal of risk for significant medical comorbidities: a primary care view. Curr Sex Health Rep. 2004;1:129–36.
66. Aruajo AB, Durante R, Feldman HA, et al. The relationship between depressive symptoms and male erectile dysfunction. Cross-sectional results from the Massachusetts male Aging Study. Psychosomatic Med. 1998;60:458–65.
67. Anderson MA, Mulhall JP. Epidemiology of erectile dysfunction. In: Mulcahy JJ, editor. Male sexual function. New York: Igaku-shoin; 2001. p. 1–11.
68. Van der Kooy K, van Hout H, Marwijk H, et al. Depression and the risk for cardiovascular disease: systematic review and meta analysis. Int J Geriatr Psychiatry. 2007;22:613–26.
69. Spertus JA, McDonell M, Woodman CL, Fihn SD. Association between depression and worse disease-specific functional status in outpatients with coronary artery disease. Am Heart J. 2000;140(1):105–10.
70. Ruo B, Rumsfeld JS, Hlaky MA, et al. Depressive symptoms and health-related quality of life: the Heart and Soul Study. JAMA. 2003;290(2):215–21.
71. Screening for Coronary Heart Disease. Recommendaiton Statement. U.S. Preventive Services Task Force. Ann Intern Med. 2004;140:569–72.

72. Wilson PW, D'Agostino RB, Levy D, et al. Prediction of coronary heart disease using risk factor categories. Circulation. 1998;97:1837–47.
73. Zoler ML. Erectile dysfunction may presage vascular dysfunction. Family Practice News. 2004;40
74. Mosher D. Sex guilt and sex myths in college men and women. J Sex Res. 1979;15:224–34.
75. Blumstein P, Schwartz P. American couples: money, work, and sex. New York: William Morrow; 1983.
76. Sprecher S, McKinney K. Sexuality. Newbury Park: Sage; 1993.
77. Selvin E, Burnett AL, Platz EA. Prevalence and risk factors for erectile dysfunction in the US. Am J Med. 2007;120:151–7.
78. Hambrecht R, Wolf A, Gielen S, et al. Effect of exercise on coronary endothelial function in patients with coronary artery disease. N Engl J Med. 2000; 342:454–60.
79. Gokce N, Vita JA, Bader DS, et al. Effect of exercise on upper and lower extremity endothelial function in patients with coronary artery disease. Am J Cardiol. 2002;90:124–32.
80. Edwards DG, Schofield RS, Lennon SL, et al. Effect of exercise training on endothelial function in men with coronary artery disease. Am J Cardiol. 2004; 93:617–20.
81. Moore BE, Rothschild AJ. Treatment of antidepressant-induced sexual dysfunction. Hosp Pract. 1999; 34:89–96.
82. Sadovsky R. Selecting patients appropriate for treatment. J Fam Pract 2005; Suppl 5–14.
83. Data on File, IMS Eli Lilly and Company 2007.
84. Bosshardt RJ, Farwerk R, Sikora R, et al. Objective measurement of the effectiveness, therapeutic success, and dynamic mechanisms of the vacuum device. Br J Urol. 1995;75:786–91.
85. Greiner KA, Weigel JW. Erectile dysfunction. Am Fam Phys. 1996;54:1675–82.
86. Rajfer J, Aronson WJ, Bush PA, Dorey FJ, Ignarro LJ. Nitric oxide as a mediator of relaxation of the corpus cavernosum in response to nonadrenergic, noncholinergic neurotransmission. N Engl J Med. 1992;326:90–4.
87. Helstrom WJG. Management recommendations for family physicians. J Fam Pract 2005; Suppl: 32–40.
88. Jiann BP, Yu CC, Su CC, Tsai JY. Compliance of sildenafil treatment for erectile dysfunction and factors affecting it. Int J Impot Res. 2006;18(2):146–9.
89. Vickers MA, Satyanarayana R. Phosphodiesterase type 5 inhibitors for the treatment of erectile dysfunction in patients with diabetes mellitus. IJIR. 2002; 14(6):466–71.
90. Montorsi F, Burnett AL. Erectile dysfunction after radical prostatectomy. BJU Int. 2004;93:404–10.
91. Carson CC, Lue TF. Phosphodiesterase type 5 inhibitors for erectile dysfunction. BJU Int. 2005;95:257–80.
92. Nusbaum MR. Therapeutic options for patients returning to sexual activity. J Am Osteopath Assoc. 2004;104(3 Suppl 4):S2–5.

# 12 Surgical Treatment for Erectile Dysfunction

Drogo K. Montague

Before the 1970s, medicine's interest in or ability to treat erectile dysfunction (ED), then known as impotence, was very limited. The development of the inflatable penile prosthesis in 1973 [1], the introduction of penile injection therapy in 1982 [2], and the advent of effective systemic therapy in 1998 [3] all expanded our ability to understand and treat this common disorder.

Sex therapy is the most appropriate treatment for men with psychogenic ED; however, this chapter will deal only with surgical treatment of organic ED. Current treatment options for organic ED are shown in Table 12.1. Two of these options, penile vascular surgery and penile prosthesis implantation are surgical; they will be reviewed in this chapter.

## Penile Vascular Surgery: Arterial Revascularization

A variety of procedures have been performed over the past 38 years in attempts to reverse ED that is primarily due to arterial insufficiency [4–7]. Although there are numerous variations on these operations, most fall into two general groups: dorsal artery revascularization and dorsal vein arterializations. Sharlip as early as 1991 questioned the reported results of these procedures [8].

D.K. Montague, MD (✉)
Center for Genitourinary Reconstruction, Glickman Urologic and Kidney Institute, Cleveland Clinic, 9500 Euclid Avenue Q10-1, Cleveland, OH 44195, USA
e-mail: montagd@ccf.org

In 2005, the American Urological Association's Guideline's Panel on the Management of Erectile Dysfunction found 31 papers on arterial revascularization, however only four of these met criteria for review. These four studies had a combined total of 50 patients; 42 with dorsal artery revascularization, and 8 with dorsal vein arterialization. Satisfactory outcomes in these 50 patients ranged from 36% to 91%. Because of the small number of patients, the panel concluded that there was insufficient evidence to determine whether penile arterial revascularization was efficacious or not. The panel did allow for this type of treatment in special circumstances by issuing the following option: "Arterial reconstructive surgery is a treatment option only in healthy individuals with recently acquired ED secondary to a focal arterial occlusion and in the absence of any evidence of generalized vascular disease" [9]. Few men meet these criteria and penile arterial revascularization is seldom performed today.

## Penile Vascular Surgery: Surgery for Veno-Occlusive ED

The same guidelines panel noted that there were many problems and uncertainties on how to accurately diagnose veno-occlusive ED and how to identify individuals who might benefit from surgical treatment for this condition. They found no evidence in the form of trials containing clearly defined diagnostic and follow-up criteria, which

D.A. Shoskes (ed.), *Urological Men's Health: A Guide for Urologists and Primary Care Physicians*, Current Clinical Urology, DOI 10.1007/978-1-61779-900-6_12,
© Springer Science+Business Media New York 2012

**Table 12.1** Treatment options for erectile dysfunction

| |
|---|
| Systemic (oral) medications |
| Intraurethral medications |
| Penile injection therapy |
| Penile vascular surgery<br>  Arterial revascularization<br>  Surgery for veno-occlusive ED |
| Penile prosthesis implantation |

documented the efficacy of procedures designed to limit the venous outflow of the corpora cavernosa. They concluded that these procedures are not recommended [9].

## Penile Prosthesis Implantation

Treatment options for organic ED traditionally have been grouped into first-, second-, and third-line options. First-line options traditionally have been the orally administered systemic therapies. Second-line options included the use of vacuum erection devices, intraurethral medication, and penile injections. Third-line treatment options were penile prosthesis implantation.

From an operational standpoint, this three-tiered system is outmoded. Unless a man is taking nitrates, nearly all men with organic ED will be given a trial of oral therapy with one or more of the currently available PDE5 inhibitors; and so it is appropriate that these remain first-line therapies. If that first line of therapy proves unsatisfactory, men go on to second-line treatment options, which should now include penile prosthesis implantation. In other words, men who are oral therapy failures are presented with all of the remaining options including penile prosthesis implantation. If they reject therapy trials with the nonsurgical second-line options (and many men do), it is appropriate to proceed next with penile prosthesis implantation.

The oldest of organic ED treatment options, penile prosthesis implantation, has continued to significantly evolve. Notable advances in recent years, which we will discuss more fully, include: girth- and length-expanding penile prostheses to produce more natural erections, antibiotic and other coatings to reduce infection, and continuous design improvements to increase device longevity.

## Types of Penile Prostheses

In broadest sense, penile prostheses are grouped into two main categories: malleable or rod prostheses and inflatable prostheses. The majority of the devices implanted in the USA (Table 12.2) are manufactured by two companies: American Medical Systems (AMS), Minnetonka, Minnesota and Coloplast Corporation, Minneapolis, Minnesota.

Malleable or rod prostheses have the following advantages: lower cost, ease of use, and low chance of mechanical failure. Disadvantages include: a constantly rigid penis which does not have the appearance of a normal erection and a higher possibility of chronic pain or device erosion through tissue [10].

Inflatable penile prostheses are divided into two-piece and three-piece devices. Two-piece devices have a pair of inflatable cylinders and a small scrotal pump. The AMS Ambicor is the only two-piece inflatable prosthesis available in the USA (Fig. 12.1). When it is deflated, a central cylinder is collapsed, and the device is not rigid. When the Ambicor is inflated, the central cylinder fills and becomes rigid. Since the central chamber does not expand, the inflated Ambicor is like a malleable prosthesis in terms of the erection it provides.

The ideal penile prosthesis would provide penile flaccidity and erection, which resemble the penis in these natural states. Only three-piece inflatable prostheses, which consist of paired expanding penile cylinders, a small scrotal pump, and a large abdominal fluid reservoir, approach this ideal. Examples of three-piece inflatable penile prostheses are AMS 700CX Inflatable Penile Prosthesis (Fig. 12.2) and Coloplast Titan Inflatable Penile Prosthesis (Fig. 12.3).

## Girth- and Length-Expanding Cylinders

The largest structures inside the penis are the paired corpora cavernosa. They are filled with smooth muscle and their outer covering, the tunica albuginea, consists of inner circular

**Table 12.2** US penile prostheses

| Prosthesis type | AMS | Coloplast |
|---|---|---|
| Malleable/rod | AMS Spectra® | Genesis® |
| Two-piece inflatable | AMS Ambicor® | |
| Three-piece inflatable reduced diameter girth expanding | AMS 700 CXR® | Coloplast Titan NB® |
| Three-piece inflatable standard diameter girth expanding | AMS 700 CX® | Coloplast Titan®<br>Coloplast Titan OTR® |
| Three-piece inflatable standard diameter girth + length expanding | AMS 700 LGX® | |

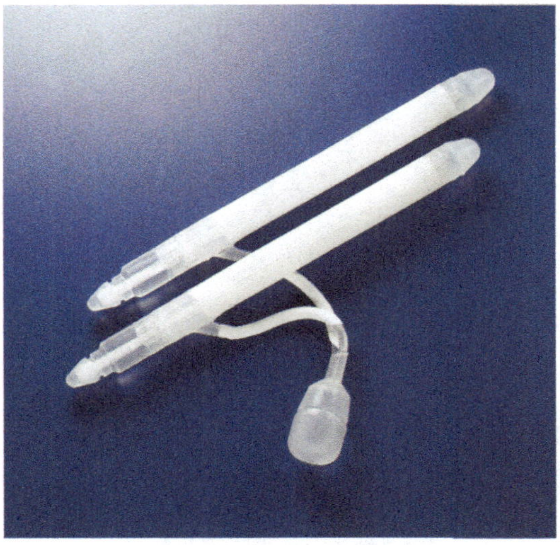

**Fig. 12.1** AMS Ambicor Penile Prosthesis®. Courtesy of American Medical Systems Minnetonka, Minnesota www.AmericanMedicalSystems.com

and outer longitudinal elastic fibers. When the corpora fill with blood to produce an erection, these elastic fibers stretch to their limits producing first penile girth and length increase and then rigidity. The ideal penile prosthesis would also do this.

All three-piece inflatable prostheses have cylinders with girth (diameter) expansion. These include the Coloplast Titan and narrow-base devices and the AMS 700 CX and smaller diameter CXR devices. The only cylinders which expand both in girth and in length are the AMS 700 LGX cylinders. Figure 12.4 shows a pair of LGX cylinders; one is deflated and the other is inflated.

The predecessors to the LGX cylinders were the Ultrex cylinders, which were introduced in 1989. These cylinders expanded in girth from 12 to 18 mm. They also provided up to 50% length expansion. We showed that this ability to expand not only in girth but also in length came at the expense of decreased cylinder survival [11]. This degree of cylinder length expansion was not needed since the limiting factor in penile length increase was tissue elasticity. In 1993, the Ultrex cylinders were modified increasing middle layer fabric strength by 61% and decreasing length expansion to 15–20%. Following this, the survival of these cylinders improved significantly [12]. Another problem noted when Ultrex cylinders were introduced was the S-shaped penile deformity [13]. This did not occur if the cylinders were sized to fit the corpora cavernosa exactly [14]. Figure 12.5 shows penile length of 11.5 cm with deflated cylinders at the conclusion of an Ultrex penile prosthesis implantation, and Fig. 12.6 shows that following inflation the penile length is now 14 cm. In 2002, the AMS 700 Ultrex prosthesis was renamed the AMS 700 LGX prosthesis.

Organic ED is sometimes associated with acquired curvature of the erect penis due to Peyronie's disease. We showed that CX cylinders, which produce girth only expansion, correct penile curvature better than Ultrex (or LGX) cylinders [15]. Other patients with small penises or with scarring due to disease or previous surgery may need smaller diameter girth-expanding cylinders (CXM now CXR) [16]. The majority of penile prosthesis recipients, however, will benefit from girth- and length-expanding LGX devices. For the Coloplast, three-piece inflatable prostheses, The Titan Inflatable Penile Prostheis is appropriate for most men; when dilation of the corpora is limited due to small penis size or scarring, the Titan Narrow-base Inflatable Prosthesis is often useful.

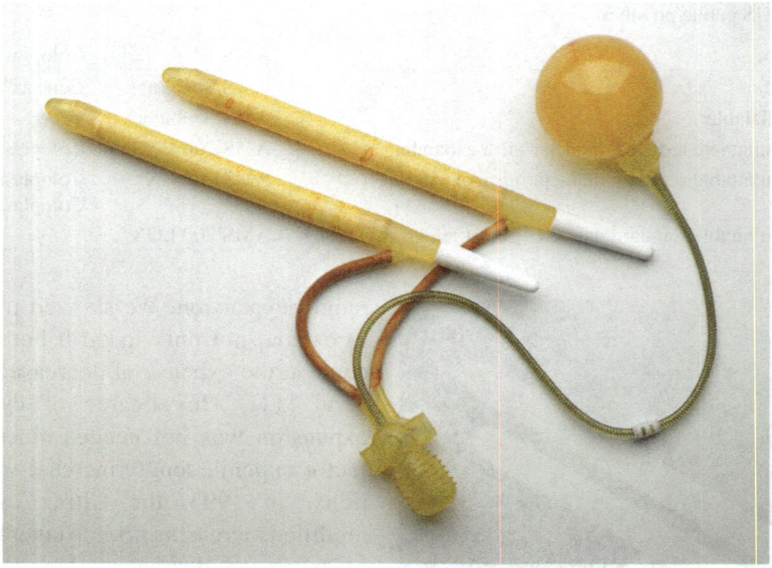

**Fig. 12.2** AMS 700 CX Inflatable Penile Prosthesis®. Courtesy of American Medical Systems Minnetonka, Minnesota www.AmericanMedicalSystems.com

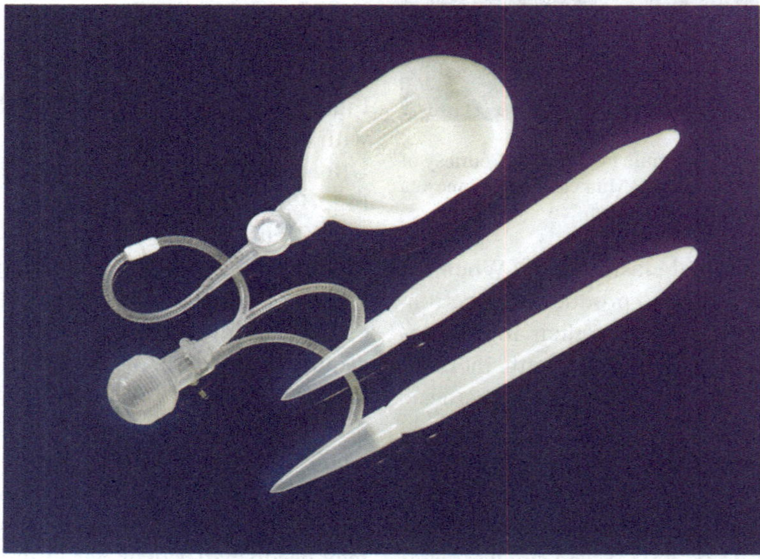

**Fig. 12.3** Coloplast Titan Inflatable Penile Prosthesis®

## Informed Consent for Penile Prosthesis Implantation

Penile prosthesis implantation is done as outpatient surgery often with an overnight 23-h stay. General or spinal anesthesia is used and the patient must be medically suitable for this elective surgery. The patient and whenever possible his partner should understand that penile prosthesis implantation produces a prosthetic erection suitable for sexual activity. Sensation following recovery from surgery is unchanged as is the ability to reach orgasm and ejaculate. However, if orgasm or ejaculation is not present prior to device implantation, they will likely be absent after. Implanting a penile

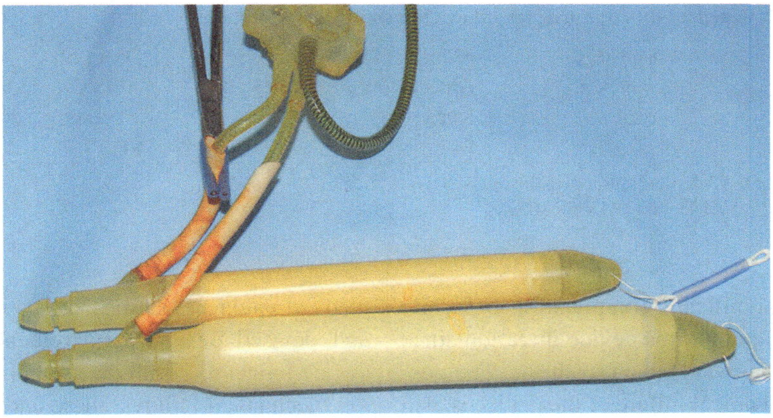

**Fig. 12.4** LGX cylinders; one deflated and one inflated

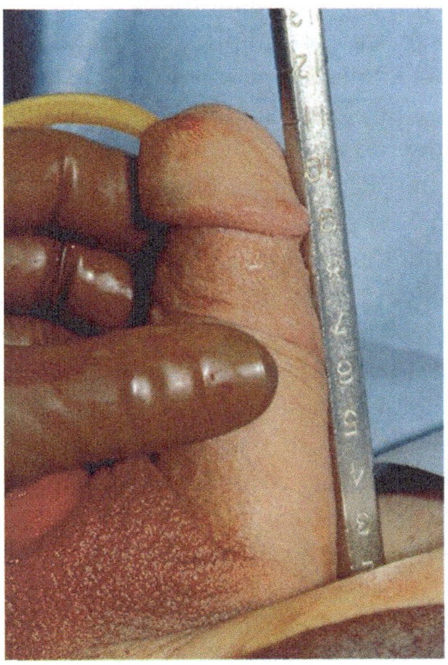

**Fig. 12.5** Ultrex cylinders deflated; penile length 11.5 cm

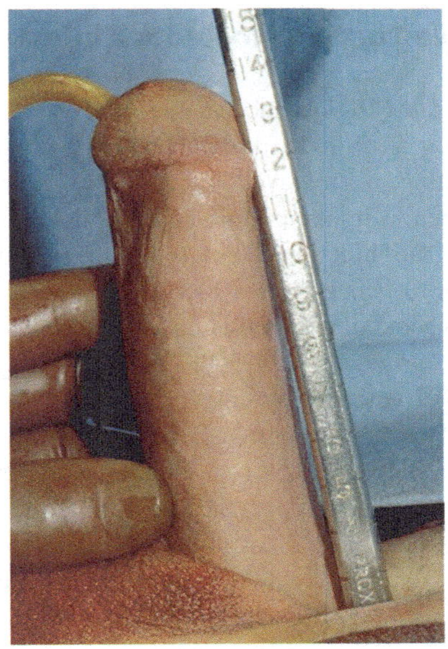

**Fig. 12.6** Ultrex cylinders inflated; penile length 14 cm

prosthesis will not restore libido unless the primary reason for decreased sexual desire is repeated failures.

The three-piece inflatable devices produce erection and flaccidity approaching that achieved naturally. Most men will feel comfortable in a locker room. We demonstrate the patient's stretched flaccid penile length and tell the patient and partner that this will be the approximate length after penile prosthesis implantation. For some men, this will be close to their erect penile length but for others it will be considerably shorter. This is particularly true after radical prostatectomy where loss of penile length has been well documented [17–19], in men with Peyronie's disease, in men who are obese, and in men with ED due to ischemic priapism or removal of a previously infected penile prosthesis. Prospective implant recipients are also told that with penile prosthesis inflation there is no increase in glans size.

**Table 12.3** Freedom from mechanical failure (Kaplan–Meier projections)

| *Reference* | Wilson [27] | Milbank [12] | Daitch [28] | Dhar [29] | Kim [30] |
|---|---|---|---|---|---|
| *Device* | Mentor Alpha-1[a] | AMS Ultrex[b] | AMS CX | AMS CX | AMS CX |
| *Follow-up* | 5 years | 5 years | 5 years | 10 years | 10 years |
| *% Freedom* | 93 | 94 | 92 | 81 | 78 |

[a]Predecessor to Coloplast Titan prosthesis
[b]Predecessor to AMS 700 LGX prosthesis

The most significant complication of penile prosthesis implantation is device infection since this requires removal of the prosthesis. The possibility of mechanical failure of the device is also discussed; infection and mechanical failure rates will be discussed later in this chapter.

## Device Coatings to Reduce Infection

In 2001, AMS introduced a dual antibiotic coating for their three-piece inflatable penile prostheses consisting of minocycline and rifampin. For first time penile implants, this coating was shown to reduce the infection rate at 6 months, when most infections occur, from 1.61% to 0.68% [20], and for revision surgeries this coating reduced infections from 2.41% to 1.36% [21]. In a study with up to 7.7 years follow-up, 1.1% of 35,737 recipients of prostheses with this dual antibiotic coating had revision for infection compared to 2.5% of 3,268 recipients of uncoated devices [22].

The Coloplast Titan prosthesis is coated with hydrophilic polyvinylpyrrolidone, which was added to the product in 2002. When this coated device is immersed in an antibiotic solution, the antibiotic is absorbed onto the surface of the device. This has been shown to reduce infections from 2.07% to 1.06% [23].

## Design Improvements to Increase Mechanical Reliability

In the early days of three-piece inflatable penile prosthesis implantation, mechanical failures were frequent occurring in 27% of patients with follow-up ranging from only 6 to 24 months [24]. Following revision surgeries, failed components were returned to the manufacturer where biomedical engineers studied the patterns of failure and devised design improvements to increase device longevity. From the standpoint of reporting mechanical failures, these early studies cited numbers of implants, the range and mean or median follow-up, and the number of mechanical failures during the study period. This method of reporting did not account for differing lengths of follow-up for each implant recipient within the study, and it did not permit different studies to be meaningfully compared. Recognizing this problem, the American Urological Association's Guidelines Panel on the Management of Erectile Dysfunction recommended using Kaplan–Meier projections to report freedom of failure from mechanical problems [9]. Current freedoms from mechanical failures expressed in terms of Kaplan–Meier projections are shown in Table 12.3. Additionally, Wilson, with four different models of three-piece inflatable penile prostheses implanted in 2,384 patients, reported 10-year and 15-year Kaplan–Meier projections of freedom from mechanical failure of 79.4% and 71.2%, respectively [25].

## Patient: Partner Satisfaction

The 1996 American Urological Guidelines Panel for Erectile Dysfunction found for multicomponent inflatable penile prostheses 12 studies on recipient satisfaction, which ranged from 83.8% to 92.5%. There were four studies which reported partner satisfaction which ranged from 74.6% to 95.9% [26]. These older studies were retrospective and did not use validated questionnaires. In their 2005 guidelines, the American Urological Association Guidelines Committee on Erectile Dysfunction recommended that future studies of satisfaction after penile prosthesis implantation be prospective, use standardized questionnaires, and include partners [9]. These new studies could also be used to compare penile prosthesis satisfaction outcomes to outcomes from other treatment options for ED. Similar study techniques could also be used to study the impact of penile prosthesis implantation on other quality life outcomes issues such as personal relationships or depression.

## Conclusions

Surgical treatment for organic ED includes penile arterial revascularization, surgery for veno-occlusive dysfunction, and penile prosthesis implantation. In the 2005 American Urological Association Erectile Dysfunction Guidelines, surgery for veno-occlusive dysfunction was not recommended, and evidence to demonstrate efficacy for penile arterial revascularization was deemed to be lacking.

When medical therapy for ED in the form of the type 5 phosphodiesterase inhibitors fails, it is now appropriate to discuss the remaining nonsurgical options, vacuum erection devices, intraurethral medications, and penile injection therapy along with penile prosthesis implantation. Men who want to proceed next with penile prosthesis implantation should be allowed to do so.

Notable advances in penile prosthesis implantation in recent years include girth- and length-expanding penile cylinders, prostheses with antibiotic and other coatings to reduce infections, and continuous design improvements to improve device survival.

## References


1. Scott FB, Bradley WE, Timm GW. Management of erectile impotence: use of implantable inflatable prosthesis. Urology. 1973;2:80–2.
2. Virag R. Intracavernous injection of papaverine for erectile failure. Letter to the editor. Lancet. 1982; 2:938.
3. Goldstein I, Lue TF, Padma-Nathan H, Rosen RC, Steers WD, Wicker PA. Oral sildenafil in the treatment of erectile dysfunction. N Engl J Med. 1998;338: 1397–404.
4. Michal V, Kramar R, Pospichal J, et al. Direct arterial anastomosis to the cavernous body in the treatment of erectile impotence. Czech Rozhledy Chir. 1973; 52:587.
5. Virag R, Zwang G, Dermange H, et al. Vasculogenic impotence: a review of 92 cases with 54 surgical operations. Vasc Surg. 1981;15:9.
6. McDougal WS, Jeffery R. Microscopic penile revascularization. J Urol. 1983;129:517.
7. Knoll LD. Penile dorsal vein arterialization in managing venogenic impotence. Tech Urol. 1995;1:157–61.
8. Sharlip ID. The incredible results of penile vascular surgery. Int J Impot Res. 1991;3:1.
9. Montague DK, Jarow JP, Broderick GA, et al. Chapter 1: The management of erectile dysfunction: an AUA update. J Urol. 2005;174:230–9.
10. Zermann DH, Kutzenberger J, Sauerwein D, Schubert J, Loeffler U. Penile prosthetic surgery in neurologically impaired patients: long-term followup. J Urol. 2006;175:1041–4.
11. Montague DK, Lakin MM. Early experience with the controlled girth and length expanding cylinder of the American Medical Systems Ultrex penile prosthesis. J Urol. 1992;148:1444–6.
12. Milbank AJ, Montague DK, Angermeier KW, et al. Mechanical failure of the American Medical Systems Ultrex inflatable penile prosthesis: before and after 1993 structural modification. J Urol. 2002;167: 2502–6.
13. Wilson SK, Cleves MA, Delk 2nd JR. Ultrex cylinders: problems with uncontrolled lengthening (the S-shaped deformity). J Urol. 1996;155:135–7.
14. Montague DK, Angermeier KW. Cylinder sizing: less is more. Int J Impot Res. 2003;15 Suppl 5:S132–3.
15. Montague DK, Angermeier KW, Lakin MM, Ingleright BJ. AMS 3-piece inflatable penile prosthesis implantation in men with Peyronie's disease: comparison of CX and Ultrex cylinders. J Urol. 1996;156: 1633–5.
16. Carbone Jr DJ, Daitch JA, Angermeier KW, Lakin MM, Montague DK. Management of severe corp[illegible] fibrosis with implantation of prosthes[illegible] verse scrotal approach. J Urol [illegible]
17. Savoie M, Kim SS, So[illegible] measuring penile le[illegible] prostatectomy for pro[illegible] 1462–4.
18. Mulhall JP. Penile leng[illegible] tatectomy. BJU Int. 200[illegible]
19. Gontero P, Di Marco M,[illegible] phase-II prospective stud[illegible] tolerability of a penile-ext[illegible] ment of 'short penis'. BJU I[illegible]
20. Carson 3rd CC. Efficacy of an[illegible] inflatable penile prostheses in [illegible] original implants. J Urol. 2004;[illegible]
21. Carson CC. Initial success wi[illegible] inflatable penile prosthesis with I[illegible] surface treatment: a retrospective [illegible] cases incidence and comparative re[illegible] treated devices. J Urol. 2004;171:S8[illegible]
22. Carson 3rd CC, Mulcahy JJ, Harsch [illegible] infection outcomes after original antibio[illegible]

inflatable penile prosthesis implants: up to 7.7 years of followup. J Urol. 2011;185:614–8.
23. Wolter CE, Hellstrom WJ. The hydrophilic-coated inflatable penile prosthesis: 1-year experience. J Sex Med. 2004;1:221–4.
24. Furlow WL. The current status of the inflatable penile prosthesis in the management of impotence: Mayo Clinic experience updated. J Urol. 1978; 119: 363–4.
25. Wilson SK, Delk JR, Salem EA, Cleves MA. Long-term survival of inflatable penile prostheses: single surgical group experience with 2,384 first-time implants spanning two decades. J Sex Med. 2007;4: 1074–9.
26. Montague DK, Barada JH, Belker AM, et al. Clinical guidelines panel on erectile dysfunction: summary report on the treatment of organic erectile dysfunction. J Urol. 1996;156:2007–11.
27. Wilson SK, Cleves MA, Delk 2nd JR. Comparison of mechanical reliability of original and enhanced Mentor Alpha I penile prosthesis. J Urol. 1999; 162:715–8.
28. Daitch JA, Angermeier KW, Lakin MM, Ingleright BJ, Montague DK. Long-term mechanical reliability of AMS 700 series inflatable penile prostheses: comparison of CX/CXM and Ultrex cylinders. J Urol. 1997;158:1400–2.
29. Dhar NB, Angermeier KW, Montague DK. Long-term mechanical reliability of AMS 700CX/CXM inflatable penile prosthesis. J Urol. 2006;176: 2599–601.
30. Kim DS, Yang KM, Chung HJ, Choi HM, Choi YD, Choi HK. AMS 700CX/CXM inflatable penile prosthesis has high mechanical reliability at long-term follow-up. J Sex Med. 2010;7:2602–7.

# 13 Managing Overactive Bladder and Urinary Incontinence in the Male

Humphrey Atiemo and J. Quentin Clemens

## Introduction

Overactive bladder (OAB), as defined by the International Continence Society (ICS), is defined by urinary urgency, usually with urinary frequency and nocturia, with or without any associated urge incontinence, in the absence of metabolic or pathologic etiology [1]. Urinary incontinence (UI) in men can be caused by functional abnormalities of the bladder (e.g., detrusor overactivity) or the urethra (e.g., stress incontinence). While men and women can be afflicted by this disease, some important differences exist in the distribution, severity and treatment approaches for UI between the genders. This chapter will explore the epidemiology, diagnosis, and treatment options regarding male OAB and UI.

## Epidemiology

Few population-based studies exist regarding the prevalence of OAB in men using the current ICS definition. However, a recent study regarding the prevalence of lower urinary tract symptoms (LUTS) in males and females provides some insight into the prevalence of OAB in males. LUTS can be divided into three groups, comprised of storage symptoms, voiding symptoms, and post-micturition symptoms. Symptoms of urinary frequency, nocturia, and urgency and urge incontinence are indicative of storage symptoms and corresponding OAB. In the "EpiLUTS" study, 30,000 participants from the USA, UK, and Sweden were randomly selected to complete a survey on LUTS. The mean age was 56 years with equal distribution of male and female participants. The prevalence of LUTS in at least "sometimes" was 72.3% for men and 76.3% for women. All voiding symptoms were more common in men. However, storage symptoms associated with OAB were more common in women. While symptoms of urgency incontinence and stress incontinence seemed to predominate in women, prevalence of frequency and nocturia shared a more equal distribution [2].

Other studies have indicated the prevalence of OAB in the USA to be 42.2 million, representing 18.6% of the adult US population. This study demonstrated 10.7% prevalence in males and 26% prevalence in females. The cost of OAB treatment was estimated to be $6.1 billion and $18 billion in men and women, respectively [3].

The epidemiology of UI has been studied much less extensively in men than in women. In general, the prevalence of UI in men is approximately half that of women [4, 5]. As in women, UI rates increase with age. Using a definition of at least one UI episode in the preceding 12 months, the prevalence increases from 4.8% in men aged 19–44 years,

H. Atiemo, MD • J.Q. Clemens, MD, FACS, MSCI (✉)
Department of Urology, University of Michigan Medical Center, 1500 East Medical Center Drive, Taubman Center 3875, Ann Arbor, MI 48109, USA
e-mail: hatiemo@umich.edu; qclemens@umich.edu

D.A. Shoskes (ed.), *Urological Men's Health: A Guide for Urologists and Primary Care Physicians*, Current Clinical Urology, DOI 10.1007/978-1-61779-900-6_13,
© Springer Science+Business Media New York 2012

to 11.2% in men aged 45–64 years, to 21.1% in men older than 65 years [6]. The prevalence of lifetime UI in older men (aged >65) is 11–34%, while the prevalence of daily UI is 2–11% [7]. The distribution of UI varies between genders, with urge UI constituting a much larger portion of total UI in men than in women. Risk factors for urge UI that are shared across genders include previous stroke, dementia, impaired mobility, constipation, diabetes, depression, pelvic radiation, urinary tract infections, and neurologic disease [5, 6]. Stress UI in men is quite rare in the absence of previous prostate surgery, pelvic trauma, or neurologic disorder. There is some evidence that the presence of UI may have a more severe quality of life impact in men than in women [8, 9].

## Pathophysiology

The pathophysiology of OAB is poorly understood. However, over the last decade, more emphasis has been placed on afferent signaling mechanism from the bladder to the spinal cord and central nervous system. These afferent mechanisms are composed of receptors and channels in the urothelium and suburothelium, which initiate the voiding reflex in normal and pathophysiologic conditions [10]. Three predominant theories exist in terms of detrusor overactivity and OAB; these are the myogenic, urotheliogenic, and neurogenic. In the myogenic hypothesis, bladder filling leads to the release of acetylcholine from non-neuronal and neuronal sources such as prostaglandins and endothelins and generate afferent nerve activation and contribute to OAB. The urotheliogenic mechanism states that changes in the coupling of urothelial and suburothelial interstitial cells may lead to involuntary bladder contractions. Adenosine triphosphate (ATP) and the P2×3 receptors have been identified to play a prominent role in suburothelial afferent conduction. Lastly, the neurogenic hypothesis states that reduced central or peripheral inhibition increases reflexive involuntary bladder contractions [11]. Current pharmacologic therapies for OAB and urinary urge incontinence are directed at reducing involuntary detrusor motor activity, and these therapies are applied to both men and women. It is hopeful that newer therapeutic agents that address afferent bladder signaling mechanisms may be developed in the near future.

It is exceedingly rare for stress UI to occur in men in the absence of prior prostate surgery, pelvic trauma, or neurologic disorder (e.g., traumatic spinal cord injury, spina bifida). By far the most common etiologic factor is prior prostate surgery. The two most frequently performed prostate surgeries are transurethral resection of the prostate (TURP) and radical prostatectomy (RP). TURP involves the resection of obstructing prostate tissue using a cystoscope. Damage to the external urethral sphincter can occur during TURP, but this is uncommon; in contemporary series, reported rates of UI following TURP are <1% [12–14]. RP involves the removal of the entire prostate, and is performed to treat prostate cancer. The urethral continence mechanism is closely approximated to the prostate apex, and therefore this structure can be compromised during the surgical dissection. Following RP, it is quite common for men to initially experience stress incontinence. However, this typically improves or resolves over a course of 12–24 months [15–18]. Up to 40% of men report some degree of long-term UI after RP, but the vast majority of this is mild and does not require treatment [19]. The rate of persistent, bothersome UI following RP is approximately 5–10% [19–23].

## Diagnosis and Initial Treatment

The diagnosis of OAB and UI in a man requires a detailed history, physical examination, and urinalysis. These are usually sufficient to guide initial therapy [24]. A 24-h voiding diary may also provide important information. It is especially helpful to discuss the goals and expectations of treatment. This initial evaluation should identify men with more "complicated" OAB or UI, including those with concomitant pain or hematuria, recurrent infections, suspected or proven poor bladder emptying, very severe symptoms, prior pelvic radiation, neurologic disease, or major pelvic surgery. These patients should be referred for specialized management. Poor bladder emptying may be suspected based on history and exam findings, or may be documented using post-void bladder ultrasound or catheterization. A history of previous prostate cancer treatment is also important, as this is a major risk factor for the presence of stress UI. OAB can be subcategorized as OAB dry (frequency, urgency, nocturia) or OAB wet (urge incontinence). Male patients with UI can then be categorized as: post-void dribbling alone, stress UI, urge UI, or mixed UI (both stress UI and urge UI symptoms).

Post-void dribbling is a common complaint in men, and is felt to be due to the retention of urine within the urethra after the bladder has completely emptied. Treatment consists of avoidance of urethral compression during voiding (such as from undergarments), and manual "milking" of the perineal urethra following micturition. Kegel exercises can also be prescribed, but evidence to support the efficacy of this treatment for post-micturition dribbling is lacking. For men with stress UI, urge UI or mixed UI, initial treatment follows the same principles as in women, and should include lifestyle advice, bladder training, pelvic floor muscle training ± biofeedback, and medications. In patients with mixed UI, it is reasonable to treat the more bothersome component (urge UI or stress UI) first.

## Behavioral Therapies (Lifestyle Advice, Bladder Training, Pelvic Floor Muscle Exercises, Biofeedback)

Behavioral therapies may be beneficial for symptoms of OAB, stress UI, or mixed UI. There is a considerable amount of scientific evidence supporting the use of behavioral therapies for the treatment of UI, but most studies are limited to women. It seems likely that urge UI symptoms would respond to behavioral therapies equally well in men and women, but this has not been subjected to study. Most of the research on behavioral therapies for UI in men has focused on post-prostatectomy stress UI. Some studies suggest that the use of behavioral therapies, either before [25] or after [26, 27] prostate cancer surgery, may hasten the recovery of urinary control and decrease postoperative UI severity. However, other studies have not demonstrated this benefit [28–31]. Based on these data, a systematic review [32] concluded that the value of the various approaches to conservative management of post-prostatectomy incontinence remains uncertain. More recently, a randomized controlled trial [33] found that behavioral therapies were effective in reducing incontinence symptoms in men with post-prostatectomy incontinence for at least 1 year following surgery.

## Medications

For OAB, or urge UI, antimuscarinic medications (oxybutynin, tolterodine, darifenacin, solifenacin, fesoterodine, trospium) are a mainstay of therapy. These medications reduce involuntary bladder contractions by partially blocking the muscarinic cholinergic receptors located on the detrusor muscle cell wall. Multiple studies have documented the efficacy of these agents in reducing OAB symptoms [34]. These studies suggest that symptom improvement is similar across genders. It appears that these medications do not cause a significant increase in post-void residual volumes when used in men. Although medical treatment of OAB seems efficacious in men one study demonstrates that only 17% of men were provided medical therapy for their symptoms [35]. Reasons for lack of treatment may include medication cost and lack of symptom improvement. In a study of compliance with OAB medication, predictors of discontinuing all OAB medication on multivariate analysis included being a smoker, not knowing whether treatment of bladder problems required taking medical several times a day, believing that side effects from medication would be severe and being bothered by the sudden urge to urinate with no warning. Patients already taking 3–4 prescription medications were less likely to discontinue medication [36].

In certain men who have OAB associated with poor bladder emptying ("overflow incontinence"), the use of an alpha adrenergic-receptor antagonist (terazosin, doxazosin, tamsulosin, alfuzosin, silodosin) may improve the UI symptoms by enhancing bladder emptying. One study has demonstrated a reduction in urge UI in men who were treated with an alpha-blocker plus an antimuscarinic agent [37]. The precise role of alpha-blocker therapy vs. antimuscarinic therapy vs. combination therapy in men with urge UI requires further investigation. Since the side effect profile of alpha blockers is low, it may be reasonable to initiate treatment with one of these agents in men with urge UI symptoms, and then add an antimuscarinic medication if the symptoms persist.

## Medications: Stress UI

There are currently no medications that have been approved in the USA for the treatment of stress UI. Duloxetine, a serotonin–norepinephrine reuptake inhibitor, is approved for this indication in many European countries. A recent systematic review of the pharmacologic treatment of male stress UI found limited evidence to support the efficacy of any medication for male SUI [38]. One randomized controlled trial ($n=112$) suggests a possible benefit of duloxetine in men with post-prostatectomy UI, but this effect quickly disappeared after discontinuation of the [39].

## Adjunctive Measures

In men, external urinary catheters (condom catheters) can be useful in managing UI. These catheters may be obtained from medical supply stores. Successful use of a condom catheter requires reliable adherence of the condom sheath to the penis, and this may not be possible in some patients (obesity, etc.). In patients with neurogenic bladder dysfunction, the use of an external catheter may be associated with progressive renal damage unless it is confirmed with urodynamics that bladder storage pressures remain low. Another option is the use of a penile incontinence clamp. A clamp is most suitable in ambulatory men with stress UI and good bladder storage function. Clamps are meant to be used on an intermittent basis. Their use in men with sensory abnormalities should be discouraged, as tissue damage from the clamp can occur with prolonged use. The treatment of UI with an indwelling catheter is usually a poor management choice.

## Specialized Management

Men with "complicated" UI and those who fail initial treatment efforts are likely to require additional diagnostic testing. The use of a 3-day bladder diary can be extremely helpful to document the frequency of UI episodes and pad use. In addition, 24-h pad weights can be used to quantify the degree of incontinence. Validated questionnaires which measure the impact of UI on quality of life can be useful to assess treatment efficacy. Other tests (renal function assessment, cystoscopy, upper urinary tract imaging) can be considered in certain patients. For instance, men with post-prostatectomy incontinence may have a concomitant bladder neck contracture (BNC) at the site of the surgical anastomosis between the bladder and urethra, and cystoscopy can identify this. It is important to treat a BNC prior to performing surgery for male stress UI, as treatment of the BNC is much more complicated after these surgeries. Urodynamic testing is not indicated in all patients with UI, but in those with "complicated" UI, it is the most useful test to identify the etiology of the symptoms [24]. The primary goal of such testing is to reproduce the patient's symptoms and to correlate them with objective measures of bladder and urethral function. Figure 13.1 demonstrates the flouro-urodynamic image of a male with urge incontinence. Note the irregular contour of the bladder (B) and the involuntary loss of urine through the urethra (red arrow). Corresponding uninhibited bladder contractions are observed on the urodynamic tracings during this study (yellow arrow) Fig. 13.2.

## Surgical Treatment: OAB

Most patients with OAB will respond adequately to nonsurgical therapies. In those who do not, a variety of surgical treatment options are available. These treatments do not differ between genders. Botulinum toxin type A injection (Botox) and

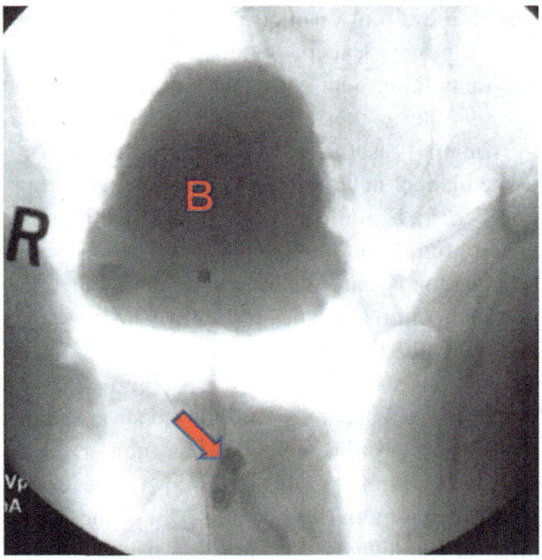


**Fig. 13.1** Flouro-urodynamic image of an overactive bladder. Note the irregular contour of the bladder (*B*) and involuntary loss of urine through the urethra (*red arrow*)

sacral neuromodulation (SNM) are the two most common surgical procedures that are performed. Botox is a neurotoxin produced by the Clostridium Botulinum bacteria. It specifically binds at the presynaptic junction of the motor endplate to prevent the release of acetylcholine at the nerve terminal. This in turn produces a paralysis of the affected muscle. For patients with urge incontinence, intradetrusor injection of Botox into the bladder via a cystoscope leads to temporary inhibition of bladder overactivity. Multiple studies have demonstrated its effectiveness in treatment of OAB regardless of age [40, 41]. The usage of intradetrusor Botox has also been associated with increased retention rates and the need for clean intermittent catheterization, quoted as 43% in one study [42]. Although evidence-based studies exist, BOTOX has not been approved for this use by the FDA, and therefore it is not typically reimbursed by insurance when used in the

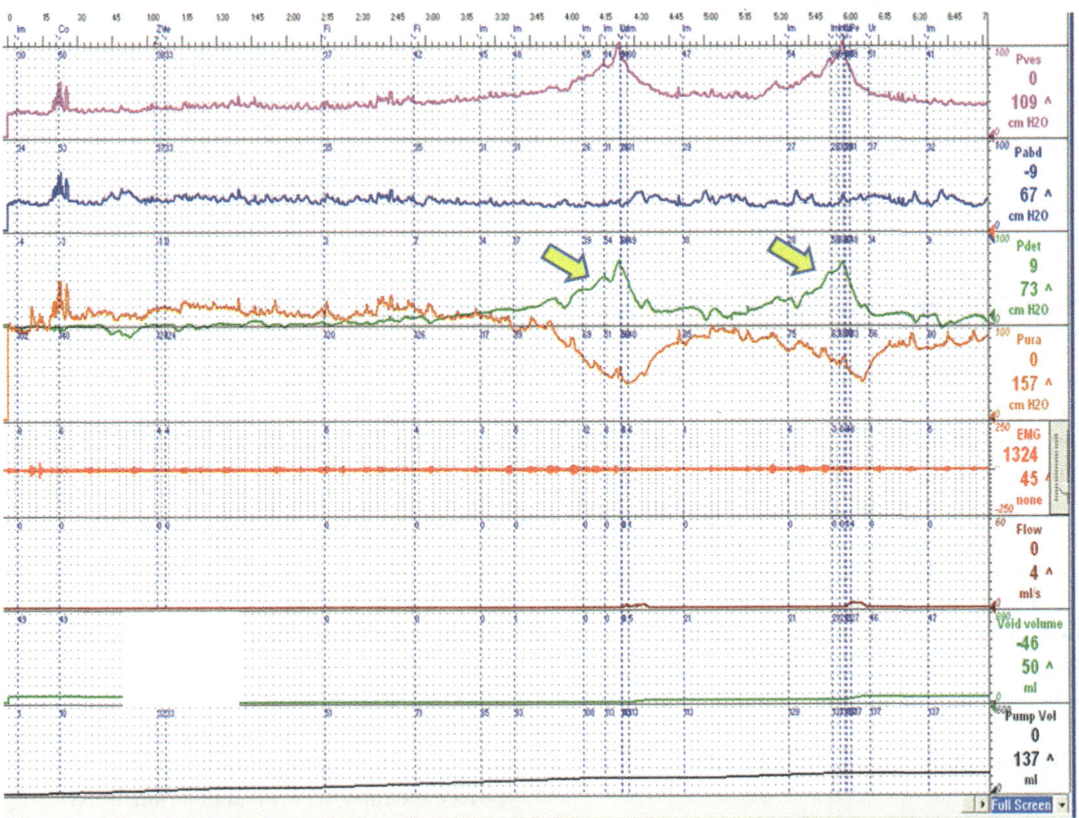


**Fig. 13.2** Urodynamic Study of an overactive bladder. Note the tracings which demonstrate uninhibited bladder contractions measured as a rise in detrusor pressure during filling of the bladder (*yellow arrows*)

USA. This has greatly limited its applicability in the USA outside of research settings.

The most common surgical treatment for OAB is SNM, which was approved by the FDA for the treatment of UI in 1997. This procedure involves placement of a small electrode into the S3 foramen to modulate the S3 nerve, which innervates the bladder. The procedure is performed in two parts, with initial placement of a lead for test stimulation using an external battery, followed by placement of a permanent subcutaneous battery if test stimulation is successful. The temporary test lead can either be placed in the office or in the operating room as an outpatient surgical procedure. If a 50% reduction on OAB symptoms is achieved during the test period, the subcutaneous battery is placed. At this time, the mechanism of action which leads to reduction of urge UI symptoms is poorly understood, but it is hypothesized that stimulation of the S3 nerve root results in a centrally mediated reflex inhibition of a detrusor contractile reflex. Cochrane reviews of randomized trials of SNM demonstrate a 50% improvement in UI symptoms in 87% of patients [43]. Cost effectiveness analysis of SNM and Botulinum Toxin A in the treatment of urge UI favor BOTOX in the first 2 years of treatment; however, it was noted that SNM was the more effective treatment [44].

## Surgical Treatment of Male Stress UI

The most commonly utilized surgical methods to treat male stress UI are transurethral bulking agents, perineal slings, and the artificial urinary sphincter (AUS). Following RP, it is generally recommended to utilize watchful waiting supplemented with conservative measures for a period of at least 6–12 months to allow for spontaneous resolution of stress UI symptoms [45, 46]. Men with persistent and bothersome stress UI are candidates for surgical therapy.

### Transurethral Bulking Agents

Various substances can be injected into the submucosal tissues of the urethra or bladder neck to improve urethral coaptation and improve stress UI symptoms. Except for collagen, data for the use of bulking agents in men are minimal. The success rates in men are lower than those reported in women, presumably due to increased scarring at the bladder neck following prostate cancer surgery. In men, multiple (up to 4) injections are usually required to achieve results, which generally last for 1 year or less, at which point an additional injection is required [47, 48]. The injections are typically performed with intravenous sedation in men, while in women it is common to utilize only local anesthesia. Reported success rates range from 36% to 69%, but few men are completely dry after this therapy [45]. However, for select men with fairly mild stress UI or those who are not candidates for more invasive surgery, injection therapy may be a reasonable treatment option. Prior injection of bulking agents does not appear to affect the postoperative results of male perineal slings [49] or AUSs [50].

### Perineal Slings

Sling techniques involving passive urethral compression have been successfully employed in the treatment of female stress UI for years. Therefore, it is not surprising that similar techniques have been adapted for use in men. Initial procedures using silicone-gel filled prostheses fastened to the corpora cavernosa were described in the 1970s [51], but these fell out of favor due to high failure rates, infectious complications, and the emergence of the AUS technique. In 1998, a bulbourethral sling technique using polytetrafluoroethylene (Gore-Tex®) was described, in which bolsters were placed under the bulbar urethra and suspended from the rectus fascia [52]. This technique, which is analogous to the retropubic pubovaginal sling technique in women, has demonstrated acceptable success rates with extended follow-up [53]. However, it is limited by prolonged perineal numbness or pain that is experienced by up to 20% of patients.

More recently, a perineal bone-anchored sling technique has been developed, and this has now become the most common sling technique used to treat male stress UI [45]. Industry-manufactured surgical sling "kits" are available, which include all the materials that are necessary for sling placement. The surgery is performed through a single perineal incision, and involves placement of 2–3 titanium bone screws into each inferior pubic ramus. The bone anchors are pre-loaded with polypropylene sutures, which are used to attach a strip of silicone-coated polyester mesh. A urethral catheter is placed to aid with identification of the urethra. The mesh sling is initially attached on one side, and then is stretched across the urethra and attached to the other side to achieve compression. Most patients are discharged the day after surgery without a urethral catheter in place, as urinary retention is quite rare.

At short-term follow-up (<12 months), stress UI cure rates following perineal bone-anchored sling placement are 60–90% [54]. Long-term data are lacking, but one study at 48 months mean follow-up reported a cure rate of 65% [55]. Male slings using nonsynthetic materials have significantly inferior results to those using synthetic mesh [56–58]. Success rates are relatively poor in men with severe stress UI symptoms [56, 59], and it is commonly accepted that this technique should be limited to men with mild-to-moderate leakage. Some authors have recommended the use of 24-h pad weights to help to identify men who are candidates for sling placement. Pad weights of 150 g [60] or 400 g [61] have been recommended as cutoff points. Complications include wound infection (0–6%), urethral erosion (0–2%), transient (< 3 month) perineal pain or numbness (16–72%) [55, 59, 61]. Postoperative urodynamic studies following male sling placement have not identified evidence of obstructive voiding [62, 63]. In general, complication following sling placement appear to be lower than those seen following AUS placement. The International Consultation on Urinary Incontinence (ICI) [45] and the UK National Institute for Health and Clinical Excellence (NICE) [64] have concluded that the current evidence supports the safety and efficacy of male slings for post-prostatectomy stress UI, but that long-term data are needed.

Recently, a new male sling technique has been described which involves placement of a mesh sling transversely through the obturator foramen [65–67]. This technique is analogous to similar "transobturator slings," which are used for female stress UI. Studies of this technique to date are limited to small numbers of patients with short duration of follow-up.

## Artificial Urinary Sphincter

Initially introduced in 1973, the AUS has been recognized for many years as the most effective long-term treatment for men with severe stress UI. Manufactured by American Medical Systems (Minnetonka, MN), the AUS has undergone a number of design changes over time; the current version is the AMS 800. The AUS consists of three silicone components—a cuff, a balloon reservoir, and a pump. Each of these components is attached to a length of silicone tubing, and this tubing is connected together during the surgical implant procedure.

## AUS Surgical Technique

The surgery is typically performed with the patient in the dorsal lithotomy position. Administration of broad-spectrum antibiotics and a thorough prep of the operative field are important to reduce postoperative wound infections. A small urethral catheter is placed to aid in identification of the urethra. A midline perineal incision is made, and the urethra is dissected circumferentially for a distance of approximately 2 cm. The AUS cuff is then placed around the bulbar urethra to provide circumferential compression. Various cuff sizes are available, and a measuring tape is used to select the correct size. Next, a lower abdominal incision is made and the balloon reservoir is placed in a small pocket beneath the rectus fascia. The reservoir is then filled with fluid (between 20 and 25 cc). A superficial plane is then developed from the abdominal incision down into the ipsilateral hemiscrotum, and the pump is placed there in a dependent position, which is easily palpable through the skin. The tubing from the cuff is then passed under the skin from the perineal incision to the abdominal incision. The tubing from the three components is then connected using proprietary connecting rings and tighteners. The AUS functions by transferring fluid from the balloon reservoir to the cuff, which causes the cuff to compress the urethra. After the tubing is connected, the device is "cycled" a few times to confirm that this fluid transfer is properly occurring, and then the AUS is deactivated (no fluid in the cuff) by pushing a button located on the pump. After the incisions are closed, the patient is typically admitted to the hospital overnight with the urethral catheter in place. The catheter is removed the following morning, and the patient is discharged home. The AUS is maintained in the deactivated state for a period of 6–8 weeks to allow for wound healing. Therefore, patients remain incontinent during the initial postoperative time period. The device is subsequently activated in the physician's office by pushing the button on the pump. When activated, fluid is present in the inflated cuff, which provides urethral compression. To urinate, the patient compresses the end of the scrotal pump, which transfers fluid from the cuff to the balloon reservoir and opens the cuff, allowing the patient to urinate. After a few minutes, the fluid automatically transfers back to the cuff to provide compression once again.

## AUS Surgical Variations

It is possible to place the entire AUS via a single scrotal incision at the base of the penis [68]. Advantages of this technique include smaller incision size, and easier pump placement. Furthermore, such an incision allows for simultaneous placement of an AUS with a penile prosthesis, if this is desired [69]. However, the transscrotal incision makes balloon reservoir placement more difficult, and continence outcomes with this technique may be inferior [70]. Regarding cuff placement, it is possible to place two cuffs next to each other around the urethra to provide additional compression. However, routine use of this technique in all men has been associated with increased complications and no clear benefit regarding incontinence outcomes [71]. The cuff can also be placed using a deeper plane of dissection, so that a portion of the penile corpora are incorporated with the dorsal portion of the urethra [72]. This technique may be useful in complicated revision surgeries, but it carries the risk of causing erectile dysfunction.

## AUS Outcomes

Success following AUS placement has typically been defined by the use of 0–1 pads per day. Using this definition, published success rates have ranged from 59% to 90%, at follow-up intervals ranging from 1 to 7.7 years [45]. Using patient-reported outcomes, patient satisfaction with this technique is quite high [73–75]. Importantly, the AUS is effective in men with very severe stress UI. Postoperative wound infection, which occurs in ≤3% of patients [54], can be a disastrous complication, as this typically requires removal of the entire device. Urethral erosion of the cuff can also occur. This is typically identified by the presence of hematuria, urinary tract infections, dysuria, or perineal pain. If urethral erosion occurs within a few weeks of surgery, iatrogenic urethral injury at the time of surgery is assumed to be the cause. A common cause of late urethral erosion is Foley catheter trauma. After AUS placement, it is vital that urethral instrumentation be kept to a minimum, as such instrumentation may weaken the urethra at the cuff site and cause erosion of the cuff. If catheterization is required, the AUS must be deactivated, a small (14 F or less) catheter should be used, and the catheter should be removed as soon as possible. If these measures are not followed, the risk of urethral erosion is high. It is often necessary to involve a urologist in this process, as most other caregivers are not familiar with the process involved in AUS deactivation. Teaching the patient to deactivate the device may be useful, as the patient may be able to take responsibility for deactivating it prior to Foley catheter placement. Some patients choose to wear a Medic-Alert bracelet or similar device to alert caregivers about the presence of the AUS. When urethral erosion occurs, the cuff must be surgically removed, and a Foley catheter is placed for a period of 2 weeks to allow the urethra to heal. Another cuff may then be placed at a later time.

To maintain long-term continence, surgical revision of the AUS is often required. Using Kaplan–Meier analyses, 5-year surgical revision rates have been estimated to be 25–50% [76–80]. Revisions may be required due to infection, urethral erosion, mechanical malfunction of the device (e.g., leak of fluid), or urethral atrophy. Mechanical malfunction has diminished with design improvements [77], so that urethral atrophy now represents the most common cause for device failure. Urethral atrophy is caused by chronic compression of the urethra, and may occur to the extent that the cuff no longer achieves adequate compression to achieve continence. A variety of techniques exist to address this problem including replacement with a smaller cuff, moving the cuff to a different location along the urethra, adding a second cuff in tandem with first one, or transcorporal cuff placement. The choice is often made intraoperatively, after inspection of the tissues. If a surgical revision is required and the device has been in place for longer than 5 years, it is common practice to replace all components. In order to prevent urethral atrophy, some patients can be taught to deactivate the AUS at bedtime and reactivate it in the morning. This typically has minimal impact on continence since most patients with stress UI are dry when in bed at night. Nighttime cuff deactivation theoretically may prolong the life of the AUS by reducing urethral atrophy, but no studies have been performed to test this theory.

## Patient Selection

For most men with persistent and bothersome stress UI, the decision involves choosing between the male sling and the artificial urinary sphincter. In men with a preceding history of a BNC or urethral stricture, it is essential to ensure that this problem has resolved. Presence of an active stricture is a contraindication to either surgery, as any treatment of a stricture following sling or AUS placement carries a high risk of damage to the continence surgery. Slings may be preferred in men with limited manual dexterity who may have difficulty manipulating the AUS, or in those with more mild incontinence (due to fewer complications associated with slings vs. the AUS). Conversely, the AUS is typically a better choice for men with previous pelvic radiation therapy or severe incontinence, as sling outcomes in these scenarios have been poor. Of note, previous AUS explantation is associated with a high rate of sling failure [59, 62], while previous sling placement does not appear to affect the outcome of AUS placement [81]. For many men, the decision between an AUS and a perineal sling is largely based on patient preference. In this situation, there are data to suggest that most men prefer a sling if given the choice [82]. Presumably, this is due to a desire to avoid a "mechanical" device to achieve continence.

## References

1. Abrams P, Artibani W, Cardozo L, et al. Reviewing the ICS 2002 terminology report: the ongoing debate. Neurourol Urodyn. 2006;25:293.
2. Coyne KS, Sexton CC, Thompson CL, et al. The prevalence of lower urinary tract symptoms (LUTS) in the USA, the UK and Sweden: results from the Epidemiology of LUTS (EpiLUTS) study. BJU Int. 2009;104(3):352–60.
3. Onukwugha E, Zuckerman I, McNally D, et al. The total economic burden of overactive bladder in the United States: a disease-specific approach. Am J Manag Care. 2009;15:S90–7.
4. Buckley BS, Lapitan MCM, Epidemiology Committee of the Fourth International Consultation on Incontinence, Paris, 2008. Prevalence of urinary incontinence in men, women, and children – current evidence: findings of the fourth International Consultation on Incontinence. Urology. 2010;76(2):265–70.
5. Stothers L, Thom DH, Calhoun EA. Urinary incontinence in men. In: Litwin MS, Saigal CS, editors. Urologic diseases in America. US Department of Health and Human Services, Public Health Service, National Institutes of Health, National Institute of Diabetes and Digestive and Kidney Diseases. Washington, DC: US Government Publishing Office; 2007. Ch. 6, p. 193–222.

6. Shamliyan TA, Wyman JF, Ping R, et al. Male urinary incontinence: prevalence, risk factors, and preventive interventions. Rev Urol. 2009;11:145.
7. Thom D. Variation in estimates of urinary incontinence prevalence in the community: effects of differences in definition, population characteristics, and study type. J Am Geriatr Soc. 1998;46:473.
8. Tennstedt SL, Chiu GR, Link CL, et al. The effects of severity of urine leakage on quality of life in Hispanic, white and black men and women: the Boston Area Community Health survey. Urology. 2010;75:27.
9. Lagro-Janssen TALM, Hilkens CJM, Klaasen RI, et al. Greater emotional and social effect of urinary incontinence in men than women. J Am Geriatr Soc. 2008;56:1779.
10. Roosen A, Chapple C, Dmochowski R, et al. A refocus on the bladder as the originator of storage lower urinary tract symptoms: a systematic review of the latest literature. Eur Urol. 2009;56:810–20.
11. Andersson KE, Gratske C, Hedlund P. The role of the transient receptor potential (TRP) superfamily if the cation-selective channels in the management of overactive bladder. BJU Int. 2010;106(8):1114–27.
12. Rieken M, Mundorff NE, Bonkat G, et al. Complications of laser prostatectomy: a review of recent data. World J Urol. 2010;28:53.
13. Thiel DD, Petrou SP. Electroresection and open surgery. Urol Clin North Am. 2009;36:461.
14. Lerner LB, Tyson MD. Holmium laser applications of the prostate. Urol Clin North Am. 2009;36:485.
15. Loughlin KR, Prasad MM. Post-prostatectomy incontinence: a confluence of 3 factors. J Urol. 2010;183:871.
16. Hammerer P, Huland H. Urodynamic evaluation of changes in urinary control after radical prostatectomy. J Urol. 1997;157:233.
17. Donnellan SM, Duncan HJ, MacGregor RJ, et al. Prospective assessment of incontinence after radical retropubic prostatectomy: objective and subjective analysis. Urology. 1997;49:225.
18. Eastham JA, Kattan MW, Rogers E, et al. Risk factors for urinary incontinence after radical prostatectomy. J Urol. 1996;156:1707.
19. Litwin MS, Hayes RD, Fink A, et al. Quality-of-life outcomes in men treated for localized prostate cancer. JAMA. 1995;273:129.
20. Penson DF, McLerran D, Feng Z, et al. 5-year urinary and sexual outcomes after radical prostatectomy: results from the prostate cancer outcomes study. J Urol. 2005;173:1701.
21. Begg CB, Riedel ER, Bach PB, et al. Variations in morbidity after radical prostatectomy. N Engl J Med. 2002;346:1138.
22. Steineck G, Helgesen F, Adolfsson J, et al. Quality of life after radical prostatectomy or watchful waiting. N Engl J Med. 2002;347:790.
23. Stanford JL, Feng Z, Hamilton AS, et al. Urinary and sexual function after radical prostatectomy for clinically localized prostate cancer: the prostate cancer outcomes study. JAMA. 2000;283:354.
24. Abrams P, Andersson KE, Birder L, et al. Fourth International Consultation on Incontinence Recommendations of the International Scientific Committee: evaluation and treatment of urinary incontinence, pelvic organ prolapse, and fecal incontinence. Neurourol Urodyn. 2010;29:213.
25. Burgio KL, Goode PS, Urban DA, et al. Preoperative biofeedback assisted behavioral training to decrease post-prostatectomy incontinence: a randomized, controlled trial. J Urol. 2006;175:196.
26. Filocamo MT, Li Marzi V, Del Popolo G, et al. Effectiveness of early pelvic floor rehabilitation treatment for post-prostatectomy incontinence. Eur Urol. 2005;48:734.
27. Van Kampen M, De Weerdt W, Van Poppel H, et al. Effect of pelvic floor re-education on duration and degree of incontinence after radical prostatectomy: a randomized controlled trial. Lancet. 2000;355:98.
28. Bales GT, Gerber GS, Minor TX, et al. Effect of preoperative biofeedback/pelvic floor training on continence in men undergoing radical prostatectomy. Urology. 2000;56:627.
29. Mathewson-Chapman M. Pelvic muscle exercise/biofeedback for urinary incontinence after prostatectomy: an education program. J Cancer Educ. 1997;12:218.
30. Franke JJ, Gilbert WB, Grier J, et al. Early post-prostatectomy pelvic floor biofeedback. J Urol. 2000; 163:191.
31. Moore KN, Griffiths D, Houghton A. Urinary incontinence after radical prostatectomy: a randomized controlled trial comparing pelvic muscle exercises with or without electrical stimulation. BJU Int. 1999;83:57.
32. Hunter KF, Moore KN, Glazener CMA. Conservative management for postprostatectomy urinary incontinence. Cochrane Database System Rev. 2007;CD001843.
33. Goode PS, Burgio KL, Johnson 2nd TM, et al. Behavioral therapy with or without biofeedback and pelvic floor electrical stimulation for persistent post-prostatectomy incontinence: a randomized controlled trial. JAMA. 2011;305:151–9.
34. Nabi G, Cody JD, Ellis G, et al. Anticholinergic drugs versus placebo for overactive bladder syndrome in adults. Cochrane Database Syst Rev. 2006;CD003781.
35. Helfand B, Evans RM, McVary KA. Comparison of the frequencies of medical therapies for overactive bladder in men and women: analysis of more than 7.2 million aging patients. Eur Urol. 2010;57:586–91.
36. Brubaker L, Fanning K, Goldberg E. Predictors of discontinuing overactive bladder medications. BJU Int. 2010;105(9):1283–90.
37. Kaplan SA, Roehrborn CG, Rovner ES, et al. Tolterodine and tamsulosin for treatment of men with lower urinary tract symptoms and overactive bladder. A randomized controlled trial. JAMA. 2006;296:2319.
38. Tsakiris P, de la Rosette JJ, Michel MC, et al. Pharmacologic treatment of male stress urinary incontinence: systematic review of the literature and levels of evidence. Eur Urol. 2008;53:53.

39. Filocamo MT, Li Marzi V, Del Popolo G, et al. Pharmacologic treatment in postprostatectomy stress urinary incontinence. Eur Urol. 2007;51:1559.
40. Schurch B, Reitz A. Botox in urology: a new treatment modality without limitations? EAU update series. 2004;2:170–8.
41. Flynn M, Amundsen C, Perevich M, et al. Outcome of a randomized double blind, placebo controlled trial of botulinum A toxin for refractory overactive bladder. J Urol. 2009;181:2608–15.
42. Khan S, Kessler T, Apostolidis A, et al. What a patient with refractory idiopathix detrusor overactivity should know about botulinum neurotoxiin type a injection. J Urol. 2009;181:1773–8.
43. Herbison GP, Arnold EP. Sacral neuromodulation with implanted devices for urinary storage and voiding dysfunction in adults. Cochrane Database Syst Rev. 2009;(2):CD004202.
44. Siddiqui N, Amundsen C, Visco A, et al. Cost-effectiveness of sacral neuromodulation versus intravesical botulinum A toxin for treatment of refractory urge incontinence. J Urol. 2009;182:2799–804.
45. Herschorn S, Bruschini H, Comier C, et al. Surgical treatment of stress incontinence in men. Neurourol Urodyn. 2010;29:179.
46. Bauer RM, Bastian PJ, Gozzi C, et al. Postprostatectomy incontinence: all about diagnosis and management. Eur Urol. 2009;55:322.
47. Smith DN, Appell RA, Rackley RR, et al. Collagen injection therapy for post-prostatectomy incontinence. J Urol. 1998;160:364.
48. Westney OL, Bevan-Thomas R, Palmer JL, et al. Transurethral collagen injections for male intrinsic sphincter deficiency: the University of Texas-Houston experience. J Urol. 2005;174:994.
49. Comiter CV. The male sling for stress urinary incontinence: a prospective study. J Urol. 2002;167:597.
50. Gomes CM, Broderick GA, Sanchez-Ortiz RF, et al. Artificial urinary sphincter for post-prostatectomy incontinence: impact of prior collagen injection on cost and clinical outcome. J Urol. 2000;163:87.
51. Kaufman JJ. A new operation for male incontinence. Surg Gynecol Obstet. 1970;131:295.
52. Schaeffer AJ, Clemens JQ, Ferrari M, et al. The male bulbourethral sling procedure for post-radical prostatectomy incontinence. J Urol. 1998;159:1510.
53. Stern JA, Clemens JQ, Tiplitsky S, et al. Long-term results of the bulbourethral sling procedure. J Urol. 2005;173:1654.
54. Comiter CV. Surgery insight: surgical management of postprostatectomy incontinence—the artificial urinary sphincter and male sling. Nat Clin Pract Urol. 2007;4:615.
55. Comiter CV. The male perineal sling: intermediate-term results. Neurourol Urodyn. 2005;24:648.
56. Onur R, Singla A. Comparison of bone-anchored male sling and collagen implant for the treatment of male incontinence. Int J Urol. 2006;13:1207.
57. Dikranian AH, Chang AH, Rhee JH, et al. The male perineal sling: comparison of sling materials. J Urol. 2004;172:608.
58. Rajpurkar AD, Onur R, Singla A. Patient satisfaction and clinical efficacy of the new perineal bone-anchored male sling. Eur Urol. 2005;47:237.
59. Castle EP, Andrews PE, Itano N, et al. The male sling for post-prostatectomy incontinence: mean followup of 18 months. J Urol. 2005;173:1657.
60. Flynn BJ, Webster GD. Evaluation and surgical management of intrinsic sphincter deficiency after radical prostatectomy. Rev Urol. 2004;6:180.
61. Fischer MC, Huckabay C, Nitti VW. The male perineal sling: assessment and prediction of outcomes. J Urol. 2007;177:1414.
62. Ullrich NF, Comiter CV. The male sling for stress urinary incontinence: urodynamic and subjective assessment. J Urol. 2004;172:204.
63. Clemens JQ, Bushman W, Schaeffer AJ. Urodynamic analysis of the bulbourethral sling procedure. J Urol. 1999;162:1977.
64. Suburethral synthetic sling insertion for stress urinary incontinence in men. National Institute for Health and Clinical Excellence. Available at http://guidance.nice.org.uk/IPG256. Accessed 12 July 2010.
65. Rehder P, Gozzi C. Transobturator sling suspension for male urinary incontinence including post-radical prostatectomy. Eur Urol. 2007;52:860.
66. Bauer RM, Mayer ME, Gratzke C, et al. Prospective evaluation of the functional sling suspension for male postprostatectomy stress urinary incontinence: results after 1 year. Eur Urol. 2009;56:928.
67. Davies TO, Bepple JL, McCammon KA. Urodynamic changes and initial results of the AdVance male sling. Urology. 2009;74:354.
68. Wilson SK, Delk JR, Henry GD, et al. New surgical technique for sphincter urinary control system using upper transverse scrotal incision. J Urol. 2003;169:261.
69. Kendrici M, Gupta S, Shaw K, et al. Synchronous prosthetic implantation through a transscrotal incision: an outcome analysis. J Urol. 2006;175:2218.
70. Henry GD, Graham SM, Cleves MA, et al. Perineal approach for artificial urinary sphincter implantation appears to control male stress incontinence better than the transscrotal approach. J Urol. 2008;179:1475.
71. O'Connor RC, Lyon MB, Guralnick MB, et al. Long-term follow-up of single versus double cuff artificial urinary sphincter insertion for the treatment of severe postprostatectomy stress urinary incontinence. Urology. 2008;71:90.
72. Guralnick ML, Miller E, Toh KL, et al. Transcorporal artificial urinary sphincter cuff placement in cases requiring revision for erosion and urethral atrophy. J Urol. 2002;167:2075.
73. Fleshner N, Herschorn S. The artificial urinary sphincter for post-radical prostatectomy incontinence: impact on urinary symptoms and quality of life. J Urol. 1996;155:1260.

74. Haab F, Trockman BA, Zimmern PE, et al. Quality of life and continence assessment of the artificial urinary sphincter in men with minimum 3.5 years of followup. J Urol. 1997;158:435.
75. Litwiller SE, Kim KB, Fone PD, et al. Post-prostatectomy incontinence and the artificial urinary sphincter: a long-term study of patient satisfaction and criteria for success. J Urol. 1996;156:1975.
76. Lai HH, Hsu EI, Teh BS, et al. 13 years of experience with artificial urinary sphincter implantation at Baylor College of Medicine. J Urol. 2007;177:1021.
77. Elliott DS, Barrett DM. Mayo Clinic long-term analysis of the functional durability of the AMS 800 artificial urinary sphincter: a review of 323 cases. J Urol. 1998;159:1206.
78. Clemens JQ, Schuster TG, Konnak JW, et al. Revision rate following artificial urinary sphincter placement for post-radical prostatectomy incontinence: actuarial analysis. J Urol. 2001;166:1372.
79. Venn SN, Greenwall TJ, Mundy AR. The long-term outcome of artificial urinary sphincters. J Urol. 2000;164:702.
80. Klijn AJ, Hop WCJ, Mickisch G, et al. The artificial urinary sphincter in men incontinent after radical prostatectomy: 5 years actuarial adequate function rates. BJU Int. 1998;82:530.
81. Fisher MB, Aggarwal N, Vuruskan H, et al. Efficacy of artificial urinary sphincter implantation after failed bone-anchored male sling for postprostatectomy incontinence. Urology. 2007;70:942.
82. Kumar A, Litt ER, Ballert KN, et al. Artificial urinary sphincter versus male sling for post-prostatectomy incontinence – what do patients choose? J Urol. 2009;181:1231.

# Treatment of Localized Prostate Cancer

14

Andrew J. Stephenson

## Introduction

In 2010, an estimated 217,730 were diagnosed with prostate cancer and 32,050 men died from this disease [1]. The introduction of PSA screening in the USA beginning in the late 1980's has led to a substantial increase in the incidence of prostate cancer (lifetime risk 7.3% in 1975 vs. 17% in 2005), particularly clinically localized disease that may be considered for curative therapy; the proportion of patients with clinically localized disease has increased from 60–70% to 85–95% while those with metastatic disease has decreased from 10–20% to less than 2% [2–4]. Since the early 1990s, a 35% reduction in age-adjusted, prostate cancer-specific mortality (PCSM) has been observed which is due, in part, to PSA screening and improvements in local therapy [5, 6].

Estimates from the United States Surveillance Epidemiology and End Results (SEER) registry and the European Randomised Screening Trial for Prostate Cancer (ERSPC) suggest that 45–70% of the reduction in PCSM since the introduction of the PSA assay is attributable to mass opportunistic screening [6]. However, screening practices have led to overdiagnosis, defined as the detection of clinically important cancers that would remain undetected over a man's lifetime in the absence of screening. Investigators from ERSPC estimate that over 50% of cancers detected through annual PSA screening in men over 55 years of age represent overdiagnosis [7]. Evidence from ERSPC also suggests that 48 men with screen-detected prostate cancer need to be treated to prevent one death from prostate cancer within 10–12 years [8].

The problem of overdiagnosis represents a major challenge to the treatment of men in North America and select European and Asian countries where mass screening is prevalent. The vast majority of men in the USA who are diagnosed with prostate cancer receive some form of definitive local therapy, even those with low-risk features and those over 75–80 years of age (including those with significant comorbid illness) [9–12]. Welch and Albertsen estimated that 1,300,000 more American men have been diagnosed with prostate cancer since the introduction of PSA in 1986, 1,000,000 more men have been treated, and 56,000 deaths have been averted (using the most optimistic assumptions of the effect of screening on reducing prostate cancer mortality) [9]. They concluded that the overwhelming majority of excess men diagnosed with prostate cancer since 1986 did not benefit from treatment. While the three standard treatment options [radical prostatectomy, external-beam radiotherapy (EBRT), and brachytherapy] are associated with overall long-term cure rates of

A.J. Stephenson, MD, FACS, FRCS(C) (✉)
Glickman Urologic and Kidney Institute, Cleveland Clinic, 9500 Euclid Avenue Q10-1, Cleveland, OH 44195, USA
e-mail: STEPHEA2@ccf.org

D.A. Shoskes (ed.), *Urological Men's Health: A Guide for Urologists and Primary Care Physicians*, Current Clinical Urology, DOI 10.1007/978-1-61779-900-6_14,
© Springer Science+Business Media New York 2012

75% or greater in appropriately selected patients and low (<10%) risks of PCSM within 10–15 years of treatment, it is uncertain whether similarly low risks of PCSM would be observed in some of these men had they been managed conservatively. Identifying those cancers that may progress, cause symptoms, and ultimately lead to a man's demise and those associated with a low-risk is critical to selecting patients for local therapy vs. observation. As all the standard treatments may negatively impact urinary, bowel, and sexual function, a policy of aggressive treatment for all patients is likely to lead to harm in the majority of cases while benefiting a relative minority.

## Natural History of Localized Prostate Cancer

Clinically localized prostate cancer is characterized by an exceptionally protracted natural history relative to other solid malignancies. In the absence of definitive local therapy, the estimated 20-year PCSM for men with clinically detected cancers (defined as palpable nodule on digital rectal examination, prostate cancer detected on transurethral prostatectomy for voiding symptoms) is 20–25%, 65–75%, and 80–90% for those with biopsy Gleason score 6 or less, 7, and 8–10 cancers, respectively [13]. Given that the lead-time associated with screening is estimated to be 5–11 years [14, 15], these risks are substantially less for men with screen-detected cancers; negligible risk of PCSM within 15 years for those with Gleason 2–6 cancers, 10–25% for Gleason 7 cancers, and 25–70% Gleason 8–10 cancers (Fig. 14.1) [16]. Men with pathological stage T3 cancers (extraprostatic extension) have a sevenfold increased risk of PCSM relative to those with pathologically organ-confined cancers [17].

Due to the protracted natural history of localized prostate cancer, prognostic factors that reflect the "treated" natural history with either surgery or radiation therapy have been based on a PSA-defined biochemical recurrence (BCR) endpoint, as it precedes PCSM by an average of 15 years [18, 19]. While BCR universally antedates metastasis progression and PCSM, it is an imprecise proxy for these endpoints due to its variable natural history; in the absence of therapy, the median time to metastasis progression is 5–8 years [20]. Clinical stage, tumor grade (biopsy Gleason score), and the PSA level before therapy are the three parameters that have consistently been shown to predict for BCR. The incremental empiric prognostic value of other factors such as systematic prostate biopsy results (number of positive and negative cores, percentage of positive cores, perineural invasion) and the rate of rise of PSA in the 1–2 years prior to therapy (known as PSA velocity or PSA doubling time) is controversial. A PSA velocity >2 ng/mL/year in the year prior to treatment was associated with PCSM in a well-publicized study, though this association has not been reproduced in several other studies [21–23].

There is evidence from randomized trials that definitive local therapy can significantly alter the natural history of prostate cancer and reduce the risk of PCSM. Scandinavian Prostate Cancer Group-4 randomized 695 men with clinically detected prostate cancer between radical prostatectomy and watchful waiting between 1989 and 1999 [17]. At 15 years, men treated by radical prostatectomy had a significantly reduced risk of all-cause mortality (HR 0.8; 95% CI: 0.6–0.9; $P=0.007$), PCSM (HR 0.6; 95% CI: 0.4–0.9; $P=0.01$), distant metastasis (HR 0.6; 95% CI: 0.5–0.8; $P<0.001$), and local progression (HR 0.4; 95% CI: 0.3–0.5; $P<0.001$) compared to those on watchful waiting, and the absolute risk reductions for these endpoints was 7%, 6%, 12%, and 22%, respectively [17, 24]. However, in an unplanned subset analysis, these benefits were restricted to men less than 65 years of age. Scandinavian Prostate Cancer Group-7 randomized 875 men with locally advanced prostate cancer (78% clinical stage T3, 40% PSA>20 ng/mL) to androgen deprivation therapy (ADT; 3 months of complete androgen blockade with LHRH agonist and oral flutamide followed by flutamide alone for 3 years) +/− three-dimensional conformal external-beam radiotherapy (3DCRT) to 70 Gy [25]. Over a median follow-up of 7 years, men in the 3DCRT arm had a significantly reduced risk of all-cause mortality (HR 0.7; 95% CI: 0.5–0.9; $P=0.004$) and PCSM (HR 0.4; 95% CI: 0.3–0.7; $P<0.001$), which

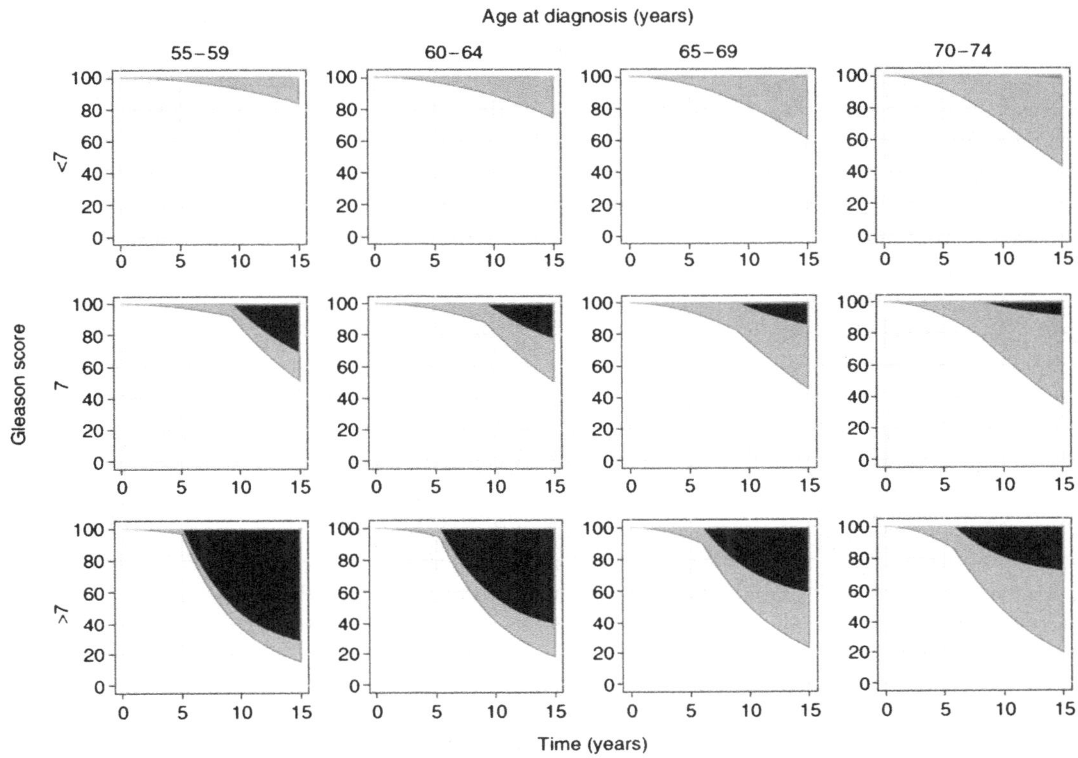


**Fig. 14.1** Survival estimates at 15 years with conservative management adjusting for the lead-time in prostate cancer diagnosis from PSA screening. [*Reprinted with permission from Parker, C., Muston, D., Melia, J., Moss, S. & Dearnaley, D. A model of the natural history of screen-detected prostate cancer, and the effect of radical treatment on overall survival. Br J Cancer 94, 1361–8 (2006).*]

translated into a 10% and 12% absolute risk reduction, respectively.

There is currently no definitive evidence from randomized trials that definitive local therapy improves the survival of patients with screen-detected prostate cancer. The only randomized trial completed to date is the PIVOT trial, which randomized 731 American men with screen-detected prostate cancer to radical prostatectomy vs. watchful waiting in a similar design to the Scandinavian Prostate Cancer Group-4 trial. In an unpublished report of this study, no significant difference in all-cause mortality or PCSM was observed at 12 years between the treatment arms [26]. No difference in all-cause mortality was observed in any of the subgroups analyzed and only high-risk patients treated by radical prostatectomy had significantly lower risk of PCSM compared to those on watchful waiting.

## Risk Stratification

As discussed, PSA, clinical stage, and biopsy Gleason score are the prime determinants of BCR and PCSM after definitive local therapy and PCSM. Numerous risk stratification tools have been developed based on these factors and others to predict BCR and PCSM. The D'Amico risk groups are the most widely used risk stratification tool due, in part, to their simplicity. By the D'Amico classification, patients are categorized as either low- (PSA < 10 ng/mL, clinical stage T1c or T2a, and biopsy Gleason score 2–6), intermediate-risk (PSA 10–20 ng/mL or clinical stage T2b or biopsy Gleason score 7), and high-risk (PSA > 20 ng/mL or clinical stage T3 or biopsy Gleason score 8–10) [27]. The Cancer of the Prostate Risk Assessment (CAPRA) score is an example of a prognostic index [28]. Patients are assigned a CAPRA score between 0 and 10 based on the points assigned for PSA (0–4), biopsy Gleason score (0–3), clinical stage (0–1), percentage of positive biopsy cores (0–1), and age (0–1). Each point on the CAPRA score corresponds with an estimated 5-year recurrence-free probability after radical prostatectomy.

An alternative method to a risk group or prognostic index is to develop continuous multivariable models called nomograms. A nomogram is a graphic representation of a mathematical formula or algorithm that incorporates several predictors modeled as continuous variables to predict a particular endpoint. Nomograms consist of sets of axes; each variable is represented by a scale, with each value of that variable corresponding to a specific number of points according to its prognostic significance. For example, the nomogram shown in Fig. 14.2 assigns each PSA level a unique point value that represents its prognostic significance [29]. In a final pair of axes, the total point value from all the variables is converted to the probability of reaching the endpoint. By using scales, nomograms calculate the *continuous* probability of a particular outcome. Nomograms have been developed to predict the risk of BCR for men treated by radical prostatectomy, EBRT, and brachytherapy, metastasis progression and PCSM for men on watchful waiting, and PCSM for men treated by radical prostatectomy [29–38].

By incorporating all relevant continuous predictive factors for individual patients, nomograms provide more accurate predictions than models based on risk-grouping and they generally surpass clinical experts at outcomes prediction by calculating probabilities in a uniform fashion [39–42]. Several studies have documented the superior performance of nomograms compared to risk-grouping schemata [42–44]. This may stem from the fact

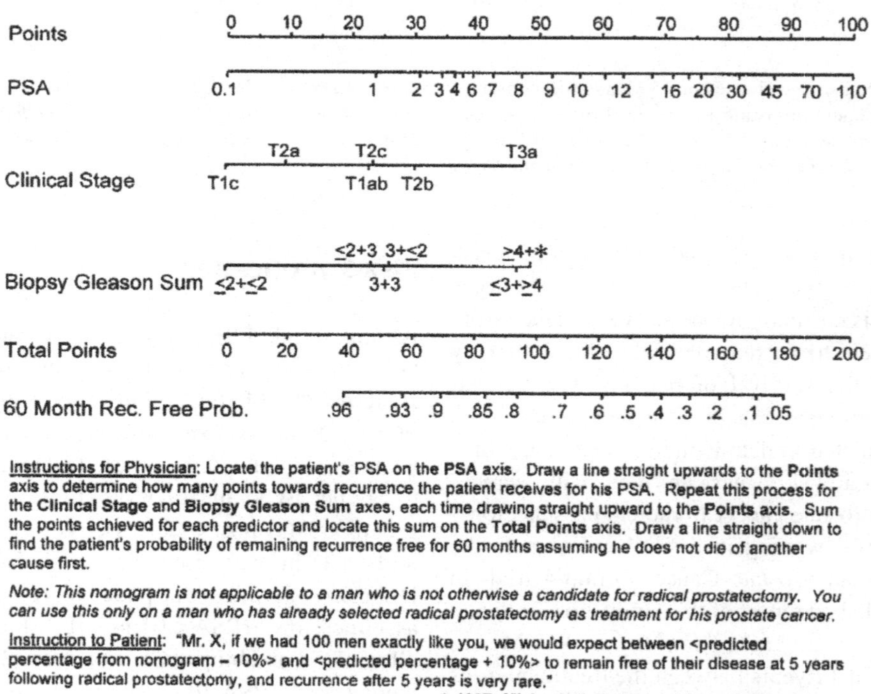


**Fig. 14.2** Preoperative nomogram predicting 5-year progression-free probability after radical prostatectomy [*Reprinted with permission from Kattan, M. W., Eastham, J. A., Stapleton, A. M., Wheeler, T. M. & Scardino, P. T. A preoperative nomogram for disease recurrence following radical prostatectomy for prostate cancer. J Natl Cancer Inst 90, 766–71 (1998).*]

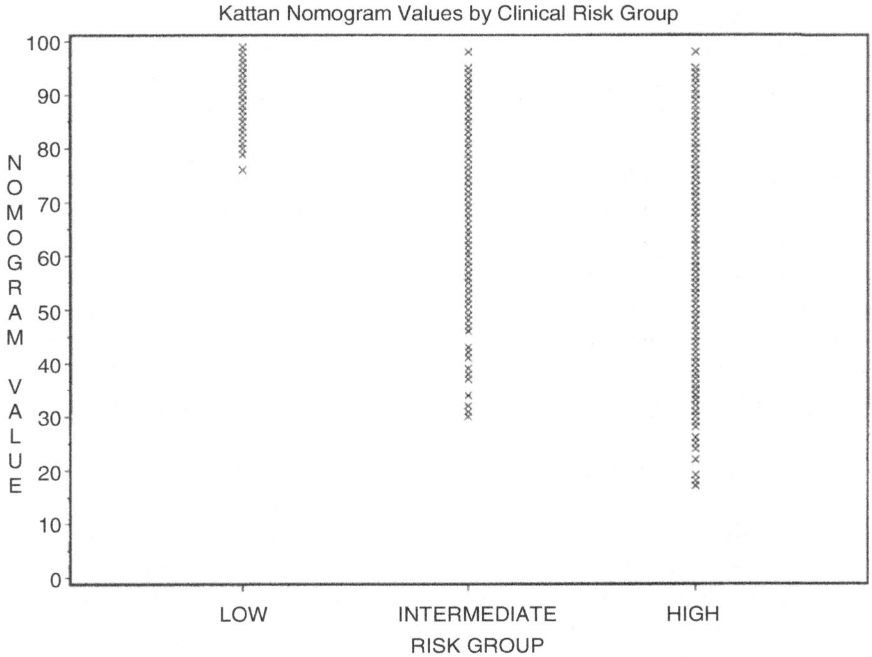


**Fig. 14.3** Estimated 5-year progression-free probability according to a validated preoperative nomogram for patients categorized as low-, intermediate-, and high-risk prostate cancer according to the D'Amico classification. [*Reprinted with permission from Mitchell, J. A. et al. Ability of 2 pretreatment risk assessment methods to predict prostate cancer recurrence after radical prostatectomy: data from CaPSURE. J Urol 173, 1126–31 (2005).*]

that risk groups consist of patients with *similar*—albeit not identical—characteristics, resulting in heterogeneity within a risk group that reduces the predictive accuracy [45, 46]. The heterogeneity inherent in risk groups is illustrated in Fig. 14.3, where the 5-year progression-free probability (PFP) after radical prostatectomy was calculated using a continuous, multivariable preoperative nomogram among patients categorized as low-, medium-, and high-risk using the criteria of D'Amico et al. [27, 47]. While low-risk patients uniformly had a high likelihood of being free of progression by the nomogram, a substantial proportion of intermediate- and even high-risk patients had a calculated 5-year PFP of 90% or more. A considerable overlap in the nomogram predictions is also evident among intermediate- and high-risk patients. While nomograms are more complex than risk groups, this added complexity results in added predictive accuracy for the both patient and physician. Nomograms have been adapted for use on personal digital assistants and personal computers to facilitate their use in the office or for research purposes. These nomograms are available in the public domain for use online (www.nomograms.org or www.clinicriskcalculators.org).

## Treatment Guidelines and Treatment Selection for Localized Prostate Cancer

The National Comprehensive Cancer Center Network (NCCN) has published guidelines for the treatment of localized prostate cancer using a modification of the D'Amico risk classification [48]. Similar treatment guidelines have also been published by other professional societies such as the American Urological Association and the European Association of Urology [49, 50]. Very low-risk patients are categorized as low-risk patients who are also T1c, <3 positive biopsy cores, 50% or less of cancer in any single core, and PSA density less than 0.15 ng/mL/g. Active surveillance is the preferred treatment for patients with life expectancy <20 years. Those with life expectancy >20 years can be treated as other low-risk patients. For low-risk patients, active surveillance is recommended to those with life expectancy <10 years and all treatments (including active surveillance, brachytherapy, EBRT, radical prostatectomy) are reasonable to consider for those with life expectancy >10 years. For intermediate-risk cancers, active surveillance and EBRT (with or without a short course of neoadjuvant-concurrent ADT) are recommended for men with life expectancy <10 years and EBRT (with or without a short course of neoadjuvant-concurrent ADT) and radical prostatectomy are recommended to men with life expectancy >10 years. For men with high-risk features, EBRT plus 2–3 years of adjuvant ADT or radical prostatectomy may be considered. Primary ADT may also be a consideration for the patient with locally advanced prostate cancer (T3b or T4). As a result of PSA screening, a stage migration has been observed over the last 2 decades in terms of the cancer risk profile. Specifically, the proportion of patients with low-risk cancers that are candidates for active surveillance has increased from 28% in the early 1990s to almost 50% in the latter part of the last decade. Likewise, the proportion of patients with high-risk features has decreased over the same time period from 46% to 25% [51].

Despite these guidelines, choosing the optimal therapy for the individual is a complex and challenging process as no treatment has been definitively proven to be superior in terms of quantity and quality of life. First, a man must choose between radical therapy and active surveillance for a cancer that may pose an uncertain threat to his longevity [13]. If an aggressive treatment approach is chosen, radical prostatectomy, EBRT, and brachytherapy are all recognized standard treatment alternatives (with the exception of brachytherapy as monotherapy for high-risk disease). Quality-of-life issues should factor into men's treatment decision as they may live decades with the sequelae of the treatments they have received.

In the absence of data from randomized trials, one must rely on observational studies, though these have the potential for bias. Four recent observational studies have reported metastasis-free, cancer-specific, and/or overall survival over 10-year follow-up among men treated by radical prostatectomy and EBRT according to contemporary treatment standards and each has reported a significant improvement in these endpoints with radical prostatectomy after adjusting for important confounders [52–55]. However, the differences in the adjusted survival between treatment modalities at 10 years were small, particularly for PCSM. As there is a recognized bias to treat older and higher risk patients with EBRT, an imbalance of confounders (known and unknown) may explain these survival differences despite the investigators' attempts to adjust for them.

Large, prospective, longitudinal quality-of-life studies using patient-reported outcomes provide important information for the impact of local therapy on functional outcomes [56–59]. What is apparent from these studies is that each of the treatments can negatively impact urinary, bowel, and sexual function to varying degrees and the nature of the side effects may differ [56]. For example, radical prostatectomy is typically associated with an increased risk of urinary stress incontinence, while EBRT and brachytherapy are typically associated with bothersome voiding symptoms such as frequency, urgency, dysuria, slow stream, and incomplete bladder emptying. Radiation treatments can cause bothersome bowel symptoms, which are uncommon after radical prostatectomy. All treatments can cause erectile dysfunction. For radical prostatectomy, the impact on erectile function is immediate and the likelihood a man will recover sexual function is influenced by his age, baseline erectile function, and the use of nerve-sparing techniques. For radiation treatments, men may experience a gradual decline in the quality of erections over 1–2 years after treatment, mainly due to the chronic effects of radiation on the penile blood supply. As with radical prostatectomy, age, baseline erectile function, and the use of ADT will impact the quality of erections after radiation therapy. Men on active surveillance are at risk of developing local symptoms (bothersome voiding symptoms, urinary retention, hematuria, pain) from local disease progression

[24]. In the Scandinavian Prostate Cancer Group-4 trial, the incidence of local progression on watchful waiting (defined as palpable transcapsular tumor growth or voiding disorder necessitating intervention) was greater than 40% at 10 years [60].

## Treatment Options

### Active Surveillance

As mentioned previously, approximately 50% of men with screen-detected prostate cancers have low-risk disease. The risk that these tumors pose to a man's longevity and quality of life appears to be very low within 10–15 years of diagnosis. Thus, active surveillance as a management option is of increased interest for these patients given the uncertain benefit of treatment in terms of improving survival but the more certain impacts of treatment on quality of life. However, acceptance rates of active surveillance in healthy men with long life expectancy are low (10% among low-risk patients in the CaPSURE series) despite accumulating evidence attesting to its safety and efficacy [11, 12].

Klotz et al. recently published an update of their active surveillance series in 450 patients diagnosed between 1995 and 2010, 72 (16%), 63 (14%), 48 (11%) of whom had biopsy Gleason 3+4, PSA > 10 ng/mL, and clinical stage T2b-T3 features, respectively [61]. Patients were followed with serial PSA measurements and repeat biopsy in year 1 and then re-biopsy every 2–3 years thereafter. Over a median follow-up of 7 years, 97 deaths were observed (5 from prostate cancer) and the 10-year overall and cancer-specific survival was 79% and 97%, respectively. The 10-year freedom from treatment was 70%, though 50% of patients undergoing definitive local therapy experienced BCR (representing 13% of the overall cohort). In the Johns Hopkins experience, 10 of 49 patients (20%) who progressed on surveillance had "noncurable" cancer at radical prostatectomy (defined as either pathological Gleason 4+3, non-organ-confined cancer, or positive surgical margins) [62, 63]. However, the classification of these patients as "noncurable" is debatable, and this rate was not significantly higher than matched patients who underwent immediate radical prostatectomy.

Despite the concerns of advanced pathological features in men with low-risk cancer by clinical criteria on (or candidates for) surveillance, intervention for men on surveillance is reported in 13–40% in most series, though one study reported a 4-year intervention rate of 73% [61, 62, 64–69]. When intervention is required, deferred therapy is highly successful. In men who undergo deferred radical prostatectomy, 85% or more have had pathologically organ-confined cancer in most series (this rate was only 65% in the Johns Hopkins series) and rates of seminal vesicle invasion and lymph node metastasis are less than 5% [65, 69–73]. With the exception of the University of Toronto series in which 50% of patients requiring eventual treatment following surveillance had progression of their disease despite deferred therapy, most series have reported successful salvage in 87% or more of patients over short-term (<5 years) follow-up [61, 65, 69, 70, 72].

Appropriate patient selection and monitoring is critical for a successful surveillance strategy. At Cleveland Clinic, all patients with low-risk prostate cancer (regardless of age and life expectancy) are counseled about the advantages and disadvantages of active surveillance and interested patients are recommended to undergo repeat biopsy within 6 months of diagnosis as several studies have reported a 21–27% re-classification to a more aggressive cancer on re-biopsy [69, 74]. Eggener et al. have also reported that the presence of cancer on the repeat biopsy was significantly associated with the need for intervention for men on surveillance [65]. Patients with low-volume Gleason 6 cancer or no cancer on repeat biopsy are offered active surveillance and patients are monitored with clinical assessment and PSA every 6 months and repeat biopsy every 2–3 years. Intervention on surveillance is recommended to patients with evidence of Gleason grade 4 cancer (3+4 or higher) or increasing cancer burden on serial biopsies, enlarging nodule on digital rectal examination, or progressive rise in serum PSA.

## Radical Prostatectomy

Radical prostatectomy is the most common intervention employed in the USA for the treatment of localized prostate cancer. Large surgical series from high-volume hospitals have reported long-term cure rates in 75% or more of patients [37]. The operation may be performed by open (including retropubic and perineal) and laparoscopic (with or without robotic assistance) approaches. Critical advances in the development of operative approaches to localized prostate cancer over the last 3 decades include the understanding of the periprostatic vasculature and cavernous nerves (which enabled the retropubic approach to be performed safely with nerve-sparing techniques for potency preservation in the 1980s) and robotic-assistance (which has enabled the widespread adoption of minimally invasive techniques among urologists over the last decade). The disadvantages of the perineal approach include the inability to perform a pelvic lymph node dissection and nerve-sparing, and an increased risk of anterior positive surgical margins.

The goals of radical prostatectomy are complete removal of the prostate and seminal vesicles with negative surgical margins, pelvic lymph node dissection, preservation of the rhabdosphincter (and its innervation) for recovery of urinary continence, and (where appropriate) preservation of the cavernous nerves for recovery of potency. Pelvic lymph node dissection may be omitted in low-risk patients as the risk of lymph node metastasis in these patients is less than 1%. Successfully accomplishing these goals is an arduous task. Even among high-volume open surgeons from centers of excellence, negative surgical margins, recovery of continence, and recovery of potency are achieved in only two-thirds of patients [75].

The popularity of robotic prostatectomy has risen dramatically over the past 5–7 years and is fueled by the potential for improved outcomes due to improved visualization, instrumentation, smaller incisions, and less blood loss. However, the only consistent advantage of robotic prostatectomy is decreased blood loss caused by the pressure of the pneumoperitoneum, though this has not resulted in a clinically meaningful reduction in the transfusion rate [76]. Perioperative outcomes such as length of hospitalization, operative time, analgesic requirements, and complication rates are not significantly different between open and minimally invasive radical prostatectomy when performed by high-volume surgeons [77–79]. Functional outcomes (continence, potency) and rates of positive surgical margins do not appear to be substantially different among high-volume open and laparoscopic surgeons [80–82]. The most critical determinant of a successful outcome is the experience and technical skill of the operating surgeon as BCR, positive surgical margins, and perioperative morbidity are all influenced by surgeon volume and individual surgeon technique [83–86].

Risk factors for cancer recurrence after radical prostatectomy include preoperative PSA level, pathological Gleason score, pathological tumor stage, positive surgical margins, and lymph node metastasis. Of these factors, pathological Gleason score 8–10 and presence of seminal vesicle invasion are the two parameters associated with the highest risk of PCSM [30]. For patients with risk factors for recurrence after surgery, postoperative radiation therapy to the prostate bed +/− pelvic lymph nodes (given as adjuvant therapy in men with undetectable postoperative PSA level or as early salvage therapy when the PSA level first reaches detectable levels) can reduce the risk of cancer progression and metastasis [87–89]. The role of postoperative ADT is controversial prior to the appearance of distant metastasis. Neoadjuvant ADT is associated with reduced risks of positive surgical margins but no impact on risk of cancer recurrence and is not considered a standard approach for patients treated with surgery [90].

## External-Beam Radiotherapy

EBRT using contemporary conformal techniques +/− neoadjuvant, concurrent, and/or adjuvant ADT is associated with similar rates of long-term cancer control compared to radical prostatectomy [91, 92]. EBRT consists of delivering high energy to the pelvic region to 50 Gy (the maximum tolerable dose to small intestine) followed by a boost to the prostate to a total of 78 Gy or more. Because of the scatter of radiation to the rectum and bladder and subsequent toxicity, the maximum dose that could be delivered to the prostate was 64–70 Gy using conventional radiation techniques. The development of 3DCRT and intensity-modulated radiotherapy (IMRT) enables delivery of high doses of radiation therapy to the prostate with a sharp drop-off in terms of the doses delivered to the surrounding pelvic organs. This permits high radiation doses to be delivered to the prostate with reduced rectal and bladder toxicity compared to conventional techniques using lower doses. A dose–response relationship has been observed with respect to local cancer control and randomized trials have shown improved cancer control in patients receiving high-dose EBRT using conformal techniques [93, 94].

Several randomized trials support the use of neoadjuvant, concurrent, and/or adjuvant ADT in combination with EBRT in intermediate- and high-risk patients. ADT may be a radio-sensitizer and increase the cytotoxic effects of EBRT on prostate cancer within the prostate and may sterilize micro-metastases (particularly long-term adjuvant ADT). ADT may also be used to reduce the gland size in men with enlarged prostates (>80–100 g) to reduce the target volume and the likelihood of bladder and rectal toxicity. For patients with high-risk features, randomized trials from Europe and North America have shown a significant survival benefit among patients receiving low-dose EBRT and 2–3 years of adjuvant ADT compared to EBRT alone [95, 96]. A recent trial attempted to determine whether a shorter course (6-month) of ADT provided similar benefits to long-term ADT but inferior survival was observed among patients receiving short-term ADT; thus, 2–3 years of adjuvant ADT remains the standard-of-care in high-risk patients. The role of short-term (≤6 months) neoadjuvant/concurrent ADT in intermediate-risk patients is controversial, with a small randomized trial showing a survival benefit [97]. Likewise, the role of whole-pelvic EBRT (treatment of the prostate and pelvic lymph nodes) is controversial and is not considered standard-of-care [98].

For patients who experience cancer recurrence after radiation therapy, patients may be considered for local salvage therapy with either radical prostatectomy or cryotherapy (freezing of the prostate) if the PSA level is low (<10 ng/mL) and a biopsy confirms the presence of recurrent prostate cancer. Both techniques are associated with favorable long-term cancer control rates but are seldom employed due to substantial risks of perioperative morbidity (including incontinence, impotence, strictures, voiding dysfunction) [99–102]. The majority of patients who receive secondary therapy after EBRT for a rising PSA level are treated with ADT.

In addition to impacts on voiding dysfunction, rectal symptoms, and erectile dysfunction, EBRT (and brachytherapy) is associated with low risks of radiation proctitis and radiation cystitis, which can cause persistent and refractory bleeding problems requiring endoscopic intervention. Likewise, EBRT (and brachytherapy) is associated with a small risk of radiation-induced pelvic malignancy [103, 104].

## Transperineal Permanent Interstitial Brachytherapy

Transperineal brachytherapy involves the insertion of radioactive iodine-125 or palladium-105 pellets within the prostate using ultrasound-guidance, which enables the delivery of high doses (up to 144 Gy) over a prolonged time period (approximately 6 months). The appeal of brachytherapy is that treatment is given in a single outpatient surgical procedure and theoretically is associated with reduced risks of rectal complications compared to EBRT. Comparative studies have shown similar long-term cancer control in appropriately selected patients treated by brachytherapy compared to EBRT and radical prostatectomy [27]. Brachytherapy is considered a standard treatment for low-risk prostate cancer and select patients with intermediate-risk disease. Brachytherapy as monotherapy is not considered a standard approach to high-risk disease due to inferior outcomes [105].

## Primary Androgen Deprivation Therapy and Watchful Waiting

Historically, primary ADT has been considered a standard approach to patients with limited life expectancy (due to advanced age and/or comorbid medical illness), though its impact on metastasis progression and PCSM is controversial [106, 107]. A European randomized trial of immediate ADT vs. observation (with deferred ADT at the time of symptomatic metastasis progression) in men with locally advanced prostate cancer showed a small improvement in overall survival with immediate ADT, but no difference in PCSM [107]. Long-term ADT is associated with substantial adverse effects on bone health (including osteoporosis and pathological fractures), metabolic syndrome, and possibly cardiovascular toxicity, which has reduced the appeal of primary ADT [108–111]. An alternative approach to men with localized prostate cancer who have limited life expectancy is close observation with deferred ADT at the time of local and/or systemic progression, termed watchful waiting. Watchful waiting differs from active surveillance as the former involves periodic clinical assessment and serial PSA testing with ADT given at the time of symptomatic progression with palliative intent. As mentioned previously, active surveillance involves intensive monitoring with serial re-biopsy to identify clinically important cancers at an asymptomatic and curable stage with definitive local therapy (radical prostatectomy, EBRT, brachytherapy) administered with curative intent.

## Summary

In the USA, mass opportunistic screening has resulted in the increased detection of prostate cancer and an increased proportion of patients who are candidates for curative therapy. Screening has also resulted in the increased detection of low-risk cancers that may pose a relatively low threat to survival and quality of life, particularly for patients with limited life expectancy. No treatment has been definitively proven to be superior to another in terms of quantity and quality of life. However, all definitive treatments (radical prostatectomy, EBRT, and brachytherapy) may negatively impact urinary, bowel, and sexual function. As there are substantial trade-offs between in terms of benefits and risks of treatments that are likely sensitive to patient preferences, it is recommended that patients be informed of all potential treatments options with adherence to published guidelines. In general, there is an underutilization of active surveillance, particularly for low-risk patients and those with limited life expectancy. The outcomes of patients undergoing definitive local therapy are favorable, particularly in terms of the low risk of clinical disease progression and serious morbidity. Outcomes appear to be sensitive to the expertise and skill of the treating urologist and oncologist.

## References

1. Jemal A, Siegel R, Xu J, Ward E. Cancer statistics, 2010. CA Cancer J Clin. 2010;60(5):277–300.
2. Hugosson J, Aus G, Lilja H, Lodding P, Pihl CG. Results of a randomized, population-based study of biennial screening using serum prostate-specific antigen measurement to detect prostate carcinoma. Cancer. 2004;100(7):1397–405.
3. Makinen T, Tammela TL, Hakama M, Stenman UH, Rannikko S, Aro J, et al. Tumor characteristics in a population-based prostate cancer screening trial with prostate-specific antigen. Clin Cancer Res. 2003;9(7): 2435–9.
4. van der Cruijsen-Koeter IW, Vis AN, Roobol MJ, Wildhagen MF, de Koning HJ, van der Kwast TH, et al. Comparison of screen detected and clinically diagnosed prostate cancer in the European randomized study of screening for prostate cancer, section rotterdam. J Urol. 2005;174(1):121–5.
5. Collin SM, Martin RM, Metcalfe C, Gunnell D, Albertsen PC, Neal D, et al. Prostate-cancer mortality in the USA and UK in 1975-2004: an ecological study. Lancet Oncol. 2008;9(5):445–52.
6. Etzioni R, Tsodikov A, Mariotto A, Szabo A, Falcon S, Wegelin J, et al. Quantifying the role of PSA screening in the US prostate cancer mortality decline. Cancer Causes Control. 2008;19(2):175–81.
7. Draisma G, Boer R, Otto SJ, van der Cruijsen IW, Damhuis RA, Schroder FH, et al. Lead times and overdetection due to prostate-specific antigen screening: estimates from the European Randomized Study of Screening for Prostate Cancer. J Natl Cancer Inst. 2003;95(12):868–78.
8. Schroder FH, Hugosson J, Roobol MJ, Tammela TL, Ciatto S, Nelen V, et al. Screening and prostate-cancer

mortality in a randomized European study. N Engl J Med. 2009;360(13):1320–8.
9. Welch HG, Albertsen PC. Prostate cancer diagnosis and treatment after the introduction of prostate-specific antigen screening: 1986-2005. J Natl Cancer Inst. 2009;101(19):1325–9.
10. Walter LC, Bertenthal D, Lindquist K, Konety BR. PSA screening among elderly men with limited life expectancies. Jama. 2006;296(19):2336–42.
11. Barocas DA, Cowan JE, Smith JA, Jr., Carroll PR. What percentage of patients with newly diagnosed carcinoma of the prostate are candidates for surveillance? An analysis of the CaPSURE database. J Urol. 2008;180(4):1330–4; discussion 4–5.
12. Harlan SR, Cooperberg MR, Elkin EP, Lubeck DP, Meng MV, Mehta SS, et al. Time trends and characteristics of men choosing watchful waiting for initial treatment of localized prostate cancer: results from CaPSURE. J Urol. 2003;170(5):1804–7.
13. Albertsen PC, Hanley JA, Fine J. 20-year outcomes following conservative management of clinically localized prostate cancer. Jama. 2005;293(17): 2095–101.
14. Etzioni R, Penson DF, Legler JM, di Tommaso D, Boer R, Gann PH, et al. Overdiagnosis due to prostate-specific antigen screening: lessons from U.S. prostate cancer incidence trends. J Natl Cancer Inst. 2002;94(13):981–90.
15. Draisma G, Etzioni R, Tsodikov A, Mariotto A, Wever E, Gulati R, et al. Lead time and overdiagnosis in prostate-specific antigen screening: importance of methods and context. J Natl Cancer Inst. 2009; 101(6):374–83.
16. Parker C, Muston D, Melia J, Moss S, Dearnaley D. A model of the natural history of screen-detected prostate cancer, and the effect of radical treatment on overall survival. Br J Cancer. 2006;94(10):1361–8.
17. Bill-Axelson A, Holmberg L, Ruutu M, Garmo H, Stark JR, Busch C, et al. Radical prostatectomy versus watchful waiting in early prostate cancer. N Engl J Med. 2011;364(18):1708–17.
18. Bianco FJ, Jr., Scardino PT, Eastham JA. Radical prostatectomy: long-term cancer control and recovery of sexual and urinary function ("trifecta"). Urology. 2005;66(5 Suppl):83–94.
19. Freedland SJ, Humphreys EB, Mangold LA, Eisenberger M, Dorey FJ, Walsh PC, et al. Risk of prostate cancer-specific mortality following biochemical recurrence after radical prostatectomy. Jama. 2005;294(4):433–9.
20. Pound CR, Partin AW, Eisenberger MA, Chan DW, Pearson JD, Walsh PC. Natural history of progression after PSA elevation following radical prostatectomy. Jama. 1999;281(17):1591–7.
21. D'Amico AV, Chen MH, Roehl KA, Catalona WJ. Preoperative PSA velocity and the risk of death from prostate cancer after radical prostatectomy. N Engl J Med. 2004;351(2):125–35.
22. Vickers AJ, Till C, Tangen CM, Lilja H, Thompson IM. An empirical evaluation of guidelines on prostate-specific antigen velocity in prostate cancer detection. J Natl Cancer Inst. 2011;103(6):462–9.
23. O'Brien MF, Cronin AM, Fearn PA, Smith B, Stasi J, Guillonneau B, et al. Pretreatment prostate-specific antigen (PSA) velocity and doubling time are associated with outcome but neither improves prediction of outcome beyond pretreatment PSA alone in patients treated with radical prostatectomy. J Clin Oncol. 2009;27(22):3591–7.
24. Bill-Axelson A, Holmberg L, Filen F, Ruutu M, Garmo H, Busch C, et al. Radical prostatectomy versus watchful waiting in localized prostate cancer: the Scandinavian prostate cancer group-4 randomized trial. J Natl Cancer Inst. 2008;100:1144–54.
25. Widmark A, Klepp O, Solberg A, Damber JE, Angelsen A, Fransson P, et al. Endocrine treatment, with or without radiotherapy, in locally advanced prostate cancer (SPCG-7/SFUO-3): an open randomised phase III trial. Lancet. 2009;373:301–8.
26. Wilt TJ, Brawer MK, Barry MJ, Jones KM, Kwon Y, Gingrich JR, et al. The Prostate cancer intervention versus observation Trial: VA/NCI/AHRQ Cooperative Studies Program #407 (PIVOT): design and baseline results of a randomized controlled trial comparing radical prostatectomy to watchful waiting for men with clinically localized prostate cancer. Contemp Clin Trials. 2009;30:81–7.
27. D'Amico AV, Whittington R, Malkowicz SB, Schultz D, Blank K, Broderick GA, et al. Biochemical outcome after radical prostatectomy, external beam radiation therapy, or interstitial radiation therapy for clinically localized prostate cancer. JAMA. 1998;280:969–74.
28. Cooperberg MR, Pasta DJ, Elkin EP, Litwin MS, Latini DM, Du Chane J, et al. The University of California, San Francisco Cancer of the Prostate Risk Assessment score: a straightforward and reliable preoperative predictor of disease recurrence after radical prostatectomy. J Urol. 2005;173:1938–42.
29. Kattan MW, Eastham JA, Stapleton AM, Wheeler TM, Scardino PT. A preoperative nomogram for disease recurrence following radical prostatectomy for prostate cancer. J Natl Cancer Inst. 1998;90:766–71.
30. Eggener SE, Scardino PT, Walsh PC, Han M, Partin AW, Trock BJ, et al. Predicting 15-year prostate cancer specific mortality after radical prostatectomy. J Urol. 2011;185:869–75.
31. Kattan MW, Cuzick J, Fisher G, Berney DM, Oliver T, Foster CS, et al. Nomogram incorporating PSA level to predict cancer-specific survival for men with clinically localized prostate cancer managed without curative intent. Cancer. 2007;112:69–74.
32. Kattan MW, Cuzick J, Fisher G, Berney DM, Oliver T, Foster CS, et al. A nomogram incorporating PSA level to predict cancer-specific survival for men with clinically localized prostate cancer managed without curative intent. Cancer. 2008;112:69–74.
33. Kattan MW, Wheeler TM, Scardino PT. Postoperative nomogram for disease recurrence after radical prostatectomy for prostate cancer. J Clin Oncol. 1999;17: 1499–507.

34. Potters L, Roach M, 3rd, Davis BJ, Stock RG, Ciezki JP, Zelefsky MJ, et al. Postoperative nomogram predicting the 9-year probability of prostate cancer recurrence after permanent prostate brachytherapy using radiation dose as a prognostic variable. Int J Radiat Oncol Biol Phys. 2010;76:1061–5.
35. Stephenson AJ, Kattan MW, Eastham JA, Bianco FJ, Jr., Yossepowitch O, Vickers AJ, et al. Prostate cancer-specific mortality after radical prostatectomy for patients treated in the prostate-specific antigen era. J Clin Oncol. 2009;27:4300–5.
36. Stephenson AJ, Scardino PT, Eastham JA, Bianco FJ, Jr., Dotan ZA, Diblasio CJ, et al. Postoperative nomogram predicting the 10-year probability of prostate cancer recurrence after radical prostatectomy. J Clin Oncol. 2005;23:7005–12.
37. Stephenson AJ, Scardino PT, Eastham JA, Bianco FJ, Jr., Dotan ZA, Fearn PA, et al. Preoperative nomogram predicting the 10-year probability of prostate cancer recurrence after radical prostatectomy. J Natl Cancer Inst. 2006;98:715–7.
38. Zelefsky MJ, Kattan MW, Fearn P, Fearon BL, Stasi JP, Shippy AM, et al. Pretreatment nomogram predicting ten-year biochemical outcome of three-dimensional conformal radiotherapy and intensity-modulated radiotherapy for prostate cancer. Urology. 2007;70:283–7.
39. Meehl PE. Causes and effects of my disturbing little book. J Pers Assess. 1986;50:370–5.
40. Kattan MW. Expert Systems in Medicine. In: Smelser NJ, Baltes PB, editors. International encyclopedia of the social & behavioral sciences. Oxford: Pergamon; 2001. p. 5135–9.
41. Ross PL, Gerigk C, Gonen M, Yossepowitch O, Cagiannos I, Sogani PC, et al. Comparisons of nomograms and urologists' predictions in prostate cancer. Semin Urol Oncol. 2002;20:82–8.
42. D'Amico AV, Whittington R, Malkowicz SB, Schultz D, Schnall M, Tomaszewski JE, et al. A multivariate analysis of clinical and pathological factors that predict for prostate specific antigen failure after radical prostatectomy for prostate cancer. J Urol. 1995;154:131–8.
43. Kattan MW, Leung DH, Brennan MF. Postoperative nomogram for 12-year sarcoma-specific death. J Clin Oncol. 2002;20:791–6.
44. Kattan MW, Zelefsky MJ, Kupelian PA, Scardino PT, Fuks Z, Leibel SA. Pretreatment nomogram for predicting the outcome of three-dimensional conformal radiotherapy in prostate cancer. J Clin Oncol. 2000;18:3352–9.
45. Kattan MW, Zelefsky MJ, Kupelian PA, Cho D, Scardino PT, Fuks Z, et al. Pretreatment nomogram that predicts 5-year probability of metastasis following three-dimensional conformal radiation therapy for localized prostate cancer. J Clin Oncol. 2003;21:4568–71.
46. Kattan MW, Reuter V, Motzer RJ, Katz J, Russo P. A postoperative prognostic nomogram for renal cell carcinoma. J Urol. 2001;166:63–7.
47. Mitchell JA, Cooperberg MR, Elkin EP, Lubeck DP, Mehta SS, Kane CJ, et al. Ability of 2 pretreatment risk assessment methods to predict prostate cancer recurrence after radical prostatectomy: data from CaPSURE. J Urol. 2005;173:1126–31.
48. Kawachi MH, Bahnson RR, Barry M, Busby JE, Carroll PR, Carter HB, et al. NCCN clinical practice guidelines in oncology: prostate cancer. J Natl Compr Canc Netw. 2010;8:162–200.
49. Heidenreich A, Aus G, Bolla M, Joniau S, Matveev VB, Schmid HP, et al. EAU guidelines on prostate cancer. Eur Urol. 2008;53:68–80.
50. Thompson I, Thrasher JB, Aus G, Burnett AL, Canby-Hagino ED, Cookson MS, et al. Guideline for the management of clinically localized prostate cancer: 2007 update. J Urol. 2007;177:2106–31.
51. Cooperberg MR, Moul JW, Carroll PR. The changing face of prostate cancer. J Clin Oncol. 2005;23:8146–51.
52. Vickers AJ, Bianco FJ, Jr., Boorjian S, Scardino PT, Eastham JA. Long-term survival after radical prostatectomy versus external-beam radiotherapy for patients with high-risk prostate cancer. Cancer. 2011;117:2883–91.
53. Cooperberg MR, Vickers AJ, Broering JM, Carroll PR. Comparative risk-adjusted mortality outcomes after primary surgery, radiotherapy, or androgen-deprivation therapy for localized prostate cancer. Cancer. 2010;116:5226–34.
54. Kibel AS, Ciezki JP, Klein EA, Reddy CA, Lubahn JD, Haslag-Minoff J, et al. Survival among men with clinically localized prostate cancer treated with radical prostatectomy or radiation therapy in the prostate specific antigen era. J Urol 2012;187(4):1259–65.
55. Zelefsky MJ, Eastham JA, Cronin AM, Fuks Z, Zhang Z, Yamada Y, et al. Metastasis after radical prostatectomy or external beam radiotherapy for patients with clinically localized prostate cancer: a comparison of clinical cohorts adjusted for case mix. J Clin Oncol. 2010;28:1508–13.
56. Sanda MG, Dunn RL, Michalski J, Sandler HM, Northouse L, Hembroff L, et al. Quality of life and satisfaction with outcome among prostate-cancer survivors. N Engl J Med. 2008;358:1250–61.
57. Litwin MS, Gore JL, Kwan L, Brandeis JM, Lee SP, Withers HR, et al. Quality of life after surgery, external beam irradiation, or brachytherapy for early-stage prostate cancer. Cancer. 2007;109:2239–47.
58. Pardo Y, Guedea F, Aguilo F, Fernandez P, Macias V, Marino A, et al. Quality-of-life impact of primary treatments for localized prostate cancer in patients without hormonal treatment. J Clin Oncol. 2010;28:4687–96.
59. Potosky AL, Davis WW, Hoffman RM, Stanford JL, Stephenson RA, Penson DF, et al. Five-year outcomes after prostatectomy or radiotherapy for prostate cancer: the prostate cancer outcomes study. J Natl Cancer Inst. 2004;96:1358–67.
60. Johansson E, Steineck G, Holmberg L, Johansson JE, Nyberg T, Ruutu M, et al. Long-term quality-of-life outcomes after radical prostatectomy or watchful waiting: the Scandinavian Prostate Cancer Group-4 randomised trial. Lancet Oncol. 2011;12:891–9.
61. Klotz L, Zhang L, Lam A, Nam R, Mamedov A, Loblaw A. Clinical results of long-term follow-up of

a large, active surveillance cohort with localized prostate cancer. J Clin Oncol. 2010;28:126–31.

62. Carter HB, Kettermann A, Warlick C, Metter EJ, Landis P, Walsh PC, et al. Expectant management of prostate cancer with curative intent: an update of the Johns Hopkins experience. J Urol. 2007;178:2359–64. discussion 2364–5.
63. Warlick C, Trock BJ, Landis P, Epstein JI, Carter HB. Delayed versus immediate surgical intervention and prostate cancer outcome. J Natl Cancer Inst. 2006;98:355–7.
64. Patel MI, De CD, Lopez-Corona E, Ohori M, Wheeler T, Scardino PT. An analysis of men with clinically localized prostate cancer who deferred definitive therapy. J Urol. 2004;171:1520–4.
65. Eggener SE, Mueller A, Berglund RK, Ayyathurai R, Soloway C, Soloway MS, et al. A multi-institutional evaluation of active surveillance for low risk prostate cancer. J Urol. 2009;181:1635–41. discussion 1641.
66. Carter CA, Donahue T, Sun L, Wu H, McLeod DG, Amling C, et al. Temporarily deferred therapy (watchful waiting) for men younger than 70 years and with low-risk localized prostate cancer in the prostate-specific antigen era. J Clin Oncol. 2003;21:4001–8.
67. van den Bergh RC, Vasarainen H, van der Poel HG, Vis-Maters JJ, Rietbergen JB, Pickles T, et al. Short-term outcomes of the prospective multicentre 'Prostate Cancer Research International: Active Surveillance' study. BJU Int. 2010;105(7):956–62.
68. van As NJ, Norman AR, Thomas K, Khoo VS, Thompson A, Huddart RA, et al. Predicting the probability of deferred radical treatment for localised prostate cancer managed by active surveillance. Eur Urol. 2008;54:1297–305.
69. Miocinovic R, Jones JS, Pujara AC, Klein EA, Stephenson AJ. Acceptance and durability of surveillance as a management choice in men with screen-detected, low-risk prostate cancer: improved outcomes with stringent enrollment criteria. Urology. 2011;77:980–4.
70. Hugosson J, Carlsson S, Aus G, Bergdahl S, Khatami A, Lodding P, et al. Mortality results from the Goteborg randomised population-based prostate-cancer screening trial. Lancet Oncol. 2011;11:725–32.
71. Soloway MS, Soloway CT, Williams S, Ayyathurai R, Kava B, Manoharan M. Active surveillance; a reasonable management alternative for patients with prostate cancer: the Miami experience. BJU Int. 2008;101:165–9.
72. van den Bergh RC, Steyerberg EW, Khatami A, Aus G, Pihl CG, Wolters T, et al. Is delayed radical prostatectomy in men with low-risk screen-detected prostate cancer associated with a higher risk of unfavorable outcomes? Cancer. 2010;116:1281–90.
73. Duffield AS, Lee TK, Miyamoto H, Carter HB, Epstein JI. Radical prostatectomy findings in patients in whom active surveillance of prostate cancer fails. J Urol. 2009;182:2274–8.
74. Berglund RK, Masterson TA, Vora KC, Eggener SE, Eastham JA, Guillonneau BD. Pathological upgrading and up staging with immediate repeat biopsy in patients eligible for active surveillance. J Urol. 2008;180:1964–7. discussion 1967–8.
75. Saranchuk JW, Kattan MW, Elkin E, Touijer AK, Scardino PT, Eastham JA. Achieving optimal outcomes after radical prostatectomy. J Clin Oncol. 2005;23:4146–51.
76. Farnham SB, Webster TM, Herrell SD, Smith Jr JA. Intraoperative blood loss and transfusion requirements for robotic-assisted radical prostatectomy versus radical retropubic prostatectomy. Urology. 2006; 67:360–3.
77. Webster TM, Herrell SD, Chang SS, Cookson MS, Baumgartner RG, Anderson LW, et al. Robotic assisted laparoscopic radical prostatectomy versus retropubic radical prostatectomy: a prospective assessment of postoperative pain. J Urol. 2005;174:912–4. discussion 914.
78. Nelson B, Kaufman M, Broughton G, Cookson MS, Chang SS, Herrell SD, et al. Comparison of length of hospital stay between radical retropubic prostatectomy and robotic assisted laparoscopic prostatectomy. J Urol. 2007;177:929–31.
79. Wood DP, Schulte R, Dunn RL, Hollenbeck BK, Saur R, Wolf JS, Jr., et al. Short-term health outcome differences between robotic and conventional radical prostatectomy. Urology. 2007;70:945–9.
80. Smith JA, Jr., Chan RC, Chang SS, Herrell SD, Clark PE, Baumgartner R, et al. A comparison of the incidence and location of positive surgical margins in robotic assisted laparoscopic radical prostatectomy and open retropubic radical prostatectomy. J Urol. 2007;178:2385–9. discussion 2389–90.
81. Touijer K, Kuroiwa K, Eastham JA, Vickers A, Reuter VE, Scardino PT, et al. Risk-adjusted analysis of positive surgical margins following laparoscopic and retropubic radical prostatectomy. Eur Urol. 2007;52:1090–6.
82. Touijer K, Eastham JA, Secin FP, Romero Otero J, Serio A, Stasi J, et al. Comprehensive prospective comparative analysis of outcomes between open and laparoscopic radical prostatectomy conducted in 2003 to 2005. J Urol. 2008;179:1811–7. discussion 1817.
83. Vickers AJ, Bianco FJ, Serio AM, Eastham JA, Schrag D, Klein EA, et al. The surgical learning curve for prostate cancer control after radical prostatectomy. J Natl Cancer Inst. 2007;99:1171–7.
84. Vickers AJ, Savage CJ, Hruza M, Tuerk I, Koenig P, Martinez-Pineiro L, et al. The surgical learning curve for laparoscopic radical prostatectomy: a retrospective cohort study. Lancet Oncol. 2009;10:475–80.
85. Eastham JA, Kattan MW, Riedel E, Begg CB, Wheeler TM, Gerigk C, et al. Variations among individual surgeons in the rate of positive surgical margins in radical prostatectomy specimens. J Urol. 2003;170:2292–5.
86. Begg CB, Riedel ER, Bach PB, Kattan MW, Schrag D, Warren JL, et al. Variations in morbidity after radical prostatectomy. N Engl J Med. 2002;346: 1138–44.
87. Thompson IM, Tangen CM, Paradelo J, Lucia MS, Miller G, Troyer D, et al. Adjuvant radiotherapy for pathological T3N0M0 prostate cancer significantly reduces risk of metastases and improves survival: long-term followup of a randomized clinical trial. J Urol. 2009;191:956–62.

88. Stephenson AJ, Shariat SF, Zelefsky MJ, Kattan MW, Butler EB, Teh BS, et al. Salvage radiotherapy for recurrent prostate cancer after radical prostatectomy. JAMA. 2004;291:1325–32.
89. Bolla M, van Poppel H, Collette L, van Cangh P, Vekemans K, Da Pozzo L, et al. Postoperative radiotherapy after radical prostatectomy: a randomised controlled trial (EORTC trial 22911). Lancet. 2005;366:572–8.
90. Klotz LH, Goldenberg SL, Jewett MA, Fradet Y, Nam R, Barkin J, et al. Long-term followup of a randomized trial of 0 versus 3 months of neoadjuvant androgen ablation before radical prostatectomy. J Urol. 2003;170:791–4.
91. Kupelian PA, Potters L, Khuntia D, Ciezki JP, Reddy CA, Reuther AM, et al. Radical prostatectomy, external beam radiotherapy <72 Gy, external beam radiotherapy > or =72 Gy, permanent seed implantation, or combined seeds/external beam radiotherapy for stage T1-T2 prostate cancer. Int J Radiat Oncol Biol Phys. 2004;58:25–33.
92. Kuban DA, Thames HD, Levy LB, Horwitz EM, Kupelian PA, Martinez AA, et al. Long-term multi-institutional analysis of stage T1-T2 prostate cancer treated with radiotherapy in the PSA era. Int J Radiat Oncol Biol Phys. 2003;57:915–28.
93. Zelefsky MJ, Leibel SA, Gaudin PB, Kutcher GJ, Fleshner NE, Venkatramen ES, et al. Dose escalation with three-dimensional conformal radiation therapy affects the outcome in prostate cancer. Int J Radiat Oncol Biol Phys. 1998;41:491–500.
94. Zietman AL, DeSilvio ML, Slater JD, Rossi CJ, Jr., Miller DW, Adams JA, et al. Comparison of conventional-dose vs high-dose conformal radiation therapy in clinically localized adenocarcinoma of the prostate: a randomized controlled trial. JAMA. 2005;294:1233–9.
95. Bolla M, Collette L, Blank L, Warde P, Dubois JB, Mirimanoff RO, et al. Long-term results with immediate androgen suppression and external irradiation in patients with locally advanced prostate cancer (an EORTC study): a phase III randomised trial. Lancet. 2002;360:103–6.
96. Hanks GE, Pajak TF, Porter A, Grignon D, Brereton H, Venkatesan V, et al. Phase III trial of long-term adjuvant androgen deprivation after neoadjuvant hormonal cytoreduction and radiotherapy in locally advanced carcinoma of the prostate: the Radiation Therapy Oncology Group Protocol 92–02. J Clin Oncol. 2003;21:3972–8.
97. D'Amico AV, Chen MH, Renshaw AA, Loffredo M, Kantoff PW. Androgen suppression and radiation vs radiation alone for prostate cancer: a randomized trial. JAMA. 2008;299:289–95.
98. Lawton CA, DeSilvio M, Roach M, 3rd, Uhl V, Kirsch R, Seider M, et al. An update of the phase III trial comparing whole pelvic to prostate only radiotherapy and neoadjuvant to adjuvant total androgen suppression: updated analysis of RTOG 94–13, with emphasis on unexpected hormone/radiation interactions. Int J Radiat Oncol Biol Phys. 2007;69:646–55.
99. Bianco FJ, Jr., Scardino PT, Stephenson AJ, Diblasio CJ, Fearn PA, Eastham JA. Long-term oncologic results of salvage radical prostatectomy for locally recurrent prostate cancer after radiotherapy. Int J Radiat Oncol Biol Phys. 2005;62:448–53.
100. Izawa JI, Madsen LT, Scott SM, Tran JP, McGuire EJ, Von Eschenbach AC, et al. Salvage cryotherapy for recurrent prostate cancer after radiotherapy: variables affecting patient outcome. J Clin Oncol. 2002; 20:2664–71.
101. Pisters LL, Rewcastle JC, Donnelly BJ, Lugnani FM, Katz AE, Jones JS. Salvage prostate cryoablation: initial results from the cryo on-line data registry. J Urol. 2008;180:559–63. discussion 563–4.
102. Stephenson AJ, Scardino PT, Bianco FJ, Jr., Diblasio CJ, Fearn PA, Eastham JA. Morbidity and functional outcomes of salvage radical prostatectomy for locally recurrent prostate cancer after radiation therapy. J Urol. 2004;172:2239–43.
103. Brenner DJ, Curtis RE, Hall EJ, Ron E. Second malignancies in prostate carcinoma patients after radiotherapy compared with surgery. Cancer. 2000; 88:398–406.
104. Moon K, Stukenborg GJ, Keim J, Theodorescu D. Cancer incidence after localized therapy for prostate cancer. Cancer. 2006;107:991–8.
105. D'Amico AV, Moran BJ, Braccioforte MH, Dosoretz D, Salenius S, Katin M, et al. Risk of death from prostate cancer after brachytherapy alone or with radiation, androgen suppression therapy, or both in men with high-risk disease. J Clin Oncol. 2009;27(24):3923–8.
106. Immediate versus deferred treatment for advanced prostatic cancer: initial results of the Medical Research Council Trial. The Medical Research Council Prostate Cancer Working Party Investigators Group. Br J Urol. 1997;79:235–46.
107. Studer UE, Whelan P, Albrecht W, Casselman J, de Reijke T, Hauri D, et al. Immediate or deferred androgen deprivation for patients with prostate cancer not suitable for local treatment with curative intent: European Organisation for Research and Treatment of Cancer (EORTC) Trial 30891. J Clin Oncol. 2006;24:1868–76.
108. Smith MR, Lee WC, Brandman J, Wang Q, Botteman M, Pashos CL. Gonadotropin-releasing hormone agonists and fracture risk: a claims-based cohort study of men with nonmetastatic prostate cancer. J Clin Oncol. 2005;23:7897–903.
109. Krupski TL, Smith MR, Chan Lee W, Pashos CL, Brandman J, Wang Q, et al. Natural history of bone complications in men with prostate carcinoma initiating androgen deprivation therapy. Cancer. 2004; 101:541–9.
110. D'Amico AV, Denham JW, Crook J, Chen MH, Goldhaber SZ, Lamb DS, et al. Influence of androgen suppression therapy for prostate cancer on the frequency and timing of fatal myocardial infarctions. J Clin Oncol. 2007;25:2420–5.
111. Nanda A, Chen MH, Braccioforte MH, Moran BJ, D'Amico AV. Hormonal therapy use for prostate cancer and mortality in men with coronary artery disease-induced congestive heart failure or myocardial infarction. JAMA. 2009;302:866–73.

# Management of Urethral Strictures in Men

**15**

Richard A. Santucci and Mang L. Chen

## Introduction

Male urethral stricture disease accounts for about 5,000 inpatient and 150,000 outpatient visits annually, leading to an estimated yearly health-care cost of greater than $6,000 per patient [1]. It has an estimated prevalence as high as 0.6% in some populations and causes significant obstructive and bothersome voiding symptoms. Management varies from minimally invasive urethral dilations and urethrotomies to complex open reconstructive surgeries.

In this chapter, we review the etiology, diagnosis, evaluation, and treatment of male urethral disease, which includes an overview of endoscopic management and detailed descriptions of open reconstructive principles and techniques.

## Urethral Anatomy

The urethra is divided into six sections: the (1) fossa navicularis, (2) pendulous or penile urethra, (3) bulbar urethra, (4) membranous urethra, (5) prostatic urethra, and (6) bladder neck. Functionally, the urethra is often divided into two segments: the anterior and posterior urethra. The anterior urethra includes the bulbar urethra, penile urethra, and fossa navicularis. The posterior urethra includes the membranous and prostatic urethra, and the bladder neck. Spongy highly vascularized tissue called the corpus spongiosum encompasses almost the entire urethra. The urethra is located eccentrically within the spongiosum: the penile urethra is in the middle of the spongiosum, but more proximally, the bulbar urethra is dorsally located [2].

The blood supply to the urethra is based on the blood supply to the corpus spongiosum, which receives its nutrients directly from the bulbar branch of the common penile artery. The common penile artery is the terminal branch of the internal pudendal artery and divides into the bulbar, cavernosal, and dorsal arteries. The paired dorsal arteries provide additional retrograde blood flow to the spongiosum and urethra at the glans penis [2].

## Etiology

Injury to the urethra or corpus spongiosum can lead to scar formation. Resultant urethral strictures may be traumatic, iatrogenic, inflammatory, or congenital in origin. In general, management depends on stricture location and length more so than etiology. Exceptions include pelvic fracture

R.A. Santucci, MD, FACS (✉)
Department of Urology, The Detroit Medical Center, 4160 John R. Suite 1017, Detroit, MI 48201, USA
e-mail: rsantucc@dmc.org

M.L. Chen, MD
Department of Urology, Detroit Receiving Hospital, Harper Professional Building, 4160 John R, suite 1017, Detroit, MI 48201, USA

D.A. Shoskes (ed.), *Urological Men's Health: A Guide for Urologists and Primary Care Physicians*, Current Clinical Urology, DOI 10.1007/978-1-61779-900-6_15,
© Springer Science+Business Media New York 2012

urethral distraction defects (PFUDDs) and inflammatory strictures associated with lichen sclerosis (see below).

## Diagnosis and Evaluation

The most common symptoms associated with urethral stricture disease include a weak urinary stream, incomplete emptying, urinary tract infections, hesitancy, and urinary retention. These obstructive urinary symptoms are also seen in men with benign prostatic hyperplasia, so an accurate diagnosis can sometimes be difficult. Performing a thorough history and physical with specific assessment of a patient's voiding symptoms, neurologic and traumatic history, and surgical history helps elucidate the diagnosis. Additional diagnostic tools are urinalysis, uroflowmetry, and bladder ultrasounds, which assess for infections, urine flow, and post-void residuals, respectively. A quick test for the presence of a urethral stricture is the passage of a 16 French Foley catheter in the clinic setting. Flexible cystoscopy quickly identifies the location and severity of urethral strictures.

With suspected urethral strictures, imaging is crucial for determination of location, number, length, and density of the stricture disease. Retrograde urethrograms reveal the location, number, and length of strictures. However, contrast can sometimes fail to show the urethra proximal to the stricture. Simultaneous voiding cystourethrograms or cystograms are performed in this situation to better delineate the urethra proximal to the stricture. Sonography has also been described as a useful modality for stricture evaluation, but this is rarely required at our institution [3].

## Treatment Overview

Management depends on the length, number, and location of the urethral stricture. It also depends on the patient's goals. For example, poor operative candidates with short strictures could be managed with urethral dilations or direct visual internal urethrotomies (DVIU) instead of open reconstruction. The procedures will ultimately fail, but they are minimally invasive and may be preferred to very elderly or unwell patients.

If the strictures are especially long or complex, cystostomy ("suprapubic") tube placement is a good option for those unwilling or too unwell to undergo definitive surgical treatment. Finally, patients who cannot tolerate or do not want complete reconstruction might elect to have a perineal urethrostomy—a surgical connection between the urethra and perineal skin several centimeters anterior to the anus, which effectively bypasses the more distal strictured urethra.

Younger and healthier patients with urethral strictures are better served with definitive surgical reconstruction. For anterior urethral strictures, excision and primary anastomosis, onlay urethroplasties, and staged Johanson urethroplasties will often suffice [4]. For more complex strictures like those seen in patients with prior hypospadias repairs, long and panurethral strictures, PFUDDs, restenosis after urethral stenting, and strictures associated with prostate cancer therapy, a more complex and flexible reconstructive approach is required [5]. As a last but often effective resort, a perineal urethrostomy can be created.

## Urethral Dilation and Internal Urethrotomy

Urethral dilation and internal urethrotomy are the least invasive surgical techniques for managing urethral strictures. Dilation can be done effectively by first placing a wire past the stricture and into the bladder followed by serial dilations with increasingly larger dilators or balloon dilating catheters. Internal urethrotomies are done with an endoscopic scalpel or a holmium laser with equal efficacy. The long-term outcomes between dilations and urethrotomies are very similar and have a high recurrence (failure) rate. Steenkamp et al. [6] prospectively evaluated 210 men with strictures who were randomized to receive either urethral dilations or internal urethrotomies and followed them every 3 months for the first year and then annually thereafter for several years. They concluded that stricture recurrence was common with a 40% recurrence rate at 12 months for short strictures, and 80% for longer strictures. Recurrence was time dependent. Most recurred within 6 months, and those who did not restricture after 12 months were stricture-free for longer periods of time. Overall, the long-term success rate of dilation or urethrotomy is low. Santucci and Eisenberg confirmed the low success rate of urethrotomy by performing a retrospective chart review of 76 patients who underwent urethrotomy [7]. They found that the stricture-free rate was 8% after the initial urethrotomy with a median time to recurrence of 7 months. The stricture-free rate was even lower at 6% for the second urethrotomy with a median time to recurrence of 9 months. Third urethrotomies had a stricture-free rate of 9% with a median time to recurrence of 3 months. Fourth and fifth urethrotomies had 0% stricture-free rates.

Given the ease of performing urethral dilations and DVIUs, they will always have a role in the initial or palliative management of urethral strictures. In fact, for younger and healthier patients with short bulbar urethral strictures, a single attempt at dilation or urethrotomy may even be a cost-effective and morbidity-minimizing way to manage initial strictures [8]. Those suffering disease recurrence can then undergo definitive open reconstruction without overtly adverse effects from their prior procedure. Stated another way, dilation and urethrotomy should be considered temporizing measures for planned definitive reconstructive surgery.

## Urethral Stents

Urethral stents treat urethral strictures and prevent stricture recurrence after dilation or internal urethrotomy. Initial reports were "good," but with longer follow-up, complications such as pain, infection, stent migration, restenosis, and encrustation or stone formation became much more prevalent. Urolume (American Medical Systems; Minnetonka, MN) is a permanent implantable urethral stent sometimes used for strictures. The North American Study Group long-term data showed that the overall success rate of stents maintaining urethral patency after 11 years without complication was less than 30% [9]. Another follow-up study from the Netherlands found that of the 15 patients implanted, only 2 had subjectively satisfactory results at 10 years [10]. Because of their ease of use, stents are often overutilized by practitioners unfamiliar with FDA requirements that they not be placed in a penile location, not be used for strictures over 3 cm, and not be used in patients under age 30. In general, urethral stents have been abandoned by most experts for bulbar urethral strictures (and were never approved for penile urethral strictures). We must also emphasize that urethral stents should never be used for urethral scarring after posterior urethral distraction defects (PFUDDs).

Despite these adverse effects, urethral stents have some utility in patients with anastomotic stricture after radical prostatectomy. Eisenberg et al. sought to further narrow the indications for urethral stent placement by analyzing their results from posterior urethral stent placement in patients with prior prostate cancer therapy [11]. They concluded that stent placement in this group of patients is reasonable but that complications are common and include stricture recurrence, pain, migration, infection, and incontinence.

## Open Reconstruction

Many operative procedures have been described for surgical management of anterior urethral strictures. However, at our institution, three main techniques are performed that satisfactorily treat most cases of anterior urethral stricture diseases: anastomotic urethroplasty, buccal mucosal graft, onlay urethroplasty, and Johanson staged urethroplasty. PFUDDs are almost universally treated by simple anastomotic urethroplasty.

Long, panurethral, and complex strictures (perhaps associated with prior hypospadias repair, prostate cancer therapy, or urethral stent restenosis) may require complex, creative approaches. Examples include Johanson urethroplasty with augmented urethral plates and combined dorsal and ventral onlay with various grafts and flaps. Even bailout perineal urethrostomy is a viable option. Many of these rare and advanced techniques are beyond the scope of this manuscript.

## Anterior Urethroplasty

### Anastomotic Urethroplasty

#### Indication

Patients ideally suited for anastomotic urethroplasty have short strictures (<2 cm) in the bulbar urethra. Anastomotic repair of long or pendulous urethral strictures can lead to chordee.

#### Surgical Technique

Patients are placed in the high lithotomy position and carefully padded. Preoperative imaging and intraopertive 22F catheters help locate the distal aspect of the stricture. The perineum is then incised to expose the bulbospongiosus muscle superficial to the stricture location. We incise this muscle longitudinally to identify the underlying corpus spongiosum and urethra. We then detubularize the urethra starting at the tip of the catheter or bougie, then through the strictured segment. An 8F feeding tube or 0.035 inch guide wire is then placed into the bladder through the proximal lumen of the stricture and we continue the incision proximally until we identify normal urethral tissue.

Prior to stricture excision, we bougie (up to 30F if possible) the nondiseased distal and proximal urethral segments to verify patency. We then mobilize these segments from surrounding tissue to ensure a tension-free anastomosis. The strictured urethral segment is subsequently removed and we spatulate the healthy urethral segments. For PFUDD, we circumferentially place 12 simple interrupted 5–0 polydiaxanone (PDS) or polyglyconate (Maxon) sutures around the spatulated urethral segments and tie them. The dorsal anastomotic sutures are tied first to allow direct visualization of final catheter placement (16F silicone). The remaining ventral anastomotic sutures are then tied. For anterior urethroplasty, we anastomose the dorsal urethra with multiple simple interrupted 5–0 PDS suture. A deep layer of ventral urethral mucosa is sewn with 5–0 PDS interrupted sutures and a second layer of tunica of the spongiosum is closed with separate 5–0 PDS sutures. This allows the spongiosum to remain in continuity, and bathe the anastomosis in oxygenated blood.

After hemostasis is obtained, we close the bulbospongiosus muscle and dartos fascia with a running polyglactin (Vicryl) suture. Local anesthesia (0.5% bupivicaine with epinephrine) is injected along the incision followed by skin closure with interrupted vertical mattress sutures of 2–0 chromic gut or fast-dissolving polyglactin suture. Drains are neither placed nor required.

#### Postoperative Care

Anastomotic urethroplasties are either outpatient procedures or overnight observations. Patients are given Celebrex (celecoxib) 400 mg in the recovery room, given an ice bag to use off and on for the first 24 h, and sent home with oral pain medication. We remind patients and nurses to avoid catheter manipulation and direct sitting pressure on the perineal wound. We prescribe prophylactic antibiotics (nitrofurantoin 100 mg by mouth twice a day) until after the catheter is removed.

Anterior anastomotic urethroplasty patients need only a short period of catheterization. PFUDD patients require 2–3 weeks. We perform a VCUG to verify that the anastomosis has healed. If extravasation is noted, a 14 or 16F coude catheter is placed carefully and we repeat the VCUG 1–2 weeks later. Further follow-ups are scheduled every 4 months for the first year and yearly after that, and include assessment of obstructive voiding symptoms, measurement of post-void residuals, and performance of uroflowmetries.

#### Complications

As with any surgery, bleeding, pain, wound infection, and skin paresthesias can be seen, but the occurrence is rare. More common and troublesome is the prevalence of erectile dysfunction and chordee that can occur after anastomotic urethroplasty, which ranges from 4% to 26% [12].

### Buccal Mucosal Graft Onlay Urethroplasty

#### Indication

Buccal mucosa is ideal for urethral reconstruction because it is hairless, resilient in a moist environment, and elastic (Fig. 15.1). Furthermore,

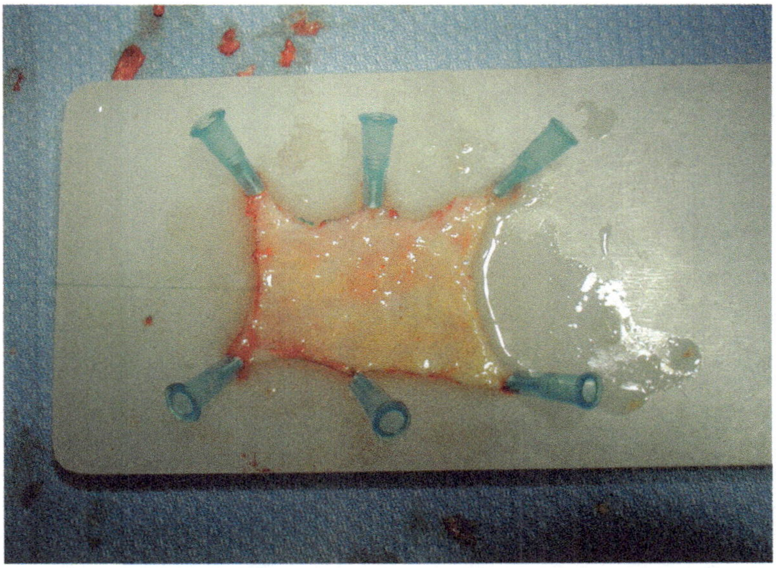

**Fig. 15.1** Harvested and defatted buccal graft

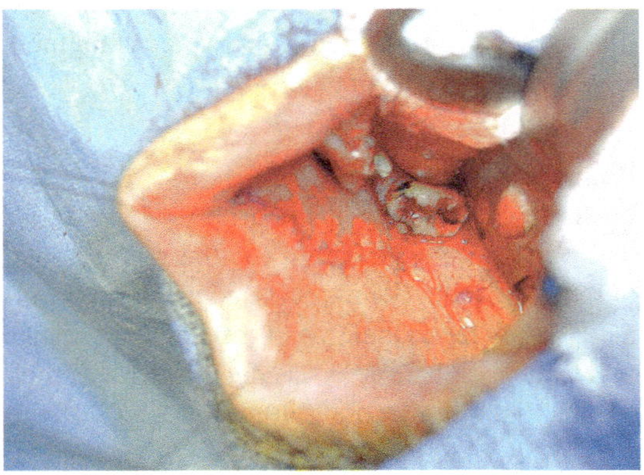

**Fig. 15.2** Buccal graft harvest surgical site

it easily assimilates to the host tissue with good graft survival rates, and it is easy to harvest with minimal morbidity to the donor site (Fig. 15.2). At our institution, buccal mucosa onlay urethroplasty is the procedure of choice for anterior urethral strictures given its high success rates and low morbidity [13–16].

## Surgical Technique

Patient preoperative workup and positioning are the same as that for anastomotic urethroplasty described earlier. The key difference arises is that the stricture is incised ventrally in the midline but not excised. Rather, we place the buccal graft in this ventral defect with the mucosa facing the urethral lumen—a ventral onlay. The buccal mucosal graft can be placed ventrally, dorsally, or laterally with near equal outcomes. However, the advantages of the ventral onlay include less dissection, decreased risk of injury to the corpora, and shorter operative times with resultant lower risks of complications. Again, a 5–0 polydioxanone or polygluconate suture is used, but for the buccal mucosal graft onlay technique, we run the suture on each side starting at each apex and lock every third stitch (Fig. 15.3). Prior to completing the watertight anastomosis, we insert a 16F silicone or silicone-coated latex catheter under direct vision. The tunica of the corpus spongiosum is then closed over the graft with a running 4–0 polyglyconate suture (Fig. 15.4) followed by closure of the bulbospongiosus muscle, dartos fascia, and skin as described before.

For more distal penile urethral stricture repairs, the surgeon must be aware that the ventral corpus spongiosum tissue is thin with less blood supply than the bulbar urethral spongiosal tissue. This decreases the ability of a ventral buccal mucosa graft to take in this area, prompting an alternative route of grafting. Dorsal buccal onlays are ideal in this situation since the vascular bed composed of the corpora cavernosa is bet-

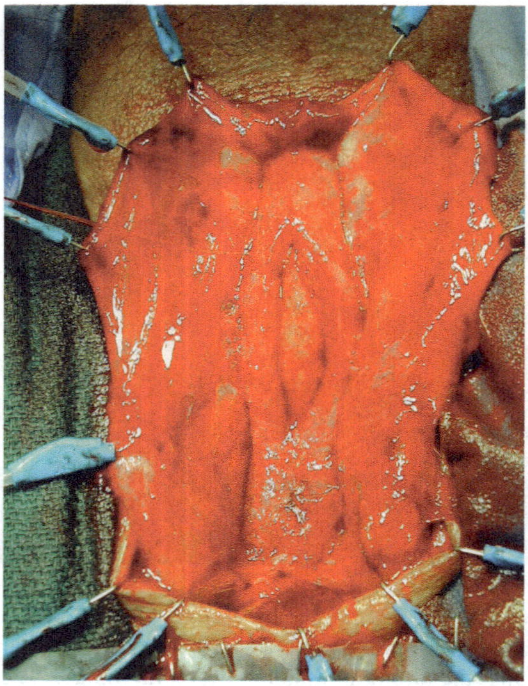

**Fig. 15.3** Ventral urethrotomy and ventral buccal graft placement

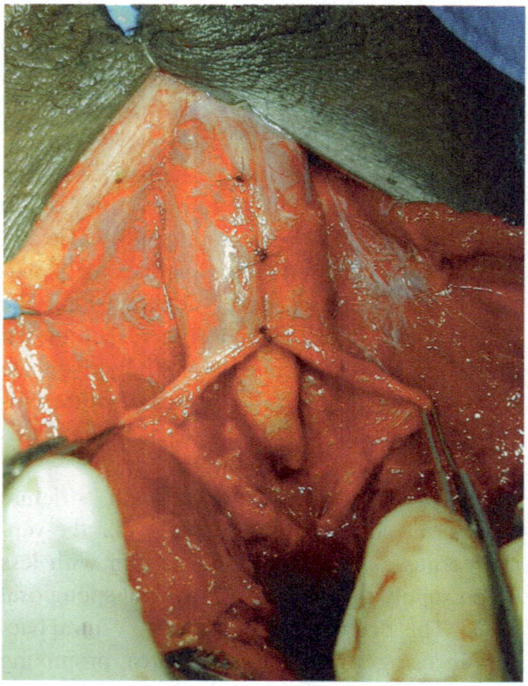

**Fig. 15.4** After closure of the tunica of the spongiosum over the ventral buccal graft

ter vascularized than the tenuous ventral corpus spongiosum at this location. To perform a dorsal buccal onlay procedure, we position the patient supine. We then deglove the penile shaft skin as proximally as possible followed by the separation of the corpora spongiosum from the corpora cavernosa. A catheter is placed to delineate the stricture site and a ventral and dorsal incision is made through the diseased urethral segment. We then secure the graft to the corpora cavernosa (the dorsal side of the urethra) with 5–0 PDS or polyglyconate. We close the ventral incision in multiple layers. However, prior to finishing the urethral-onlay anastomosis, a 16F catheter is placed under direct vision, alternatively, an Asopa technique (where a ventral urethrotomy is made to allow access to place a dorsal graft, then closed). We subsequently obtain hemostasis and close the skin with interrupted 3–0 or 4–0 chromic sutures. Local anesthesia by way of a penile block can augment postoperative pain control.

## Postoperative Care

Postoperative care is identical to that of anastomotic urethroplasty except for the management of the donor site. We instruct patients to intermittently apply ice to their face for the first 24 h, take oral pain medication as needed, and rinse their mouth four times a day with chlorhexidine gluconate after every meal for 1 week postoperatively. Diet restrictions include clear liquids on the day of surgery, full liquids the day after, and a regular diet thereafter.

## Complications

Complications from this procedure are very similar to those of anastomotic urethroplasty. The main difference and advantage of this procedure is that there is a lower risk of developing erectile dysfunction and chordee. Complications for the buccal mucosa donor site include bleeding, pain, bite contracture, facial swelling, and injury to Stensen's duct, but these complications are exceedingly rare. The most common complaint is bite contracture—a temporary nuisance that typically resolves within 3 months.

## Johanson Urethroplasty

### Indication

For patients with long anterior urethral strictures, anastomotic and buccal onlay urethroplasties are often insufficient. These strictures are therefore managed with a two-stage Johanson urethroplasty: the first stage is creation of a dorsal urethral plate; the second stage is tubularization of the dorsal plate. Specifically, adult patients with urethral stricture after childhood hypospadias repair and patients with lichen sclerosis of the penis do poorly with one-stage techniques and are excellent candidates for the two-stage Johanson technique.

### Surgical Technique

The urethra is intubated with a catheter if possible, and a ventral longitudinal incision is made through the skin and urethra to detubularize the urethra proximally until normal tissue is encountered. We then sew the edges of the urethra to the skin edges to recreate a hairless dorsal urethral plate. On occasion, when a 3 cm width urethral plate cannot be created due to insufficient native urethra and penile skin, a dorsal buccal graft onlay is used in the first stage (Fig. 15.5).

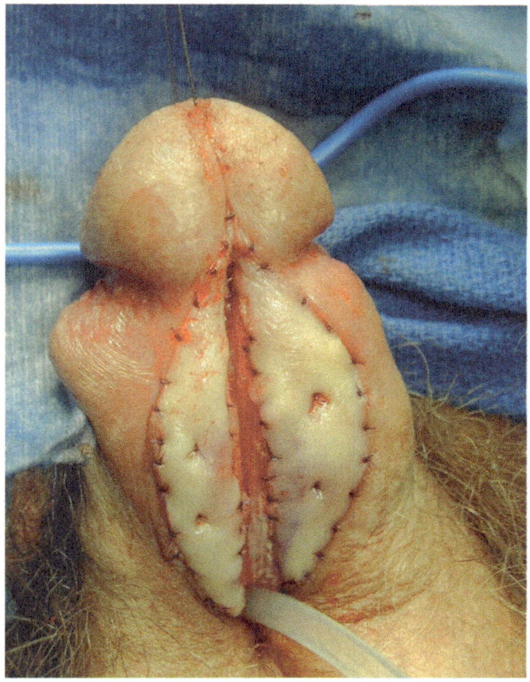

**Fig. 15.5** Johanson urethroplasty with buccal graft

We reevaluate the patient 5 months later to assess his candidacy for the second-stage procedure. If the urethral plate is 3 cm or wider, the patient is scheduled for retubularization (Fig. 15.6). At this time, the urethral plate edges are demarcated, incised, and dissected free. Care is taken not to thin the urethral plate so much as to put the tissue at risk for devascularization. We then retubularize the plate over a 16F catheter in multiple layers with fine absorbable suture (Fig. 15.7). In addition, we purposefully create a large meatus to avoid stricture recurrence at the fossa navicularis. Sometimes we encounter a dorsal urethral plate that is inadequate for the second-stage Johanson urethroplasty. If buccal mucosal graft was not used before, we add a buccal mucosal graft onlay and have the patient return 6 months later for reassessment of the plate and schedule a third-stage urethral retubularization procedure.

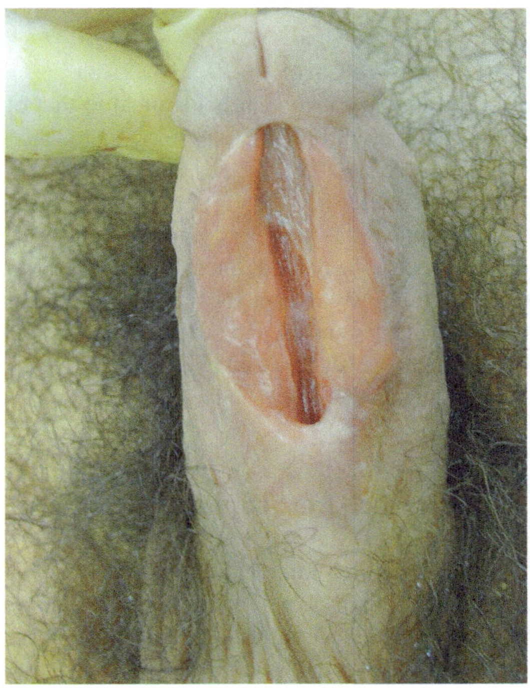

**Fig. 15.6** After healing, Johanson urethroplasty with buccal graft

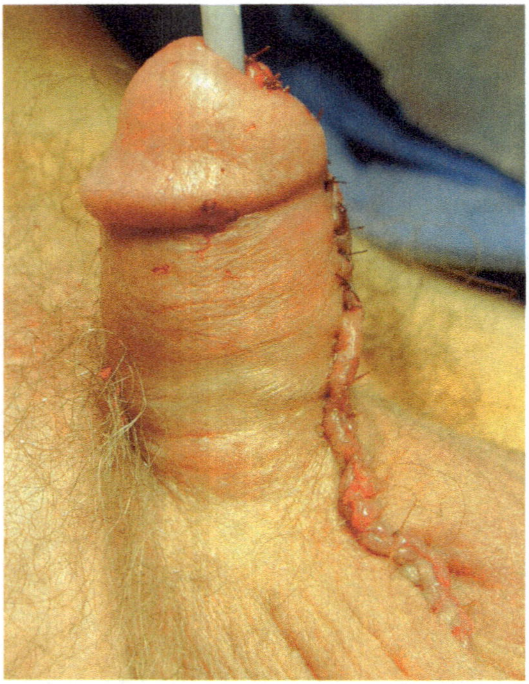

**Fig. 15.7** After second-stage Johanson urethroplasty

### Postoperative Care

Postoperative management is identical to that of anastomotic urethroplasty.

### Complications

The complications are very similar to anastomotic urethroplasty and buccal mucosal graft only urethroplasty except for the slightly higher risk of meatal stenosis and stricture recurrence. Meatal stenosis is decreased by purposefully creating a megameatus.

## Complicated Urethroplasty

Urethral strictures after childhood hypospadias repair, long bulbar and panurethral strictures, PFUDDS, restenosis after urethral stent placement, and strictures associated with prostatic cancer therapy require complex urethroplasties for appropriate management. Surgeons must therefore be flexible in their approach.

### Urethral Stricture After Hypospadias Repair

Hypospadias repair is a relatively common pediatric urologic procedure. Hypospadias has an incidence of 8 in 1,000, making it one of the most common congenital urethral defects [17]. Surgical repair in infancy and childhood has a good short-term success rate, but the long-term complication rates are as high as 30% [18]. Adults with complications present at various ages and with various symptoms often related to bladder outlet obstruction including a weak stream, frequency, incomplete emptying, epididymitis, and prostatitis. Rarely, an adult will present with renal failure from a decompensated bladder [19]. Other complications include chordee, residual hypospadias, intraurethral hair, urethral diverticula, and urethral stones.

Meatal stenosis after childhood hypospadias repair is perhaps the simplest complication to correct because dilation and/or outpatient meatotomy are easily performed. However, for more complex urethral strictures, a one- or multiple-staged approach with a Johanson-type urethroplasty is often warranted. The goal is to create a usable dorsal urethral plate by ventrally incising the entire urethral stricture followed by retubularization with or without the aid of a buccal or skin graft. If the plate is not at least 3 cm in width, we supplement it with buccal mucosa dorsal onlays. We retubularize the dorsal plate 5–6 months later. Of note, local genital skin flaps are often not usable for urethral plate augmentation due to the poor vascularity associated with penile skin from prior hypospadias repair.

Some surgeons believe that single-stage repairs have higher success rates than multistage repairs, and that buccal grafts fare better than penile skin grafts [20]. The overall success rate for single- and multistage repair was 75% after a mean follow-up of almost 3 years. However, given the complexity and length of most hypospadias-associated urethral stricture disease, we found that a multistage approach often works better. A confirmatory study by Meeks et al. reported an overall 86% success rate with multistaged repair of long urethral strictures after a median follow-up of 23 months. Furthermore, a recent review by Mangera et al. [21] looked at graft augmentation urethroplasties for anterior urethral strictures. The authors found that two-stage urethroplasty for penile urethral strictures had a higher success rate (91% vs. 76%) than the single-stage procedure [22].

## Long Bulbar and Panurethral Strictures

A long bulbar stricture is typically >7 cm and cannot be treated with a single buccal mucosal graft. Therefore, panurethral and long bulbar strictures require multiple grafts, including two in-line buccal grafts, a buccal graft combined with a local genital skin flap, or other graft combinations. Reconstruction can also be a single procedure or a staged repair. Local skin flaps can be obtained from scrotal or penile skin, and free skin grafts from the abdomen, flank, thigh, or postauricular region (we prefer hairless flank skin as a donor). Mucosal free grafts can be obtained from the mouth (buccal, lingual). We avoid lower lip grafts assiduously because of unacceptably high complication rates (lip scarring, lip anesthesia). Bladder or colon grafts have been described, but donor site morbidity and difficulty in harvesting these tissues have eliminated their use in our practice.

For long strictures treated with a ventral buccal onlay, we suspect higher failure rates than with shorter strictures (<4 cm). In this case, we perform a "double graft" technique. We place a dorsal skin graft followed by a ventral buccal graft (Fig. 15.8). Palminteri et al. described this technique in their management of 48 patients with inadequate urethral plates and stenotic rings [23]. After incising the strictured urethra ventrally to expose the lumen, the authors described three techniques to augment the dorsal urethral plate. The first was transversely incising the urethral plate and freeing the edges from the underlying tunica followed by suturing a buccal graft to the tunica and the edges of the urethral tissue. The second was making a longitudinal incision in the dorsal urethral plate with incorporation of a

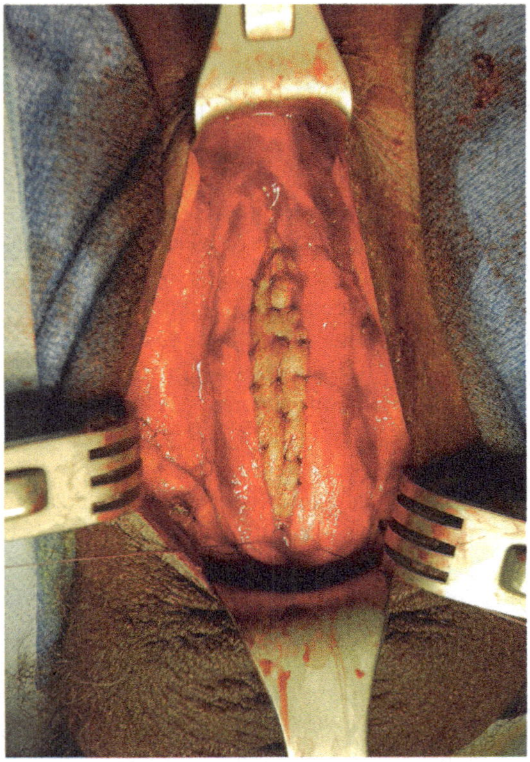

**Fig. 15.8** Double graft technique for long bulbar urethral stricture, with dorsal full thickness skin graft and simultaneous ventral onlay buccal graft

buccal mucosal graft to reconstruct the urethral plate. The third option for forming an adequate dorsal urethral plate includes excising up to 1 cm of atretic urethral mucosa, leaving the underlying spongiosum tissue intact, and sewing the distal and proximal ends together. (I call this a "modified augmented roof strip anastomotic urethroplasty.") Once the dorsal plate was adequately constructed, a ventral graft or flap of either buccal mucosal tissue or local penile skin was used to complete the urethroplasty. This simultaneous single stage dorsal and ventral graft technique has a success rate of 89% at 22 months follow-up.

Another option for long strictures is the combined use of buccal grafts and genital skin island flaps, as described by Berglund and Angermeier [24]. In their series of 18 patients with a mean stricture length of 15 cm, they described using depilated genital skin and buccal mucosal grafts to reconstruct extensive anterior urethral strictures in a single procedure. Their success rate was 83% with only 3 of the 18 patients having stricture recurrence. However, we are concerned about the use of depilated scrotal skin because hair re-growth eventually occurs in all patients, and can cause complications of urethral stones or obstruction by a tangled hairball in the urethra.

If buccal mucosa and genital skin flaps are unavailable, other graft options include split thickness or full thickness skin, tunica albuginea, and colonic/bladder mucosa. Dalpiaz et al. reviewed their series of 27 patients who had urethral stricture recurrence after prior urethroplasty [25]. They describe using split thickness skin grafts (STSG) from the thigh for dorsal onlay urethroplasty with a success rate of 93% after mean follow-up of 32 months. (We remain skeptical about split skin grafts because of their tendency toward contraction, and would likely use a full thickness skin graft harvested from the hairless flank area.) Mathur and Sharma reviewed 86 patients with panurethral strictures who had tunica albuginea grafts [26]. Their mean follow-up was 36 months with a reported success rate of 89.5%. Xu et al. reviewed their experience with end-to-end anastomosis with tubularized colonic grafts after excising the diseased urethral segment [27]. The reported success rate was 86% with a mean follow-up of 54 months. The obvious disadvantage for this technique is the need for colon resection and its associated risks and morbidity, but it appears to be a viable alternative for complex urethral reconstruction in patients who desire restoration of normal voiding.

In patients with prior failed urethroplasties or with multiple medical comorbidities with no desire to undergo a complex urethral reconstruction procedure, a perineal urethrostomy is a good option with high satisfaction rates [28]. Perineal urethrostomies should be performed in a side-to-side fashion much like in first-stage Johanson urethroplasties. For more proximal strictures, the surrounding skin may need to be mobilized to expose the unaffected bulbar urethra, which is done through creation of a "U" flap from inferior perineal skin.

## Pelvic Fracture Urethral Distraction Defects

Urethral defects associated with pelvic trauma are oftentimes avulsion injuries with a resultant cylinder of scar bridging the disconnected urethral tissue. They are commonly referred to as posterior urethral strictures, but these strictures are not always posterior and are not true strictures. Therefore, the more accurate term is pelvic fracture urethral distraction defects, or PFUDDs.

Initial management is urethral realignment followed by delayed urethroplasty via scar excision and primary anastomosis, which—depending on scar location and length—usually does not require pubectomy or urethral lengthening procedures. Cooperberg et al. examined 134 patients who underwent removal of fibrotic scar tissue followed by tension-free anastomosis [29]. The success rate was 84% over a median follow-up of 11 months. Recurrent stricture occurred in 17 patients: 12 were managed endoscopically and 5 required repeat anastomotic urethroplasty. Shenfeld et al. favor repeat excision with primary anastomosis for stricture recurrence from prior PFUDDs repair [30].

We strongly favor direct anastomosis for PFUDDs and have never failed to achieve a tensionless anastomosis. However, if somehow primary tension-free anastomosis cannot be performed, another modality for treatment of PFUDDS is excision of the scar and mobilization and advancement of the distal bulbar urethra proximally to the prostatic urethra and bladder neck. Wang and colleagues reviewed their findings from 113 patients who underwent this urethral pull-through operation [31]. About a quarter of these patients had prior urethroplasty, and there were only four patients who suffered stricture recurrence during follow-up of 48.5 months. We emphasize that most experts are able to achieve a tensionless anastomosis even in redo cases and would favor a standard anastomotic urethroplasty instead of a pull-through operation. It is important to note that seldom or ever should a graft or flap urethroplasty be required after a PFUDD; the treatment modality of choice is simple anastomosis.

### Surgical Technique

The patient is placed in the high lithotomy position in Candy cane stirrups and thoroughly padded. Urethral catheter insertion then delineates the urethral course, guiding our midline perineal incision. We then use the Jordan retractor system (J Hugh Knight Instrument company; Slidell, LA; http://jhughknightinstruments.com/), a specialty add-on to the Bookwalter retractor, for optimal exposure. For perineal surgery, the Jordan retractor is far superior to handheld retractors and the Lone Star retractor. We dissect the distal urethral segment completely off the corpus carvernosa up to the penoscrotal junction and carefully retract it out of the way. The proximal urethral segment dissection is facilitated by placing a metal sound into the bladder neck via the suprapubic tube tract. The distal scar is sharply removed to free the urethral stump completely, followed by placement of 12 interrupted 5–0 absorbable monofilament anastomotic sutures (Fig. 15.9). We then place these sutures in their corresponding location in the distal urethral segment followed by insertion of a 16F silicone catheter through the distal and proximal urethral segments (Fig. 15.10). The sutures are subsequently tied down to bring the urethral segments together. On the rare occasion that we cannot appose the urethral segments, the corpus cavernosa are split to provide a shorter path to the urethral stump.

### Postoperative Care

As in anastomotic urethroplasty, above.

### Complications

Urethral anastomotic stricture, incontinence, and impotence are complications specific to this procedure that are fortunately rare. There may already be baseline incontinence and impotence from the inciting pelvic trauma. Furthermore, the neural control of micturition is sometimes disrupted from the original injury, resulting in a preexisting neurogenic bladder, which is appreciated only after the patient attempts to void through their newly patient urethra.

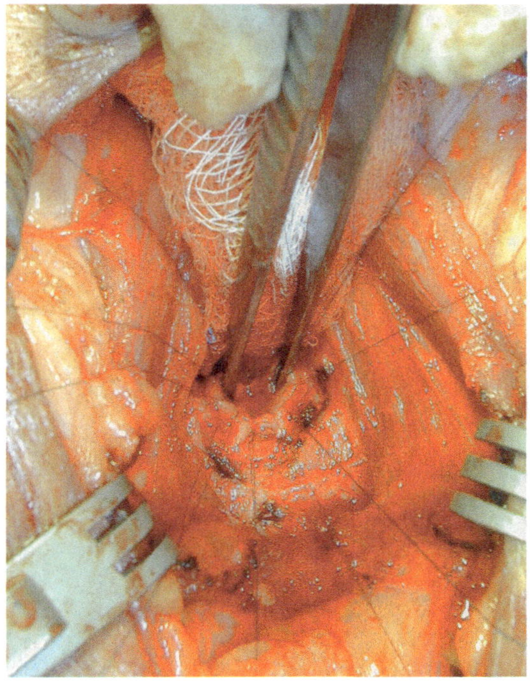

**Fig. 15.9** PFUDD, after complete dissection of the bulbar urethra (which is tucked away under the scrotal skin) and removal of the intervening scar tissue blocking the proximal urethral stump

## Restenosis After Urethral Stent Placement

Early enthusiasm for urethral stents has led to an overzealous use of stents for stricture disease that may have been better treated alternatively, especially since new evidence has shown that long-term stent stricture recurrence rate is unacceptably high [32]. Patients also suffer from other stent complications: pain, stent migration, encrustation, and infections, which might require their removal. Eisenberg et al. retrospectively reviewed 22 patients who were treated for restenosis after urethral stent placement [33]. Ten patients had anterior urethral stricture and 11 had posterior stricture; one patient had both, equating to a total 11 anterior strictures and 12 posterior strictures. They performed open repair for 9 of 11 anterior strictures and 4 of 12 posterior strictures with or

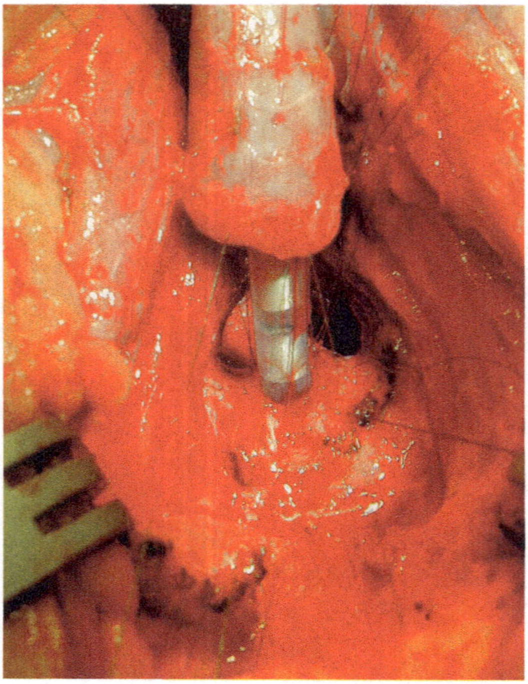

**Fig. 15.10** PFUDD, anastomosis using 12 fine sutures to ensure a wide-open watertight anastomosis

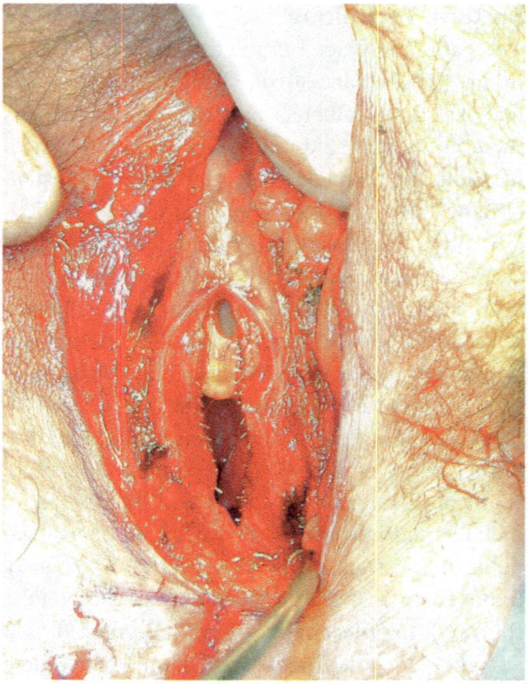

**Fig. 15.11** Urolume stent which has been cut in the ventral midline and now can be removed wire by wire

without removal of the urethral stents and wide excision of the local fibrotic scar. Their overall success rate was 67% for posterior urethral strictures and 82% for anterior strictures over a mean follow-up period of 30 months. We have had excellent success performing a standard ventral buccal onlay procedure after incising and removing the wires that make up the stent (Fig. 15.11) [34]. Gelman and Rodriguez, Jr. also report good results with one-stage urethral reconstruction for patients with stent-associated restenosis [35]. They removed the urethral stent in all their patients and performed either an anastomotic urethroplasty or various combinations of dorsal and ventral buccal graft onlays. They report no stricture recurrence at a median follow-up of 51.2 months.

## Strictures Associated with Prostate Cancer Therapy

The incidence of urethral stricture disease requiring treatment after prostate cancer therapy was determined to be 5% based on the CaPSURE (Cancer of the Prostate Strategic Urologic Research Endeavor) database. Radical prostatectomy had a higher risk than radiation therapy for stricture formation, and strictures tended to occur during the first 24 months versus later for radiation treatments [36]. Management of these strictures requires flexible and individualized approaches as poor tissue vascularization and scarring inevitably complicate surgical repair.

Radiation-associated urethral strictures are difficult to manage primarily because of local damage to urethral tissue leading to poor vascularization and resultant poor wound healing. For patients treated with brachytherapy, about 8% will develop strictures, and 92% of these strictures will be in the bulbo-membranous urethra [37]. These patients can be managed endoscopically with dilation and direct visual urethrotomies, but half will have disease recurrence over the following 3 years. Elliott et al. looked at 32 patients with urethral strictures after treatment for their prostate cancer [38]. Eleven had radical prostatectomy and 21 received radiation, and treatment depended on disease location and length. For patients with anterior strictures that were short bulbar strictures, an anastomotic urethroplasty or buccal mucosa graft onlay procedure was performed. For long or penile urethral strictures, management depended on whether patients received radiation: those who had radiation underwent a perineal urethrostomy and those with healthier nonirradiated tissue had a two-stage Johanson reconstruction or a fasciocutaneous graft repair.

Management of patients with posterior urethral strictures was stratified based on whether the prostate was present. Patients who still had their prostate and who were found to have a membranous or prostatic urethral stricture or bladder neck contracture were managed with stenting or complex open reconstruction with prostatectomy and anastomotic urethroplasty to the bladder neck. Patients with posterior strictures after prostate removal could also be managed with stenting if the stricture was short or undergo stenosis excision and bladder neck-to-urethra anastomotic urethroplasty. Their overall success rate given this treatment algorithm was 73% (23/32) with anastomotic urethroplasty in 19 cases, urethral stent in 9, flap urethroplasty in 2, and perineal urethrostomy in 2. It should be noted that urethral stenting or open urethroplasty can cause total incontinence in some patients, and that care at a center with extensive reconstructive experience is recommended. If repair will likely create incontinence, some patients are offered and treated with suprapubic tubes alone. Suprapubic drainage is also a viable option for those with intractable strictures, especially after radiation.

## Conclusions

There are many varieties and etiologies of urethral strictures that must all be taken into account when planning for reconstruction. Management can vary from minimally invasive dilation and optical urethrotomy to complicated open reconstruction. Critical to patient and practitioner satisfaction is an adaptable and individualized outlook on treatment of each type of urethral stricture disease since life expectancy, goals, and expectations will vary from patient to patient.

In general, short annular strictures can be treated with dilation and/or optical urethrotomy, with the expectation that most will eventually fail and require surgery. Patients seeking permanent solutions with lower restenosis rates benefit from open urethral reconstruction. A majority of patients with anterior urethral strictures can be managed with anastomotic urethroplasties, buccal mucosal graft onlays, or Johansson urethroplasties. Those stricture patients with prior hypospadias repair should generally be treated with staged Johanson urethroplasty. More complex cases like long stricture with inadequate dorsal urethral plates can be managed with combined procedures like a dorsal and ventral onlay buccal graft urethroplasty or a Johanson urethroplasty with or without graft and flap augmentation. Bailout perineal urethrostomy is also an option with overall high satisfaction rates. Strictures that occur after the treatment of prostate diseases are often complex and should be treated by experts in the field.

Patients suffering from PFUDDs and stent restenosis can generally be managed with scar and stent excision followed by primary reanastomosis with acceptable success rates.

## References

1. Santucci RA, Joyce GF, Wise M. Male urethral stricture disease. J Urol. 2007;177:1667–74.
2. Jordan GH, Schlossberg SM. Surgery of the penis and urethra. In: Wein AJ, Kavoussi LR, Novick AC, Partin AW, Peters CA, editors. Campbell-Walsh urology. 9th ed. Philadelphia: Saunders Elsevier; 2007. p. 1054–75.
3. Morey AF, McAninch JW. Sonographic staging of anterior urethral strictures. J Urol. 2000;163:1070–5.
4. Zimmerman WB, Santucci RA. A simplified and unified approach to anterior urethroplasty. Nature. 2010;7:386–91.
5. Burks FN, Santucci RA. Complicated urethroplasty: a guide for surgeons. Nature. 2010;7:521–8.
6. Steenkamp JW, Heyns CF, DeKock MLS. Internal urethrotomy versus dilation as treatment for male urethral strictures: a prospective randomized comparison. J Urol. 1997;157:98–101.
7. Santucci RA, Eisenberg L. Urethrotomy has a much lower success rate than previously reported. J Urol. 2010;183:1859–62.

8. Wright JL, Wessells H, Nathens AB, Hollingworth W. What is the most cost-effective treatment of 1 to 2 cm bulbar urethral strictures: societal approach using decision analysis. Urology. 2006;67:889–93.
9. Shah DK, Paul EM, Badlani GH. North American Study Group: 11-year outcome analysis of endourethral prosthesis for the treatment of recurrent bulbar urethral stricture. J Urol. 2003;170:1255–8.
10. De Vocht TF, van Venrooij GE, Boon TA. Self-expanding stent insertion for urethral strictures: a 10-year follow-up. BJU Int. 2003;91:627–30.
11. Eisenberg ML, Elliott SP, McAninch JW. Preservation of lower urinary tract function in posterior urethral stenosis: selection of appropriate patients for urethral stenosis. J Urol. 2007;178:245–2461.
12. Coursey JW, Morey AF, McAninch JW. Erectile function after anterior urethroplasty. J Urol. 2001;166:2273–6.
13. Barbagli G, Palminteri E, Rizzo M. Dorsal onlay graft urethroplasty using penile skin or buccal mucosa in adult bulbourethral strictures. J Urol. 1998;160:1307–9.
14. Elliott SP, Metro MJ, McAninch JW. Long-term follow-up of the ventrally placed buccal mucosa onlay graft in bulbar urethral reconstruction. J Urol. 2003;169:1754–7.
15. Iselin CE, Webster GW. Dorsal onlay urethroplasty for urethral stricture repair. World J Urol. 1998;16:181–5.
16. Kellner DS, Fracchia JA, Armenakas NA. Ventral onlay buccal mucosal grafts for anterior urethral strictures: long-term follow-up. J Urol. 2004;171:726–9.
17. Paoluzzi LJ. Is hypospadias an 'environmental' birth defect? Dial Pediatr Urol. 2000;23:2–4.
18. Chrzan R, Dik P, Klijn AJ, de Jong TP. Quality assessment of hypospadias repair with emphasis on techniques used and experience of pediatric urologic surgeons. Urology. 2007;70:148–52.
19. Tang SH, Hammer CC, Doumanian L, Santucci RA. Adult urethral stricture disease after childhood hypospadias repair. Adv Urol. 2008;10:1503–15.
20. Barbagli G, De Angelis M, Palminteri E, Lazzeri M. Failed hypospadias repair presenting in adults. Eur Urol. 2006;49:887–94.
21. Meeks JJ, Erickson BA, Gonzalez CM. Staged reconstruction of long segment urethral strictures in men with previous hypospadias repair. J Urol. 2009;181:685–9.
22. Mangera A, Patterson JM, Chapple CR. A systematic review of graft augmentation urethroplasty techniques for the treatment of anterior urethral strictures. Eur Urol. 2011;59:797–814.
23. Palminteri E, Manzoni G, Berdondini E. Combined dorsal plus ventral double buccal mucosa graft in bulbar urethral reconstruction. Eur Urol. 2008;53:81–90.
24. Berglund RK, Angermeier KW. Combined buccal mucosa graft and genital skin flap for reconstruction of extensive anterior urethral strictures. Urology. 2006;68:707–10.
25. Dalpiaz O, Kerschbaumer A, Pelzer A. Single-stage dorsal inlay split-skin graft for salvage anterior urethral reconstruction. BJU Int. 2008;101:1565–70.
26. Mathur RK, Sharma A. Tunica albuginea urethroplasty for panurethral strictures. Urol J. 2010;7:120–4.
27. Xu YM, Qiao Y, Sa YL. Urethral reconstruction using colonic mucosa graft for complex strictures. J Urol. 2009;182:1040–3.
28. Burks FN, Santucci RA. Complicated urethroplasty: a guide for surgeons. Nat Rev Urol. 2010;7:521–8.
29. Cooperberg MR, McAninch JW, Alsikafi NF. Posterior urethral reconstruction for traumatic posterior urethral disruption: outcomes of a 25-year experience. J Urol. 2007;178:2006–10.
30. Shenfeld OZ, Gofrit ON, Gdor Y. Anastomotic urethroplasty for failed previously treated membranous urethral rupture. Urology. 2004;63:837–40.
31. Wang P, Fan M, Zhang Y. Modified urethral pull-though operation for posterior urethral stricture and long-term outcome. J Urol. 2008;180:2479–85.
32. Hussain M, Greenwell TJ, Shah J. Long-term results of a self-expanding wallstent in the treatment of urethral stricture. BJU Int. 2004;94:1037–41.
33. Eisenberg ML, Elliott SP, McAninch JW. Management of restenosis after urethral stent placement. J Urol. 2008;179:991–5.
34. Fisher MB, Santucci RA. Extraction of UroLume endoprosthesis with one-stage urethral reconstruction using buccal mucosa. Urology. 2006;67:9–10.
35. Gelman J, Rodriguez Jr E. One-stage urethral reconstruction for stricture recurrence after urethral stent placement. J Urol. 2007;177:188–91.
36. Elliott SP, Meng MV, Elkin EP. Incidence of urethral stricture after primary treatment for prostate cancer: data from CaPSURE. J Urol. 2007;178:529–34.
37. Sullivan L, Williams SG, Tai KH. Urethral stricture following high dose rate brachytherapy for prostate cancer. Radiother Oncol. 2009;91:232–6.
38. Elliot SP, McAninch JW, Chi T. Management of severe urethral complications of prostate cancer therapy. J Urol. 2006;176:2508–13.

# Medical and Surgical Interventions in Male Fertility

16

Kevin Chandler and Edmund Sabanegh Jr.

## Introduction

Infertility, defined as the failure to conceive after 1 year of unprotected intercourse, affects about 15% of reproductive age couples. Over the years, treatment of infertility has become increasingly more successful, and this has largely been dependent on interdisciplinary interactions among a number of specialties. With joint efforts between primary care physicians, obstetricians, urologists, geneticists, endocrinologists, and andrologists, couples are now able to undergo comprehensive stepwise evaluations that allow their physicians to determine the cause of infertility, provide evidence-based advice regarding prognoses, and determine the best approach toward achieving pregnancy or family planning.

In this chapter, we focus on the male infertility evaluation, and the medical and surgical treatment options available, both alone and in combination with assisted reproductive techniques (ART). It is our goal to discuss the thought process behind the evaluation and when to proceed with each type of intervention. Ultimately, this chapter will assist in the identification of tests to initiate the infertility evaluation, recognize criteria for subspecialty referral, and assist with patient counseling. In addition, it can serve as a general framework to help urologists and infertility specialists formulate plans for evaluation and treatment of their infertility patients.

Even though only male infertility is discussed here, it is important to emphasize that a thorough infertility evaluation, to truly be effective, requires evaluation of both the male and female partner. The practice of evaluating only the female partner, which is often the case at least initially, is not efficient since a male factor alone is responsible for infertility in 20% of cases and an additional 30–40% of cases involve both male and female factors [1, 2].

## Presentation

Detailed histories and physical exams are essential to the male infertility evaluation and will guide an efficient, focused workup. When a history of infertility or concern about conception is obtained, the evaluating physician should inquire about the duration in addition to other factors that could warrant further investigation. Table 16.1 lists pertinent history and exam findings that are keys to the male fertility evaluation. When a male factor is involved, there are certain aspects of the history that can point to an anatomic or functional abnormality. A history of low-volume or absent ejaculate in a patient could signal ejaculatory duct obstruction or retrograde ejaculation. Similarly, this history in conjunction with obstructive voiding complaints may suggest the possibility of urethral stricture. The history should include

K. Chandler, MD • E. Sabanegh Jr., MD (✉)
Department of Urology, Cleveland Clinic,
9500 Euclid Avenue Q10, Cleveland OH 44195, USA
e-mail: chandlk@ccf.org; sabanee@ccf.org

D.A. Shoskes (ed.), *Urological Men's Health: A Guide for Urologists and Primary Care Physicians*,
Current Clinical Urology, DOI 10.1007/978-1-61779-900-6_16,
© Springer Science+Business Media New York 2012

**Table 16.1** Pertinent history and exam findings

| | |
|---|---|
| Infertility/sexual history | • Duration of infertility<br>• Pregnancy with prior partner<br>• Prior infertility therapy<br>• Partner's fertility status<br>• Decreased amount of semen volume/dry ejaculations<br>• Decreased libido or erectile dysfunction<br>• Timing and frequency of intercourse<br>• Use of lubricants |
| Past medical history | • Cryptorchidism<br>• Mumps orchitis<br>• Recurrent childhood respiratory or sinus infections<br>• History of neoplasms such as testis cancer<br>• Personal/family history of cystic fibrosis or infertility<br>• Diabetes<br>• Hypospadias<br>• STDs (HIV, gonorrhea, chlamydia)<br>• Neurologic disease (i.e., MS, spinal cord injury)<br>• Recent febrile illness |
| Past surgical/trauma history | • Scrotal/pelvic trauma<br>• Orchiopexy/orchiectomy<br>• Testicular torsion<br>• Vasectomy<br>• Inguinal hernia repair<br>• Endourologic procedures (specifically bladder neck surgery)<br>• RPLND |
| Social history | • Tobacco<br>• Illicit drug use<br>• Exogenous steroids |
| Medications | • Alpha blockers<br>• Androgen therapy<br>• Chemotherapy/pelvic radiation<br>• Antidepressants<br>• 5α- reductase inhibitors<br>• Anti-androgen therapy<br>• GnRH analogs |
| Physical exam | • Testes<br>– Size, consistency?<br>– Cryptorchid?<br>• Varicocele(s)<br>• Presence and consistency of vasa deferentia<br>• Location and appearance of urethral meatus<br>• Midline prostate nodules/cystic lesions<br>• Incomplete/partial virilization<br>• Gynecomastia<br>• Body habitus (i.e., obese, eunuchoid) |

*MS* multiple sclerosis, *RPLND* retroperitoneal lymph node dissection, *GnRH* gonadotropin-releasing hormone

a thorough medical and surgical history; a review of medications or supplements (prescription and nonprescription) and allergies; a review of lifestyle exposures and a review of systems; family and personal reproductive history; and a survey of past infections such as sexually transmitted diseases and respiratory infections.

Equally important as the history is the physical exam. Key areas that should be assessed include body habitus (i.e., eunuchoid, muscular, etc.), presence of gynecomastia, and hair distribution. On the genitourinary exam, special attention should be paid to testicular size, as well as their location and consistency. The presence of scrotal/testicular lesions including varicoceles should be noted and the presence and consistency of the vasa deferentia should be established. Last, the appearance of the urethral meatus should be noted and a digital rectal exam should be performed.

## Workup

The male infertility workup can be initiated by the patient's primary care provider or the infertility specialist. The initial evaluation begins with a thorough history and physical examination as well as a semen analysis. The American Urological Association recommends the following standards for semen collection: a period of abstinence of two to three days prior to collection; collection by masturbation or by intercourse using semen collection condoms that do not contain substances detrimental to sperm; and semen storage at room or body temperature during transport and examination within one hour of collection [3]. It is recommended that at least two specimens be examined over a period of several weeks due to marked physiologic variability in semen parameters. Febrile illnesses can negatively affect semen parameters for a period of months and therefore semen analysis should be deferred for 2–3 months after resolution of the illness to allow better assessment of he patient's baseline semen parameters [4].

Evaluation of the hypothalamic–pituitary–gonadal axis generally follows if abnormalities are observed on the semen analysis. In a retrospective review of 1,035 patients who had undergone an infertility evaluation, 9.6% had

**Table 16.2** Causes of male infertility by category

| Diagnostic category | Specific cause | Key signs/symptoms |
|---|---|---|
| Endocrine abnormalities | Congenital hypogonadotropic hypogonadism (CHH) | Absent/incomplete puberty, decreased libido, erectile dysfunction, eunuchoid body habitus, decreased muscle mass, scant axillary and pubic hair, prepubertal testes, small penis |
| | Kallman's syndrome | Symptoms same as CHH + anosmia |
| | Androgen excess | Failure of testicular development (if condition present prior to puberty), hirsutism, acne, weight gain, gynecomastia |
| | Estrogen excess | Decreased libido, erectile dysfunction, gynecomastia, obesity |
| | Hyperprolactinemia | Decreased libido, erectile dysfunction, gynecomastia, headaches or vision changes (prolactinoma) |
| | Prader–Willi syndrome | Decreased mental capacity, insatiable appetite, almond-shaped eyes, obesity, decreased muscle tone |
| Disorders of spermatogenesis | Klinefelter's syndrome (XXY male) | Phenotypic male with small firm testes, gynecomastia, eunuchoid body habitus |
| | Y chromosome microdeletions | Asymptomatic |
| | Cryptorchidism | Elicited from pediatric history – if status post orchiopexy, the cryptorchid testis may be small compared to the other; empty hemiscrotum if untreated |
| | Testicular torsion | Empty hemiscrotum if status post orchiectomy; if status post orchiopexy, the torsed testis may be small compared to the other |
| | Varicocele | Usually painless swelling within the scrotum that feels like a "bag of worms" |
| | Mumps orchitis | Painful and inflamed at the time of infection; testicle may be atrophic if infection was remote |
| Disorders of sperm delivery | Vasal obstruction (secondary to congenital bilateral absence of vas deferens, cystic fibrosis, iatrogenic injury, vasectomy) | Low-volume ejaculate; no ejaculate |
| | Ejaculatory duct obstruction | Low-volume ejaculate; dry ejaculation |
| | Retrograde ejaculation | Low-volume ejaculate |
| Disorders of sperm function | Antisperm antibodies | Asymptomatic; usually have a history of testicular surgery or trauma |
| | Cilia defects | Often associated with respiratory cilia defects, leading to chronic sinus infections and bronchiectasis |

endocrine abnormalities, but only 1.7% were found to have a clinically significant endocrinopathy that altered disease management [5]. Despite the historically low yield of the endocrine workup, it is essential that it be performed to rule out any endocrinopathies that may have other health consequences in addition to infertility. Specific indications for initiating an endocrine workup include (1) an abnormal semen analysis, (2) impaired sexual function; or (3) other clinical findings suggestive of a specific endocrinopathy. The initial endocrine evaluation should include at minimum a serum total testosterone and follicle-stimulating hormone (FSH). Serum luteinizing hormone (LH) and prolactin levels, as well as repeat testosterone (total and free) levels, are obtained if the first testosterone level is low. These studies round out the extent of the endocrine workup and may identify diagnoses such as congenital hypogonadotropic hypogonadism, acquired hypogonadotropic hypogonadism (HH) secondary to hyperprolactinemia, or exogenous androgen use. Additional diagnostic studies that may be useful in specific patients include: transrectal ultrasonography (TRUS), post-ejaculatory urinalysis, and genetic testing with karyotype, y-chromosome microdeletions, and cystic fibrosis transmembrane conductance regulator (CFTR) genes.

The goal of the male infertility workup is to classify the patient into a specific diagnostic category and tailor a treatment plan based upon it. Categories include endocrine abnormalities, disorders of spermatogenesis, sperm delivery disorders, and sperm function disorders. Table 16.2

lists the different conditions within each category that can lead to problems with fertility. Even after extensive workup it is not always possible to identify a specific cause with which to attribute infertility. These cases are termed idiopathic and approximately 23% of male infertility patients fall into this category [6].

## Treatment

Treatment of male infertility has evolved over the past 20 years thanks to advances in medical management and ART. In general, there are three options for treating male infertility (Fig. 16.1). The first is to treat the underlying male factor where possible to give the couple the best chance at natural conception. This assumes that there is no female factor contributing to infertility, or if there is, that it can be corrected. Alternatively, ART can be employed as first-line therapy, either in combination with attempts at treating the male factor or alone. When given the option between these treatment approaches, the first is generally preferred as it avoids placing too much of the burden on the female partner. Targeted treatment of the underlying male factor also tends to be less costly than ART. In the event that neither targeted therapy nor ART lead to conception the practitioner should counsel the couple on donor insemination or adoption. In the next two sections, we discuss the various medical and surgical approaches that are employed alone or in combination with ART in treating male factor causes of infertility.

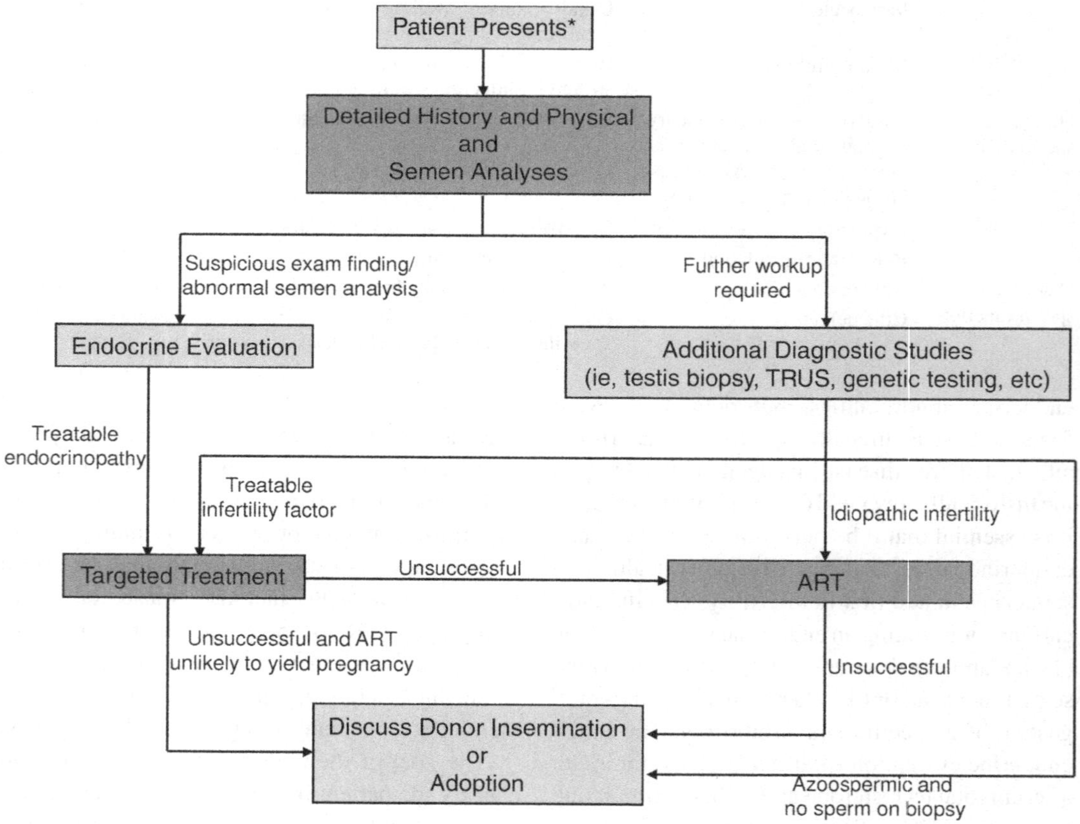


**Fig. 16.1** Algorithm for the workup and treatment of male infertility. *TRUS* transrectal ultrasonagraphy, *ART* assisted reproductive techniques. *The partner should be referred for infertility evaluation if not already initiated

## Medical Treatments

There are many medical therapies employed in the treatment of male infertility.

In order to discuss the various medical treatments available in the treatment of infertility, a brief overview of the conditions in which they are used must first be given. There are four categories of male factor infertility: endocrine dysfunction, disorders of spermatogenesis, disorders of sperm delivery, and abnormalities of sperm function. Of these categories, endocrine causes tend to be more amenable to medical therapy whereas in most cases disorders of sperm delivery and function are less likely to be resolved with medical therapy alone. Disorders of spermatogenesis are usually difficult to treat with medical or surgical interventions, and often surgical sperm harvest with ART offers the only chance of conception. Below we highlight causes of male factor infertility and discuss the medical therapies used in their treatment.

### Endocrine Causes of Male Infertility and Their Medical Therapies

The majority of endocrine causes of infertility result from congenital or acquired hypogonadotropic hypogonadism (HH). As the name implies, male infertility resulting from HH is due to insufficient secretion of the gonadotropins luteinizing hormone (LH) and/or follicle-stimulating hormone (FSH), from the anterior pituitary. In contrast to primary hypogonadism, the problem is not with the gonad, but instead is a result of conditions affecting the hypothalamic–pituitary portion of the axis, leading to decreased secretion of LH or FSH. When there is a hypothalamic cause, decreased levels of gonadotropin-releasing hormone (GnRH) lead to decreased stimulation of the anterior pituitary to secrete LH and FSH. Pituitary causes directly affect the secretion of LH, FSH, or both, and in some cases other pituitary hormones as well. Pathology that interferes with the hypothalamic–pituitary–gonadal axis can lead to HH.

Medical therapy for infertility secondary to HH is aimed at supplementing the hypothalamic–pituitary–gonadal axis or counteracting hormones that are inhibiting it through negative feedback. Agents used for treatment of hypothalamic dysfunction include gonadotropin-releasing hormone (GnRH) via SQ injections or pulsatile infusion pumps, or gonadotropin therapy with human chorionic gonadotropin (hCG), recombinant FSH, or human menopausal gonadotropin (hMG), a formulation containing both LH and FSH. With the exception of GnRH, these same agents are employed when the defect is localized to the pituitary. It is important to note that testosterone therapy may be employed to induce virilization in patients with prepubertal HH, but should not be utilized for infertility purposes as it has a detrimental effect on spermatogenesis due to its negative feedback on the hypothalamic–pituitary–gonadal axis.

Androgen excess causes HH by feedback inhibition of the hypothalamic–pituitary–gonadal axis. Anabolic steroid use, androgen-producing tumors, or processes such as congenital adrenal hyperplasia (CAH) lead to androgen excess and resultant infertility from HH. Exposure to exogenous androgens actually serves more as a contraceptive instead of augmenting fertility potential due to the systemic (target tissue) versus local (gonadal) actions of androgens. Testosterone stimulates sperm production as a result of local action on seminiferous tubules secondary to the supra-serum concentrations made possible by secretion within the testicle by Leydig cells. These cells also secrete testosterone systemically to act on target tissues. It is during systemic secretion that testosterone effects it major inhibitory action on the hypothalamic–pituitary–gonadal axis. Any androgen that originates outside the testes (i.e., exogenous or from androgen-secreting tumor) effects its action mostly systemically and only minimally within the testes as testosterone levels do not reach the supra-serum intratesticular concentrations that are normally seen as a result of Leydig cell production. These systemic androgens therefore activate negative feedback without ever stimulating spermatogenesis by the seminiferous tubules. Treatment of these conditions relies on decreasing systemic levels of androgen. For conditions such as CAH, where the primary enzymatic defect results in decreased cortisol production, glucocorticoid therapy is the treatment. This normalizes serum levels of adrenocorticotropic hormone (ACTH), resulting in decreased androgen production from the adrenal gland. This has shown to be effective in the treatment of infertility in men with CAH [7]. Unlike CAH, there is no medical treatment for androgen excess secondary to androgen-secreting tumor. This requires surgical excision, which should result in resolution of HH upon normalization of serum androgen levels.

Hyperprolactinemia is another endocrine abnormality that has been associated with male infertility by inducing HH [8]. Elevations in prolactin may stem from a multitude of causes, including pituitary tumors, medications (i.e., antipsychotics, antiemetics, and antidepressants), medical illnesses, or it may be idiopathic. Clinical signs of hyperprolactinemia include decreased libido, ejaculatory dysfunction, gynecomastia, and galactorrhea. The primary treatment of hyperprolactinemia in infertile men involves medical therapy with dopamine agonists such as bromocriptine or cabergoline, both of which have been shown to improve semen parameters and potency [9]. These medications also induce reduction in size of prolactinomas, which usually obviates the need for surgical resection. It is important to note that dopamine agonists do not cure prolactinomas and that withdrawal from therapy results in recurrent hyperprolactinemia in 80–90% of patients [10]. In contrast, it is reasonable to periodically stop treatment in patients with idiopathic hyperprolactinemia to see whether normalization of prolactin levels can be sustained.

Similar to androgens, high concentrations of peripheral estrogens can suppress pituitary gonadotropin secretion. Estrogen excess can be seen in patients with estrogen-secreting adrenal or testicular tumors, or in morbidly obese patients secondary to increased conversion of testosterone to estrogen from high peripheral levels of aromatase. With the exception of the presence of testicular atrophy, signs of estrogen excess can be similar to that of hyperprolactinemia. Treatment of these individuals is aimed at correcting the underlying abnormality, which should normalize serum estrogen levels, and remove pituitary inhibition. Anastrozole, a nonsteroidal aromatase inhibitor, is sometimes utilized to accomplish this goal in patients with aromatase excess.

Overall, the approach to management of infertility secondary to congenital or acquired HH is relatively straightforward. In almost all cases, medical treatments are available for hormonal replacement or counteracting feedback inhibition, and in some cases, treatment simply requires removing the causative agent (i.e., exogenous testosterone or hyperprolactinemia-inducing medication).

## Other Targets of Medical Therapy

Other factors that may affect male fertility for which there are targeted medical treatments include antisperm antibodies and ejaculatory dysfunction. Therapies directed at these factors are often utilized, but unfortunately may not be as successful at treating male infertility as the therapies used for HH.

Antisperm antibodies represent the main immunologic association with infertility. The body's primary mechanism to prevent testicular antigen recognition and formation of antisperm antibodies is the blood–testis barrier. Tight junctions between Sertoli cells in the seminiferous tubules prevent the immune system from contact with surface antigens present on postmeiotic germ cells. Any condition that can potentially violate the blood–testis barrier risks the formation of antisperm antibodies. Ductal obstruction, congenital bilateral absence of the vas deferens (CBAVD), and vasectomy have all been associated with antisperm antibody formation. It is believed that antisperm antibodies affect fertility by multiple mechanisms, but the most frequent is reduced sperm motility [11]. Medical treatment of infertility presumably secondary to antisperm antibodies is directed at preventing their formation. Corticosteroids, the main class of medication utilized to prevent antisperm antibody formation, have been shown to decrease antisperm antibody levels in seminal plasma, but the use of them alone has been shown by most studies to result in low pregnancy rates. ART is often required to achieve pregnancy in these patients [12, 13].

Retrograde ejaculation is another factor in which medical therapy is utilized to improve fertility. Any patient with low semen volume or absent ejaculate, especially with a prior history of normal semen volume, should be suspected of having retrograde ejaculation. It is diagnosed by the finding of sperm (greater than 10–15 sperm/HPF) on a post-ejaculatory urinalysis. Anatomic causes of retrograde ejaculation include bladder neck surgery and transurethral resection of the prostate, while functional causes include neurologic abnormalities secondary to diabetes mellitus, multiple sclerosis, and retroperitoneal surgery. Medications such as alpha blockers can also lead to functional retrograde ejaculation. All of these causes may produce an incompetent internal sphincter at the bladder neck that does not close during seminal emission. The first step in treatment should be to remove any potential offending agents, such as alpha blockers. Specific therapies include alpha agonists such as phenylpropanolamine, ephedrine, or pseudoephedrine, and certain antidepressants such as imipramine. The goal of therapy is to increase the sympathetic tone of the internal sphincter, or decrease parasympathetic activity, and thus keep the sphincter closed during seminal emission. A literature review by Kamischke and colleagues cited a 50% success rate with medical treatment of retrograde ejaculation, regardless of the underlying cause [14]. Given these numbers, medical therapy is the first-line treatment for retrograde ejaculation. In cases where medical therapy fails to achieve antegrade ejaculation, efforts can be made to alkalinize the urine to create a less hostile environment for sperm. The sperm are then recovered from the urine and used for future artificial insemination.

Empiric medical therapies are used when no specific underlying cause of infertility or abnormal semen parameters can be identified. Common agents used either alone or in combination to treat idiopathic infertility include antiestrogens, aromatase inhibitors, gonadotropins, L-carnitine, antioxidants, vitamins, kallikrein, indomethacin, pentoxifylline, low-dose corticosteroids, androgens, and zinc. Strong evidence of their effectiveness in treating idiopathic infertility is lacking, but their limited use may be justified by their low side effect profile and cost [15].

Altogether, there are a variety of medical therapies employed in the treatment of male infertility. Those that are geared at treating the several different causes of both congenital and acquired HH tend to be the most effective. Others, such as therapies for antisperm antibodies or retrograde ejaculation, may not be as effective, but when these fail there are many additional avenues available through surgical sperm retrieval techniques and ART.

## Surgical Treatments

Surgical procedures for male infertility serve to accomplish at least one of three goals: aid in diagnosis and sperm retrieval, improve sperm delivery, or improve sperm production. Diagnostic procedures include testis biopsies and seminal vesicle aspiration, while those aimed at improving sperm delivery include microsurgical reconstructions with vasovasostomy or vasoepididymostomy or resection of ejaculatory duct obstruction. The most common procedure performed to improve sperm production is varicocelectomy. Below we discuss the surgical procedures commonly utilized in the treatment of male infertility.

### Procedures for Diagnosis and Sperm Retrieval

Testicular biopsies can be done for both diagnostic and therapeutic purposes. A diagnostic testicular biopsy is indicated in azoospermic patients with normal levels of FSH and normal testicular size and consistency. This will help differentiate azoospermia secondary to obstruction versus spermatogenic failure. If sperm are found on biopsy, they can be cryopreserved and utilized for future intracytoplasmic sperm injection (ICSI), thus making it a therapeutic procedure as well. A single biopsy of one testis may not be indicative of the spermatogenic process in the remainder of that testis or the contralateral testis [16–18]. Therefore, multiple biopsies of both testes may be necessary for adequate sampling for both diagnostic purposes and to maximize the chances of successful sperm retrieval.

There are both open and percutaneous approaches for performing testicular biopsy. Both have their respective advantages and disadvantages. Open biopsy can be carried out under local, spinal, or general anesthesia, and is generally associated with more pain and morbidity. Percutaneous testicular biopsy can be performed with local anesthesia in an office-based setting, and even though it maybe less morbid to the patient, it usually yields less seminiferous tubules for examination. In addition, percutaneous biopsy carries with it the risks associated with blind needle insertion, including risk of injury to the testicular artery or epididymis. These risks aside, a high correlation has been demonstrated between diagnoses obtained from percutaneous and open surgical biopsy specimens [19, 20].

Sperm retrieval can be accomplished by epididymal aspiration as well. This can be done via a percutaneous (PESA) or microsurgical (MESA) approach. PESA is easier to perform as it does not require the microsurgical skills necessary for MESA, but it is associated with less sperm retrieval [21]. TRUS-guided seminal vesicle aspiration is often performed for diagnostic purposes, but sperm retrieved during the procedure can be cryopreserved and utilized for future ICSI as well. The finding of numerous sperm on seminal vesicle aspiration of an azoospermic patient is diagnostic of ejaculatory duct obstruction and indicates the presence of active spermatogenesis, thus obviating the need for testicular biopsy [22]. Any of these methods of sperm retrieval are reasonable to pursue as none offers any clear advantage over the others in regards to pregnancy rates.

## Procedures for Improving Sperm Delivery

Vasovasostomy, the anastomosis of two separate segments of vas deferens, is the most common procedure undertaken to improve sperm delivery. Indications for this procedure include a desire for vasectomy reversal and infertility in a man with vasal obstruction. Nearly 6% of men who have undergone vasectomy will subsequently request a vasectomy reversal [23]. Vasovasostomy is normally utilized to accomplish this, but when secondary epididymal obstruction is observed, the area of obstruction is bypassed by anastomosing the distal vas segment to the epididymis via vasoepididymostomy. Patency and pregnancy rates after vasovasostomy can reach as high as 97% and 76%, respectively, depending on the time interval since the vasectomy [24]. Older age of the female partner can be a negative predictive factor in achieving pregnancy after vasovasostomy. Despite this, it has been shown that vasectomy reversal still offers success rates comparable to that of a single cycle of IVF with ICSI when the female partner is 35 or older, and therefore it remains an excellent option for patients with partners around this age [25].

When performed for nonvasectomy-related obstructive causes, such as that caused by injury to the vas deferens during inguinal surgery, vasovasostomy and vasoepididymostomy tend not to be as good as that performed for vasectomy reversal. In their series of 13 patients, Pasqualotto and colleagues reported patency rates of 60% and 80% for vasovasostomy and vasoepididymostomy, respectively [26]. Not surprisingly, the majority of the patients in this particular study were many years out from herniorrhaphy, and this likely explains the lower patency rates. This paper further demonstrated that patency rates are inversely related to the time interval from the onset of obstruction to reversal, regardless of cause of obstruction.

The only other procedure utilized to improve sperm delivery is transurethral resection of the ejaculatory duct (TURED), which is employed for treating ejaculatory duct obstruction. Unlike patients with vasal obstruction, those with ejaculatory duct obstruction often present with low-volume ejaculate or dry ejaculate (feeling of ejaculation without urethral extrusion of semen). TURED is performed with a standard resection loop at the midline of the verumontanum and has been shown to be effective at improving ejaculation, sensation of orgasm, semen values, and fertility [27].

Procedures aimed at improving sperm delivery offer infertile men with normal spermatogenesis the chance of natural conception with their

**Table 16.3** Varicocele grading system

| Grade | Physical Exam Finding |
|---|---|
| 1 | Palpable only with the Valsalva maneuver |
| 2 | Palpable without the Valsalva maneuver |
| 3 | Visible through the scrotal skin |

partners. When these procedures fail to provide conception, ART is an appropriate option.

## Procedures to Improve Sperm Production

Surgical treatments of varicoceles represent the majority of the procedures that are performed to improve sperm function. Varicoceles, which are an abnormal tortuosity and dilatation of the testicular veins within the spermatic cord, are believed to affect testicular function by increasing intratesticular temperature, although the exact pathophysiology remains controversial. They are an underlying cause in up to 70% of patients with secondary infertility [28]. Consequently, varicocele repair remains the most commonly performed surgical procedure in the treatment of male infertility.

A thorough physical exam is the most important part in the diagnosis of a varicocele. Table 16.3 lists the different varicocele grades based on physical exam findings. Per AUA guidelines, varicocele repair is indicated for infertility purposes if all of the following criteria are met: the couple has known infertility; the female partner has normal fertility or a potentially treatable cause of infertility; the varicocele is palpable on physical examination, or if it is suspected, the varicocele is corroborated by ultrasound examination; and the male partner has an abnormal semen analysis [29]. Additionally, most urologists consider a reduction in ipsilateral testicular volume in an adolescent male another indication for varicocele repair.

There are different surgical approaches available for varicocele repair including retroperitoneal, laparoscopic, inguinal, or subinguinal. In addition, percutaneous embolization of the spermatic vein may be obtained with interventional radiology. Given the risk of damage to nearby structures, some of the surgical approaches are less favored than others. Most reproductive urologists today employ microsurgical techniques via inguinal or subinguinal approaches to preserve the internal spermatic arteries and lymphatics. When varicoceles recur or persist after attempted ligation, percutaneous embolization is especially useful as it allows radiographic clarification of the anatomy.

Success of varicocele repair is measured by resolution of the varicocele and improvement in semen parameters and pregnancy rates. Grade 3 varicoceles are more likely to be associated with impairment in semen quality. Therefore, repair of larger varicoceles results in significantly greater improvement in semen quality, whereas repair of subclinical, nonpalpable varicoceles has not been of proven benefit [30, 31]. Overall, repair of clinical varicoceles has been moderately effective in improving semen parameters and is therefore recognized as a legitimate treatment for male factor infertility [32].

In summary, surgical procedures for male fertility are performed to either aid in diagnosis, sperm delivery, or sperm function. The different procedures utilized to accomplish these goals can be very efficacious depending on the underlying condition of the patient and baseline fertility of their partner. When the therapeutic procedures fail to aid in achieving pregnancy, or if there are multiple factors contributing to infertility, ART may be undertaken.

## Assisted Reproductive Techniques

Assisted reproductive techniques (ART) include specialized procedures that involve the manipulation of sperm or oocytes or both to improve the chance of conception and resultant live birth rates. Examples of ART include intrauterine insemination (IUI), and in-vitro fertilization (IVF) with or without intracytoplasmic sperm injection (ICSI). Indications for ART include idiopathic male infertility or failure of other treatments to result in pregnancy. ART can be very successful, but on occasion has been overutilized, or prematurely utilized in the treatment of male infertility. Most of the previously discussed procedures, including vasovasostomy/vasoepididymostomy for vasectomy reversal and varicocele repair, have all been shown by different studies to be more cost-effective than ART [33–35]. ART should be employed as part of a stepwise approach to the evaluation and treatment of male infertility, and is best utilized in idiopathic cases, or when targeted therapies fail to overcome identified causes of infertility.

ART is usually associated with controlled ovarian hyperstimulation, a process that involves hormonal stimulation of the female to induce the simultaneous development of multiple oocytes. Commonly used medications to accomplish this include clomiphene citrate (an oral medication) or gonadotropins (usually subcutaneously). As evident from above, by employing ART, the treatment burden is shifted to the female partner, even when only a male factor for infertility has been identified. This is important given the stress it can place on the female partner as well as on the couple's relationship. It once again emphasizes the significance of exhausting targeted therapies prior to undertaking ART.

In general, the approach to ART should be to provide the minimal amount of assistance to allow conception by as close to natural means as possible. Therefore, IUI is often performed first, followed by IVF with or without ICSI if unsuccessful. IUI is performed by injecting processed sperm through the cervix into the uterine cavity and is indicated for cervical mucus abnormalities, anatomic abnormalities that prevent normal deposition of sperm at the cervical os (i.e., hypospadias, retrograde ejaculation, erectile dysfunction), as well as idiopathic infertility with relatively normal bulk semen parameters. With IVF, multiple oocytes are recruited each cycle with the use of controlled ovarian hyperstimulation. They are then harvested by ultrasound-guided transvaginal needle aspiration and in-vitro insemination is performed by mixing processed sperm with recovered oocytes. The embryos are incubated for 2–3 days and then placed transcervically to allow for possible implantation. For IVF with ICSI, a single sperm is injected into an individual ovum. This method is therefore indicated for patients with severe oligospermia, in couples with prior failed or poor fertilization during regular IVF cycles, or in cases in which the sperm demonstrate significant fertilizing ability defects.

Overall, success rates with ART are dependent upon the technique utilized and the specific factors contributing to infertility with each couple. Live birth rates after IUI have been reported by some studies to range from 9% to 12% in patients under the age of 40 [36, 37]. If deliveries are not achieved with IUI, it is often reasonable to proceed with IVF/IVF with ICSI. In a cohort study in which 10,656 ART cycles were reported to the Canadian ART Register in 2003, clinical pregnancy rates and live birth rates per cycle of IVF/IVF with ICSI were 31.2% and 23.9%, respectively. Of cycles with oocytes retrieved, IVF was performed in 44% and ICSI in 56%, with similar outcomes between the two procedures [38]. Pregnancy and live birth rates with IVF or IVF with ICSI are largely dependent upon the age of the female partner, with decreased success being associated with more advanced age. When ART and all other means of achieving pregnancy have failed, the practitioner should feel comfortable counseling the couple on other options such as donor insemination or adoption. While not as attractive to some couples as having their own genetic-related child, these options can be very gratifying for couples looking to expand and complete their family.

## Summary

Infertility can have multiple causes and in some cases they can be coexistent, making for a very challenging entity to manage. Like many other medical conditions, it requires a systematic approach for an efficient evaluation and management. It is important to remember that the end-goal is to achieve pregnancy, and in order to maximize the probability of this happening, both partners should be evaluated concurrently to identify potential factors that could be contributing to infertility.

At the foundation of the male evaluation are a thorough history and physical examination, and semen testing. Information gained from these can help guide subsequent workup and management.

Some causes of male factor infertility are amenable to medical therapy, while others such as ductal obstruction or varicoceles require surgical procedures for treatment. All of these therapies have the potential to be very successful dependent on the severity of infertility and any additional female factors. When these fail, ART can be employed and gives many couples an opportunity for conception that would not have been available 30 years ago. Lastly, additional options that are available to couples include donor insemination or adoption. With joint efforts by practitioners from many specialties, these treatments are constantly being refined and will continue to offer even more promising diagnostic strategies and therapies for infertility.

## References


1. Mosher WD, Pratt WF. Fecundity and infertility in the United States: incidence and trends. Fertil Steril. 1991;56:192–3.
2. Thonneau P, Marchand S, Tallec A, et al. Incidence and main causes of infertility in a resident population (1,850,000) of three French regions (1988-1989). Hum Reprod. 1991;6:811–6.
3. The Optimal Evaluation of the Infertile Male: Best Practice Statement, Revised 2010. http://www.auanet.org/content/media/optimalevaluation2010.pdf. Accessed 13 May 2011.
4. Carlsen E, Andersson AM, Petersen JH, et al. History of febrile illness and variation in semen quality. Hum Reprod. 2003;18:2089–92.
5. Sigman M, Jarow JP. Endocrine evaluation of infertile men. Urology. 1997;50:659–64.
6. Sigman M, Jarow JP. Male Infertility. In: Wein AJ, Kavoussi LR, Novick AC, Partin AW, Peters CA, editors. Campbell-Walsh urology. 9th ed. Philadelphia, Pa: Saunders Elsevier; 2007. p. 609–53.
7. Augarten A, Weissenberg R, Pariente C, et al. Reversible male infertility in late onset congenital adrenal hyperplasia. J Endocrinol Invest. 1991;14:237–40.
8. Segal S, Yaffe H, Laufer N, et al. Male hyperprolactinemia:effects on fertility. Fertil Steril. 1979;32:556–61.
9. De Rosa M, Colao A, Di Sarno A, et al. Cabergoline treatment rapidly improves gonadal function in hyperprolactinemic males: a comparison with bromocriptine. Eur J Endocrinol. 1998;138:286–93.
10. van't Verlaat JW, Croughs RJ. Withdrawal of bromocriptine after long-term therapy for macroprolactinomas; effect on plasma prolactin and tumour size. Clin Endocrinol (Oxf). 1991;34:175–8.
11. Mathur S, Williamson HO, Baker ME, et al. Sperm motility on postcoital testing correlates with male autoimmunity to sperm. Fertil Steril. 1984;41:81–7.
12. Robinson JN, Forman RG, Nicholson SC, et al. A comparison of intrauterine insemination in superovulated cycles to intercourse in couples where the male is receiving steroids for the treatment of autoimmune infertility. Fertil Steril. 1995;63:1260–6.
13. Lähteenmäki A, Räsänen M, Hovatta O. Low-dose prednisolone does not improve the outcome of in-vitro fertilization in male immunological infertility. Hum Reprod. 1995;10:3124–9.
14. Kamischke A, Nieschlag E. Treatment of retrograde ejaculation and anejaculation. Hum Reprod Update. 1999;5:448–74.
15. Ghanem H, Shamloul R. An evidence-based perspective to the medical treatment of male infertility: a short review. Urol Int. 2009;82:125–9.
16. Skakkebaek NE, Hammen R, Philip J, et al. Quantification of human seminiferous epithelium. 3. Histologicalstudies in 44 infertile men with normal chromosome complements. Acta Pathol Microbiol Scand A. 1973;81:97–111.
17. Kahraman S, Ozgur S, Aksoy S, et al. High implantation and pregnancy rates with testicular sperm extraction and intracytoplasmic sperm injection in obstructive and non-obstructive azoospermia. Hum Reprod. 1996;11:673–6.
18. Yoshida A, Miura K, Shirai M. Evaluation of seminiferous tubule scores obtained through testicular biopsy examinations of nonobstructive azoospermic men. Fertil Steril. 1997;68:514–8.
19. Kessaris DN, Wasserman P, Mellinger BC. Histopathological and cytopathological correlations of percutaneous testis biopsy and open testis biopsy in infertile men. J Urol. 1995;153:1151–5.
20. Carpi A, Agarwal A, Sabanegh E, et al. Percutaneous biopsy of the testicle: a mini review with a proposal flow chart for non-obstructive azoospermia. Ann Med. 2011;43:83–9.
21. Sheynkin YR, Ye Z, Menendez S, et al. Controlled comparison of percutaneous and microsurgical sperm retrieval in men with obstructive azoospermia. Hum Reprod. 1998;13:3086–9.
22. Jarow JP. Transrectal ultrasonography in the diagnosis and management of ejaculatory duct obstruction. J Androl. 1996;17:467–72.
23. Potts JM, Pasqualotto FF, Nelson D, et al. Patient characteristics associated with vasectomy reversal. J Urol. 1999;161:1835–9.
24. Belker AM, Thomas Jr AJ, Fuchs EF, et al. Results of 1,469 microsurgical vasectomy reversals by the vasovasostomy study group. J Urol. 1991;145:505–11.
25. Kolettis PN, Sabanegh ES, Nalesnik JG, et al. Pregnancy outcomes after vasectomy reversal for female partners 35 years old or older. J Urol. 2003;169:2250–2.
26. Pasqualotto FF, Pasqualotto EB, Ågarwal A, et al. Results of microsurgical anastomosis in men with

seminal tract obstruction due to inguinal herniorrhaphy. Rev Hosp Clin Fac Med Sao Paulo. 2003; 58:305–9.
27. Johnson CW, Bingham JB, Goluboff ET, et al. Transurethral resection of the ejaculatory ducts for treating ejaculatory symptoms. BJU Int. 2005;95: 117–9.
28. Witt MA, Lipshultz LI. Varicocele: a progressive or static lesion? Urology. 1993;42:541–3.
29. Report on Varicocele and Infertility: An AUA Best Practice Policy and ASRM Practice Committee Report, Reviewed and Validity Confirmed 2010. www.auanet.org/resources.cfm?ID=466. Accessed 12 June 2011.
30. Steckel J, Dicker AP, Goldstein M. Relationship between varicocele size and response to varicocelectomy. J Urol. 1993;149:769–71.
31. Jarow JP, Ogle SR, Eskew LA. Seminal improvement following repair of ultrasound detected subclinical varicoceles. J Urol. 1996;155:1287–90.
32. Agarwal A, Deepinder F, Cocuzza M, et al. Efficacy of varicocelectomy in improving semen parameters: new meta-analytical approach. Urology. 2007;70:532–8.
33. Kolettis PN, Thomas Jr AJ. Vasoepididymostomy for vasectomy reversal: a critical assessment in the era of intracytoplasmic sperm injection. J Urol. 1997;158: 467–70.
34. Lee R, Li PS, Goldstein M, et al. A decision analysis of treatments for obstructive azoospermia. Hum Reprod. 2008;23:2043–9.
35. Meng MV, Greene KL, Turek PJ. Surgery or assisted reproduction? A decision analysis of treatment costs in male infertility. J Urol. 2005;174:1926–31.
36. de Mouzon J, Goossens V, Bhattacharya S, et al. Assisted reproductive technology in Europe, 2006: results generated from European registers by ESHRE. Hum Reprod. 2010;25:1851–62.
37. Bagis T, Haydardedeoglu B, Kilicdag EB, et al. Single versus double intrauterine insemination in multi-follicular ovarian hyperstimulation cycles: a randomized trial. Hum Reprod. 2010;25:1684–90.
38. Gunby J, Daya S. IVF Directors Group of the Canadian Fertility and Andrology Society. Assisted reproductive technologies (ART) in Canada: 2003 results from the Canadian ART Register. Fertil Steril. 2007;88:550–9.

# Evaluation and Therapy of Chronic Scrotal Content Pain and Epididymitis

17

Jonas S. Benson and Laurence A. Levine

## Introduction

Chronic orchialgia is a problem seen commonly by urologists, but remains a treatment dilemma due to its frequent idiopathic etiology, patient distress and physician frustration with caring for the condition. When encountered in the primary care setting, identifying the etiology and subsequent management can be difficult. Chronic orchialgia is defined as intermittent or constant testicular pain, 3 months or longer in duration that significantly interferes with the daily activities of the patient [1]. The term chronic orchialgia is frequently used to describe pain actually originating from other structures within the scrotum all of which fall under the umbrella term, *chronic scrotal content pain*. The structures that can be involved include the testicle, paratesticular structures, spermatic cord, and the epididymis. An inflammatory condition specifically located within the epididymis is by definition, epididymitis. Inflammation of the epididymis can be classified into acute, subacute and chronic based on the duration of symptoms. Acute epididymitis usually consists of pain and swelling of the epididymitis for less than 6 weeks. Subacute persists for 6 weeks to 3 months, while chronic epididymitis is primarily associated with pain and no swelling that lasts longer than 3 months [2]. Chronic epididymitis can further be classified into inflammatory chronic epididymitis, obstructive chronic epididymitis, and chronic epididymalgia [3]. The focus of this chapter will be chronic scrotal content pain, which includes chronic epididymitis as well as acute epididymitis.

J.S. Benson, MD
Department of Urology, Rush University Medical Center, 1725 W. Harrison, Suite 348, Chicago, IL 60612, USA
e-mail: Jonas_benson@rush.edu

L.A. Levine, MD (✉)
Department of Urology, Ruch University Medical Center, Professional Building, 1725 W. Harrison Street, Suite 352, Chicago, IL 60612, USA
e-mail: drlevine@hotmail.com

## Epidemiology, Etiology, and Pathophysiology

Chronic scrotal content pain can be due to direct sources, including infection, torsion, tumor, obstruction, varicoceles, spermatoceles, rarely hydroceles and can follow direct trauma as well as iatrogenic injury after vasectomy or inguinal hernia repair (see Tables 17.1 and 17.2). Indirect pain, also called referred pain, can occur as a result of a ureteral stone, indirect inguinal hernia, aortic or common iliac artery aneurysms, lower back disorders, and nerve entrapment due to perineural fibrosis. In a study by Davis et al., 50% of patients may present with generalized scrotal content pain that is idiopathic in origin without a specific inciting event [1]. Urologists are more likely to see a specific subset of chronic scrotal content pain called post-vasectomy pain syndrome, which is uncommon but nonetheless

D.A. Shoskes (ed.), *Urological Men's Health: A Guide for Urologists and Primary Care Physicians*, Current Clinical Urology, DOI 10.1007/978-1-61779-900-6_17,
© Springer Science+Business Media New York 2012

**Table 17.1** Differential diagnosis for chronic scrotal content pain

| |
|---|
| Chronic infection |
| Testicular torsion |
| Testicular or paratesticular tumor |
| Vas deferens or epididymal obstruction |
| Varicocele |
| Spermatocele |
| Hydrocele |
| Trauma |
| Post-vasectomy pain syndrome |
| Post-inguinal hernia repair |
| Referred pain from ureteral stone, indirect inguinal hernia, aortic or common iliac artery aneurysms, lower back disorders |
| Chronic pelvic pain/chronic prostatitis, interstitial cystitis, fibromyalgia |
| Idiopathic |

**Table 17.2** Potential inciting event contributing to or resulting in chronic scrotal content pain

| |
|---|
| Idiopathic (found in a high as 50% of patients) |
| Scrotal content infection, single or multiple (epididymitis, orchitis, sexually transmitted diseases) |
| Trauma |
| Prior scrotal content surgery for pathologic or benign condition (vasectomy, correction of varicocele, spermatocele, hydrocele or hernia) |
| Vas deferens or epididymal obstruction |
| Post-inguinal hernia repair |
| Referred pain from ureteral stone, indirect inguinal hernia, aortic or common iliac artery aneurysms, lower back disorders |

distressing to the patient. This syndrome presents anywhere from shortly after the vasectomy to as long as 7 years after the procedure [4]. The etiology of post-vasectomy pain syndrome is thought to be due to congestive epididymitis, sperm granuloma, or nerve entrapment. Psychiatric issues, as well as secondary gain with malingering must also be considered in the differential diagnosis of men presenting with chronic pain.

According to the National Center for Health Statistics, 1 in 144 outpatient visits in men age 18–50 years old are for epididymitis or orchitis. Among the inflammatory conditions within the scrotum, epididymitis is the most common. Pathogens usually enter the epididymitis via a retrograde ascent. Historically, chemical irritation from refluxing urine was believed to be the primary cause of epididymitis. In 1979, a study showed that bacteria of various types were the primary cause of epididymitis [5]. The origin and type of bacteria appear to be age specific. There are noninfectious causes of epididymitis and have been shown to be a result of medications (Amiodarone) and vasculitis-associated conditions [6]. Acute epididymitis in young sexually active men (less than age 35) is most frequently caused by *Chlamydia trachomatis* and *Neisseria gonorrhoeae*. Enteric organisms such as *Escherichia coli* and *Pseudomonas* have also been reported to occur among men who are the insertive partner during anal intercourse. When obtained via sexual intercourse, epididymitis is typically associated with asymptomatic urethritis. Sexually transmitted epididymitis is uncommon in men >35 years old. Nonsexually transmitted epididymitis is associated with obstructive uropathy from benign prostatic hyperplasia, urinary tract instrumentation, systemic disease, and/or those who are immunocompromised. Chronic epididymitis can be a granulomatous reaction related to mycobacterium tuberculosis, which is the most common granulomatous disease affecting the epididymis with up to 25% of patients having bilateral disease [7]. The granulomatous reaction can also be caused by the administration of Bacillus Calmette-Guerin (BCG) to treat bladder cancer [8]. Epididymitis in children has been linked with post-infectious inflammatory reaction such as recent infections from *Mycoplasma pneumonia*, enteroviruses, and adenoviruses.

## Diagnosis

Initial evaluation of the patient with chronic scrotal content pain should include ruling out medically important and reversible causes including tumor, torsion, infection, and varicocele. History should focus on pain onset, duration, severity (graded on a 0–10 scale), location and referral of pain. There is not a gold standard for reporting on pain. Simply asking the question "How would you rate your pain on a scale of 0–10?" is typically done. The Visual Analog Scale (cartoon scale from 0 to 10) is also commonly used. These two methods are simple and easily reproduced from visit to visit. They also allow comparison of pretreatment and post-treatment perception of pain [9]. Although other pain scales are available, they have not been adopted for this pain problem. Identifying other associated factors such as prior surgery, trauma or an infectious process is important. One should ascertain whether certain activities exacerbate or ameliorate the pain. These can include voiding, bowel movements/valsalva, sexual activity, prolonged sitting, physical activity or exercise. Obtaining a past surgical history is essential with particular attention to back, inguinal, scrotal, transurethral, pelvis or retroperitoneal surgery as they can all result in chronic scrotal content pain. Psychosocial questions should identify potential secondary gain or malingering. Associated conditions such as depression or substance abuse should be identified as well as a history of other areas of chronic pain, including prostatitis, interstitial cystitis, or fibromyalgia. In addition, it has been recognized that chronic genital pain may be associated with a history of sexual abuse.

A detailed and focused urologic physical exam is of utmost importance. The patient should be examined supine and standing, starting the genital exam on the nonpainful or less-painful side if bilateral. Thorough examination of the testes, epididymis, and vas deferens is indicated. A digital rectal exam should also be performed. With epididymitis, the epididymis is tender, indurated, and swollen. Laboratory evaluation includes a urinalysis, urine culture/gram stain, and semen culture if indicated. A polymerase chain reaction assay for *C. trachomatis* and *N. gonorrhoeae* should be performed if epididymitis is suspected or when there is a history of sexually transmitted disease. The diagnosis of urethritis is confirmed with a Gram stain which is a rapid, highly sensitive, and specific diagnostic test. Urethral secretions which demonstrate ≥5 white blood cells (WBC) per high powered magnification field are diagnostic. Gonococcal infection is confirmed when WBCs contain Gram-negative diplococci. Other diagnostic tests that can be used to diagnose urethritis are positive leukocyte esterase test on first-void urine or microscopic examination of a voided urine specimen with ≥10 WBCs per high power field [7]. All patients presenting with scrotal content pain should undergo a duplex scrotal ultrasound. The duplex ultrasound has the benefit of being noninvasive and allows assessment of perfusion to the testis and anatomy of the scrotal contents. When epididymitis is present there will be an enlarged, thick epididymis with increased Doppler wave signal suggesting enhanced blood flow. The lack of blood flow to the testis in the acute setting is nearly diagnostic for testicular torsion and immediate surgical exploration is indicated. In the pediatric population Doppler ultrasound has a sensitivity of 82% and a specificity of 100% for testicular torsion, with a 70% sensitivity and 88% specificity for epididymitis [10].

## Treatment

The treatment of acute epididymitis and chronic scrotal content pain has little overlap and will be discussed separately within this section. The initial treatment for acute epididymitis is empiric in nature and should be based on the patient's age, medical and social history. Laboratory workup and cultures should be obtained, but the treatment can be initiated based on the likely bacteria. Those under the age of 14 or over the age of 35 should be treated for enteric organisms with a quinolone for 10 days. There is a low incidence of urinary tract infection in boys with epididymitis thus in prepubertal patients antibiotic therapy can be reserved for young infants and those with pyuria or positive urine culture findings. Urine cultures should be obtained on all pediatric patients with epididymitis [11]. The antibiotic choices for the pediatric population include trimethoprim and sulfamethoxazole, amoxicillin and potassium clavulanate, ciprofloxacin, and levofloxacin. The role of quinolones in the treatment of urologic infection in children is currently being investigated [12]. Treatment should be provided for 10–14 days and be tailored to culture results.

**Table 17.3** Recommended treatment for acute epididymitis [2,7,11,13]

| |
|---|
| All patients should have the following for symptomatic relief while acute symptoms of fever and local inflammation present: bed rest, scrotal elevation, cold packs, NSAIDs, and analgesics |
| If likely cause by enteric organisms (*Escherichia coli* and *Pseudomonas* spp.) |
| Levofloxacin 500 mg orally once daily for 10 days |
| OR |
| Ofloxacin 300 mg orally two times a day for 10 days |
| If sexually active with age between 14 and 35 (likely cause *C. trachomatis* or *N. gonorrhoeae*) |
| Ceftriaxone 250 mg intramuscular one time dose |
| AND |
| Doxycycline 100 mg orally two times a day for 10 days |
| Azithromycin 1 g orally one time dose may be substituted for doxycycline if treatment compliance is questionable |
| Additional therapy with a fluoroquinolone if *C. trachomatis* or *N. gonorrhoeae* not found on diagnostic testing resulting in the most likely caused by enteric organisms |
| Pediatric population |
| Treat patients with evidence of urinary tract infection with antibacterial agents, otherwise symptomatic relief is needed |
| Potential antibiotics for treatment in pediatric population, treat 10–14 days: trimethoprim and sulfamethoxazole, amoxicillin and potassium clavulanate, ciprofloxacin, or levofloxacin. Adjust antibiotic according to urine culture results |

A summary of treatment options for acute epididymitis is shown in Table 17.3.

If chlamydial or gonococcal infection is identified (age 14–35), the goals of treatment are microbiologic cure of infection, improve the patients symptoms, prevent transmission of sexually transmitted diseases to partners, and decrease the likelihood of complications. Treatment is with ceftriaxone 250 mg intramuscularly and single 1-g dose of azithromycin or doxycycline 100 mg two times a day for 10 days. Those who are immunocompromised with human deficiency virus or on prednisone are treated in the same way [7]. Symptomatic treatment is also necessary for acute epididymitis. Analgesics as needed, nonsteroidal anti-inflammatories, scrotal elevation, limited activity, and applying cold packs to the affected side will all help alleviate the discomfort and reduce the inflammation associated with the pain and swelling. Systemic or worsening local symptoms should be monitored which include sepsis, abscess, chronic scrotal area pain, or extension of the infection into adjacent structures (e.g. spermatic cord, scrotal wall or testis). Along with chronic pain, infertility is also a possible long-term consequence of acute epididymitis. Acute epididymitis treatment is typically done as an outpatient with close follow-up. On occasion the patient will not be able to tolerate oral medication due to emesis and will require intravenous antibiotics and pain control. Systemic symptoms consistent with sepsis should also be managed in an inpatient setting as well as those patients who will be poorly compliant. Patients should be instructed to have early follow-up if their symptoms fail to improve within 2 days. Failure of resolution of symptoms should prompt further workup with the differential diagnosis including tumor, testis infarction, tuberculosis, fungal infection, or abscess.

Treatment for chronic scrotal content pain is a dilemma and not well described. An algorithm describing a basic workup for chronic scrotal content pain is shown in Fig. 17.1. Initial management should be simple and noninvasive. Medications including nonsteroidal anti-inflammatory drugs and antibiotics are first-line treatment particularly when there is evidence of infection. Flouroquinolones and tetracyclines are best, as they appear to have the highest penetration into the structures within the scrotum. Treatment can be given for 4–6 weeks when indicated. Other oral medications include antidepressants, such as amitrptyline or nortriptyline. These medications inhibit norepinephrine release at first- and second-order neurons. Initially developed as an anticonvulsant medication, gabapentin has neuropathic pain properties as well. The drug works via calcium channel modulation in the central nervous system to reduce neuropathic pain [13]. A review by Sinclair et al. in 2007 demonstrated little benefit with these drugs for post-vasectomy pain syndrome [14]. Although there are no published reports, the authors do recommend external and internal pelvic physical therapy when there is no indication of infection. This has been

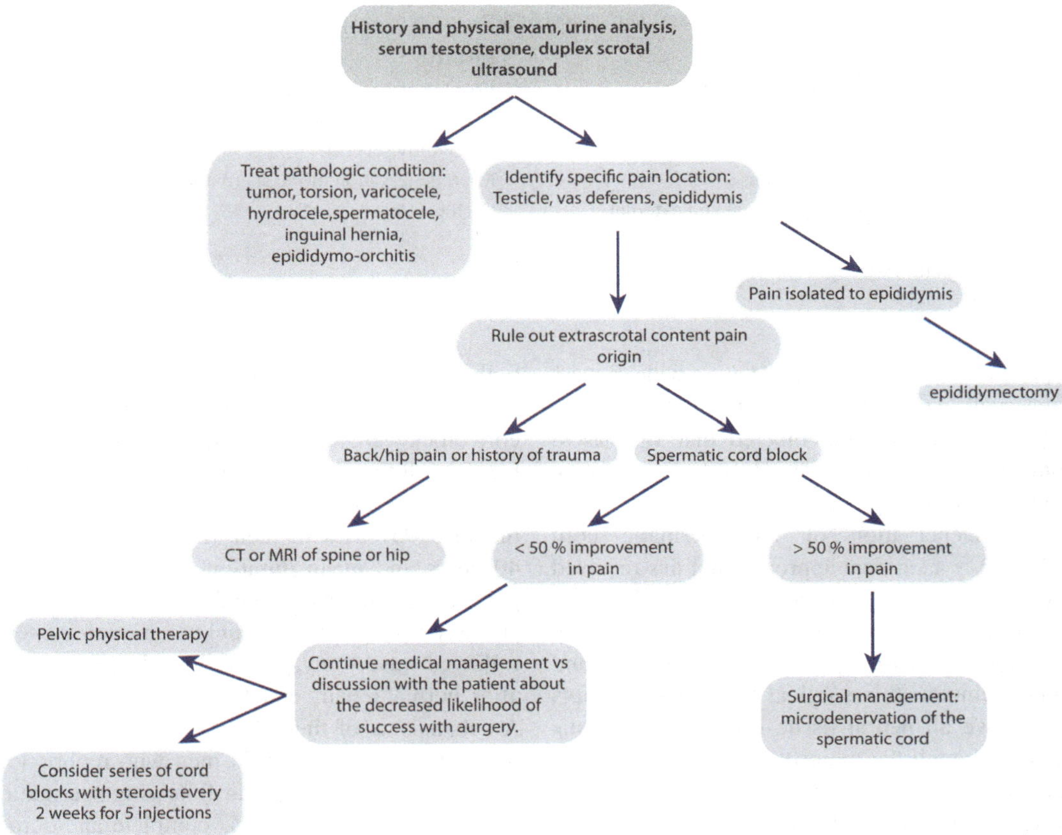


**Fig. 17.1** Algorithm for scrotal content pain

used successfully and should be considered particularly when there is a history of chronic pain elsewhere or there are urinary tract symptoms. A recently introduced form of noninvasive treatment is known as TMR®, which is a delivery system for focused, painless, topical, high-intensity pulsed electromagnetic energy. Initial trials with TMR® are ongoing with encouraging results. Nerve blocks as a single or a series of injections have also been used to treat chronic scrotal content pain. A long-lasting local anesthetic such as bupivacaine with or without steroid injections can be done in an attempt to break the pain cycle. This tends to be most successful when the pain has a duration of less than 6 months. Psychological counseling may be beneficial to help the patient deal with the pain, but when medical and less invasive approaches fail, surgery is frequently the next option as summarized in Table 17.4.

## Surgical Management for Chronic Scrotal Content Pain

When scrotal content pain is localized just to the epididymis, an epididymectomy is indicated. There is a wide range of published outcomes studies reporting success rates with epididymectomy ranging from 10% to 80% [15]. The best results for epididymectomy are those with post-vasectomy pain syndrome [16]. Multiple case series have shown poor results with epididymectomy when the pain is more diffuse, involving the cord and/or the testicle. Vasectomy reversal has also been performed either open ended historically or by vasovasostomy. The largest series evaluating vasovasostomy for chronic pain was a 10-year experience with 45 men where they reported a 75% complete relief of pain, 10% partial pain relief, and 10% failed to improve [17]. Smaller

**Table 17.4** Chronic scrotal content pain treatment options

| Noninvasive | Invasive |
|---|---|
| Nonsteroidal anti-inflammatory drugs | Local anesthetic injection with/without steroids |
| Antibiotics when indicated (4–6 weeks) | Epididymectomy (when localized pain) |
| Antidepressants | Vasectomy reversal |
| Neuropathic pain medications | Microdenervation of the spermatic cord |
| Pelvic physical therapy internal and external | Orchiectomy |
| TMR | |
| Acupuncture | |

reports on vasectomy reversal have a wide success range with pain relief ranging from 69% to 84% [18]. It should be remembered that vasovasostomy is costly and when successful it reverses the prior sterilization process.

Microdenervation of the spermatic cord (MDSC) is a surgical approach that has received increased attention due to several articles published over the past decade [19–21]. Initially described as a case report in 1978 by Devine and Schellhammer, this surgical technique attempts to remove all neural tissue supplying the testis [22]. Although the majority of MDSC surgeries are performed with microscope magnification, recent advances in technology have allowed new surgical approaches. Parekattil et al. reviewed their experience with 230 robotic-assisted MDSC procedures performed between October 2008 and September 2010. They had a relatively short median follow-up of 8 months and reported a 77% complete resolution of pain with an additional 8% having at least a 50% decrease in pain [23]. Regardless of the technique utilized to perform MDSC, the goal continues to be to divide all structures, which may be carrying neural fibers while preserving the testicular, cremasteric, and deferential arteries. Several lymphatics are also preserved to reduce the likelihood of hydrocele. The vas deferens is divided if vasectomy was previously performed to ensure that there are no residual vasal or perivasal nerves. The primary advantage of MDSC is sparing the testicle for both psychological and physiological reasons. Those considering an MDSC for chronic scrotal content pain should undergo a spermatic cord block with a long-acting local anesthetic such as bupivacaine. In a recently presented study, men with chronic scrotal content pain who had complete albeit temporary relief from the spermatic cord block were more likely to have durable complete resolution of pain after undergoing MDSC [24]. A recent published report on MDSC included 95 cases in men with a mean age of 40 years and mean duration of scrotal content pain for 62 months (range 5–252 months). Pain etiology varied: 43% had unknown etiology, 8% followed vasectomy, 7% followed trauma, 9% after hernia repair, and 9% after epididymitis. A subanalysis of these MDSC cases performed between 2007 and 2009 in men who reported a 90–100% reduction of pain following spermatic cord block revealed an 88% complete and durable response after surgery. Thus, it appears the spermatic cord block can provide useful information for selecting men who are most apt to have surgical success. For those men who had no benefit from MDSC, several explanations exist, including: central nervous system sensitization had already occurred, sensory nerves were missed, a posterior or pudendal source carried the pain stimuli, and malingering must be considered. Interestingly, 40% of the men who had complete pain resolution noted immediate postoperative relief, but this may take up to 6 months to occur. Mean follow-up in this patient population was 20 months with a range of 1–102 months. There were two men who experienced testicular atrophy with complete pain resolution, and there was no hypogonadism. There was one hydrocele which resolved spontaneously in 6 months [19].

Orchiectomy remains an option for surgical correction of chronic orchialgia. Yet, reported success rates are not encouraging at 20–70%. This may be due to central sensitization or failure to divide the sensory nerve input. Pain resolution appears to be better with inguinal versus a scrotal approach [1].

## Conclusions

Properly ruling out other pathologies within the scrotum in the acute and chronic setting is of utmost importance. Once the diagnosis of acute epididymitis is made, the medical management has a structured path that is well established within the literature. The management of chronic scrotal content pain is evolving to identify the optimal diagnosis and treatment methods to obtain the best patient outcomes. More elegant and successful treatment options are likely to emerge as large-scale, multi-center, randomized control trials are undertaken. A multidisciplinary approach including pain services, physical therapists, and psychologists may be beneficial before considering surgical management. When surgical management is required, MDSC provides testicular sparing surgery with complete and durable resolution of pain reported in the 71–89% range.

## References

1. Davis BE, Novle MJ, Weigel JW, et al. Analysis and management of chronic testicular pain. J Urol. 1990;143:936–9.
2. Trojian TH, Lishnak TS, Heiman D. Epididymitis and orchitis: an overview. Am Fam Phys. 2009;79(7): 583–7.
3. Nickel JC, Siemens DR, Nickel KR, et al. The patient with chronic epididymitis: characterization of an enigmatic syndrome. J Urol. 2002;167:1701–4.
4. McMahon AJ, Buckley J, Taylor A, et al. Chronic testicular pain following vasectomy. Br J Urol. 1992; 157:518.
5. Berger RE, Alexander ER, Harnisch JP, et al. Etiology, manifestations and therapy of acute epididymitits: prospective study of 50 case. J Urol. 1979;121(6):750–4.
6. Nikolaou M, Idonomidis I, Lekakis I, et al. Amiodarone-induced epididymitis: a case report and review of the literature. Int J Cardiol. 2007;121(1): 15–6.
7. National Center for Health Statistics. Sexually transmitted disease treatment guidelines. 2010. http://www.cdc.gov/std/treatment/2010/epididymitis.htm. Accessed 6 Oct 2011.
8. Rischmann P, Desgrandchamps F, Malavaud B, Chopin DK. BCG intravesical instillations: recommendations for side-effects management. Eur Urol. 2000;37 Suppl 1:33–6.
9. Rabah DM, Fabrozio MD. Postoperative pain: current management concepts. Conep Urol. 2003;15:15–29.
10. Stehr M, Hoehm R. Critical validation of colour Doppler ultrasound in diagnostics of acute scrotum in children. Eur J Pediatr Surg. 2003;13(6):386–92.
11. Santillanes G, Gausche-Hill M, Lewis RJ. Are antibiotics necessary for pediatric epididymitis? Pediatr Emerg Care. 2011;27(3):174–8.
12. Richman MN, Bukowski TP. Pediatric epididymitis: pathophysiology, diagnosis, and management. Medscape. http://www.medscape.com/viewarticle/410234. Accessed 6 Oct 2011.
13. Brown JT, Randall A. Gabapentin fails to alter P/Q-type Ca2+ channel-mediated synaptic transmission in the hippocampus in vitro. Synapse. 2005;55(4): 262–9.
14. Sinclair AM, Miller B, Lee LK. Chronic orchialigia: consider gabapentin or nortriptyline before considering surgery. Int J Urol. 2007;14:622–5.
15. Siu W, Ohl DA, Schuster TG. Long-term follow-up after epididymectomy for chronic epididymal pain. Urology. 2007;70:333–5.
16. Hori S, Sengupta A, Shukla CJ, et al. Long-term outcome of epididymectomy for the management of chronic epididymal pain. J Urol. 2009;182:1407–12.
17. Werthman P. Vasectomy reversal for post-vasectomy pain syndrome: a ten year experience. J Urol. 2010;183 (Suppl):e752.
18. Myers SA, Merson CE, Fuchs EF. Vasectomy reversal for the treatment of the post-vasectomy pain syndrome. J Urol. 1997;157:518.
19. Strom KH, Levine LA. Microsurgical denervation of the spermatic cord for chronic orchialgia: long-term results from a single center. J Urol. 2008;180: 949–53.
20. Heidenreich A, Olbert P, Engelmann UH. Management of chronic testalgia by microsurgical testicular denervation. Eur Urol. 2002;41:392–7.
21. Levine LA, Matkov TG. Microsurgical denervation of the spermatic cord as primary surgical treatment of chronic orchialgia. J Urol. 2001;165:1927–9.
22. Devine CJ, Schellhammer PF. The use of microsurgical denervation of the spermatic cord for orchalgia. Trans Am Assoc Genitourin Surg. 1978;70:149.
23. Parekattil SJ, Cohen MS. Robotic microsurgery 2011: male infertility, chronic testicular pain, postvasectomy pain, sports hernia pain and phantom pain. Curr Opin Urol. 2011;21:121–6.
24. Benson JS, Larsen SM, Abern MR, Levine LA. Microdenervation of the spermatic cord: single institution review on preoperative cord block predicting surgical outcome. Presented as part of 85th North Central Section of American Urologic Association, Rancho Mirage, CA, USA, 18–22 October 2011.

# Psychosocial Factors in Painful Urogenital Conditions in Men

18

Dean A. Tripp and Jessica Ginting

## Psychosocial Factors in Painful Urogenital Conditions in Men

Pain is often a mystery to patients. Pain is an alarming, fear-raising, life-altering experience that demands our attention, but this is usually a good thing! Pain is of tremendous survival and diagnostic value but yet it remains an ambiguous entity to many in health care. Pain, which can be described as "an unpleasant sensory and emotional experience associated with actual or potential tissue damage, or described in terms of such damage" [1], is the most commonly reported motivation for physician consultation in the USA [2]. Further, other reports show that pain is the primary motivator for emergency department usage in over half of patients [3] and exists in almost one third of primary care usage [4].

Pain is not only a major presenting symptom in a variety of medical conditions, but it is also significantly associated with diminished quality of life (QoL) and in particular poorer general communal functioning [5]. The classic distinction in pain has been between the *acute* and *chronic* pains, which have been set by arbitrary time intervals from pain inception. The two most common cut points for describing pain as acute or chronic has been 3 and 6 months since pain onset [6], but some suggest the modification from acute to chronic is the 12-month mark [7]. Further, depending on other sources, subacute pain is suggested to exist from 1 to 6 months [8] and a substitute definition of chronic pain suggests that it has no solid timeframe, but is "pain that extends beyond the expected period of healing" [6]. Chronic pain may also be classified as malignant or benign depending on the concurrent disease process [8].

## Pain and the Biomedical Model

There is little doubt that pain is an important feature of disease, but for some health-care practitioners, psychosocial factors have no place in pain management. This type of thinking is a great misstep in patient management and is likely due to the small amount of direct "pain" training afforded to medical students in the present curriculums. A historical review of the pain literature shows the current concepts of pain and differences in pain perception have been formed by cultural and scientific shifts associated with the advance of medicine, philosophy, and psychology.

Pain has always played a valuable role in medicine, such as diagnosing and treating illness.

D.A. Tripp, PhD (✉)
Departments of Psychology, Anesthesiology & Urology, Queen's University, 62 Arch Street, Humphrey Hall, Kingston, ON K7L 3N6, Canada
e-mail: Dean.Tripp@queensu.ca

J. Ginting, MSc
Department of Psychology, Queen's University, 62 Arch Street, Humphrey Hall, Kingston, ON K7L 3N6, Canada
e-mail: jginting@gmail.com

D.A. Shoskes (ed.), *Urological Men's Health: A Guide for Urologists and Primary Care Physicians*, Current Clinical Urology, DOI 10.1007/978-1-61779-900-6_18,
© Springer Science+Business Media New York 2012

However, centuries ago, and actually today in some cultures, pain was believed to be the manifestation of a supernatural presence or spiritual possession, a personality fault, or a warning to others of impending social malevolence [9]. Although pain models can be traced back to the stone ages, such as Chinese acupuncture, or Grecian medicine, many scholars consider Rene Descartes' dualistic conceptualization of pain and its associated mechanisms a cornerstone or turning point in our understanding of pain [9]. Descartes' biomedical (or mechanistic) pain model assumed that pain was reported as equivalent to the amount of observable physical pathology. Indeed, he proposed that the mind held no influence on such bodily processes and that pain was experienced within a "straight-through" physical system [9]. Interestingly, in his "Passions of the Soul" Decartes suggested that a human being was comparable to a watch [10]. According to Decartes, human beings could be described as an automaton, and when wounded they moved as a device with principle, but when broken (i.e., deceased) they were a piece without purpose or movement. His directive anatomical works were important because they ranked among several important lines of thinking in the 1600s that provided a significant departure from the spiritual and philosophical roots developed to explain pain and human suffering.

With the expanding practice of medical research and the advances it provided through the 17th and 1800s, a growing dissatisfaction developed around the mechanistic Descartesian model of pain. For example, the pattern theory of pain proposed by Goldscheider in 1894 was based on findings suggesting that certain patterns of stimulation (i.e., skin) would respond by the summation of sensory inputs into the dorsal horn of the central nervous system [11]. Further, research developments of the mid-1950s argued for the growing consensus that the emotional state of the patient was as predictive of outcomes as the function aspects of their presentation. Hill et al. showed that individuals with high anxiety also reported significantly greater pain [12]. Further, Beecher [13] illustrated how powerful suffering and mental relief from fear can be in regard to pain and pain treatment. His observations of battle-injured soldiers showed that the in-hospital pain medication requests from these soldiers during treatment of their wounds were significantly lower than civilians having undergone similar clinical procedures. Beecher went on to suggest that such differences may be explained by the soldiers' psychological dynamics of fear associated with their war experiences and their associated relief of being free from war.

To disentangle the complexity of pain from the physical and mental state, the "Gate Control Theory" of pain was adapted to outline the clinical experience of pain, addressing the impact of cognitive influences on pain experience and expression [14]. The gate theory suggested that physiological pain pathways in the central nervous system were the center of neural activity that either augmented or reduced subjective pain experiences. Based on decades of clinical observation, research, and treatment, the gate model suggested there was indeed a mind–body interface to pain. The mechanisms of pain were centered on pain signaling coming in over the C-fibers that were modulated by the presynaptic inhibition arriving from the incoming beta-fibers (i.e., pain) in the substantia gelatinosa of the dorsal horn. The thin fibers (i.e., pain) impede the inhibitory cells of the dorsal horn tending to leave the pain gate open, while the large diameter fibers (i.e., C-fibers: touch, pressure to skin) can excite the inhibitory cells and tend to close the pain gate.

In sum, the greater the large C-fiber activation relative to thin pain fiber activity experienced at the inhibitory cells, the pain is reduced at the experience level. This type of gating was suggested as to why we might rub a painful area. This type of pain "gating" is dependent upon the quality and type of signaling occurring in these associated structures for sensation and ultimately pain. Interestingly, the gate model not only presented a pain signal traveling from the injury site to the dorsal horns inhibition or transmission cells and then up the spinal cord to the brain, but also suggested that a signal also traveled directly in the CNS to the brain bypassing the inhibitory and transmission cells in the dorsal horn. Depending on the emotional state at that time, this signal could trigger a top-down signal along the spinal cord to modulate inhibitory cell activity, thus, increasing or decreasing the intensity of pain signaling.

The basic "pain gating" model has been discussed and researched for years with much of it discounted but the concept of competition at the central nervous system by central mechanisms and external stimuli have promoted significant advancements in pain understanding. Indeed, pathways in the nervous system have been suggested to assist pain signals, whereas the neurophysiological influence of emotional and cognitive activity travels down the spinal cord, modulating incoming signals at the dorsal horn in such a pain gate. This proposal has basically suggested that strong negative emotional states act to increase subjective reports of pain through facilitated sensory processing, while positive emotions may decrease subjective pain through decreased afferent processing in varying degrees [15].

For the most part, our society views acute pains as warning signals of disease or injury in people or in animals, but chronic pain is known for its ability to ruin the lives of the patients and that of the people closest to them. Chronic or refractory pain is not considered to be a warning to prevent an injury or help in identifying an emerging disease. In fact, chronic pain is often referred to as a disease onto itself. Chronic pain is described now to be a disease state of the central nervous system, a system in which the usual function of neural mechanisms have been significantly altered. The neuromatrix concept suggests that the dysfunction of various brain mechanisms may underlie some kinds of chronic pain and points to new forms of treatment.

Melzack [16] proposed a Neuromatrix pain model where people are suggested to have a genetic/characteristic patterns of nerve impulses activated by either sensory input or central input often independent of peripheral activation. The Neuromatrix model suggests that there is an anatomical, widespread network of motor and sensation neurons that are part of extensive recursive feedback loops in association with the thalamus and cortex, and cortex and limbic system. Natural acute events such as injuries or the threat of injury alter bodily homeostasis stressing the organism to initiate neural, hormonal, and behavioral activation to achieve a normal baseline state. Whether physiological or psychological, stress activates the limbic system and its functions of emotional processing. In chronic activation, a predisposition for central nervous system sensitization to repeated stimulation patterns might act in the development of chronic pain states. Thus, the Neuromatrix model can be considered a diathesis-stress process wherein physiological predispositions interact with the acute stressors ultimately manifesting a person's experience with pain [17]. Pain in this model can therefore be conceptualized as a "stress" that reduces bodily homeostasis. The presence of persistent pain creates a constant physiological activation and heavy physiological loads or helplessness or anxiety, can reduce bodily homeostasis, further augmenting the pain experience. Several underlying neuroanatomical pathways, neurophysiological mechanisms, and several well-known psychosocial factors can therefore be involved in pain experience [18].

Current models of pain suggest that pain is not entirely a sensory experience and that identical painful stimulation (i.e., same experimental pain applied by pressure or temperature) does not produce identical reports of pain and distress across research participants and clinical patients alike. Pain varies between people; influenced by their subjective meanings of situation, attention, and other personal appraisals [19]. Further, cognitive-bio-behavioral pain models add consideration of environmental factors to individual cognitive factors. For example, if someone believes they have poor coping skills (i.e., inability to self-manage a particular situation or physical sensation), or that the environment is not supportive in some manner to assisting them in managing their pain (i.e., medical staff or significant other not present or available), such factors may manifest various degrees of anxiety. In turn, anxiety may be associated with appraisals of helplessness and stress that exacerbates the pain experience.

Research shows that pain appraisals (i.e., pain catastrophizing) are prominent in predicting poor experimental and clinical pain outcomes [19].

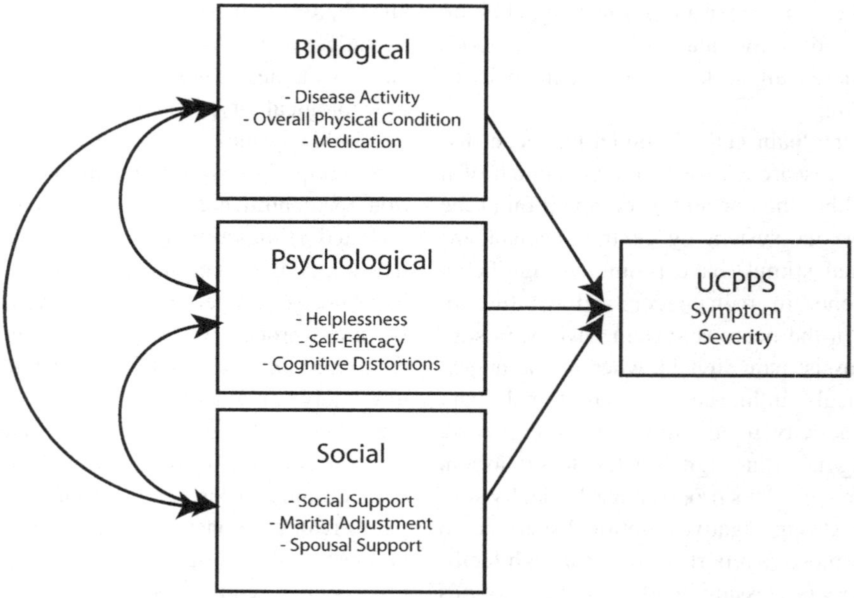


**Fig. 18.1** Diagram of biopsychosocial relations

Further, a biopsychosocial model of pain asserts that biological aspects of chronic illness (e.g., changes in muscles, joints, or nerves generating nociceptive input) affect psychological factors (e.g., catastrophizing, helplessness) and the social context of the individual (e.g., social activity, activity of daily living, interpersonal relationships) (see Fig. 18.1) [20]. It is clear that following nociceptive input, the perception or interpretation of pain occurs, making individual patient characteristics central components of their adaptive and/or maladaptive pain interpretation, which is often prejudiced by long-held core beliefs about one's ability to manage pain.

## A Focus on Urogenital Pain?

In the broadest sense, urologic chronic pelvic pain syndromes (UCPPS) are a significant healthcare issue. This chapter focuses primarily on the research examining a prevalent urogenital pain condition of chronic prostatitis/chronic pelvic pain syndrome (CP/CPPS) and discusses the widespread role of psychosocial risk factors in determining symptom severity and patient QoL. Primary care physicians and urologists alike must recognize important psychosocial factors to optimize therapeutic strategies for UCPPS management, because these types of syndromes are not cured by traditional treatments. As indicated earlier in this chapter, physicians should remember that patient reported stress, catastrophizing, and social support are key concerns for patients with pain, disability, and QoL. Due to the focus of this chapter on particular male patient outcomes in CP/CPPS, other areas of clinical interest for patients suffering from UCPPs should not be interpreted as unimportant management targets (e.g., impact of genitourinary pain conditions on sexual functioning).

Prostatitis, which is the umbrella term wherein CP/CPPS fits, can be either bacterial or abacterial and bacterial prostatitis is characterized by symptoms of a urinary tract infection usually caused by *Escherichia coli*, another Gram-negative organism, or enterococcus [21]. Symptoms such as chills, fever, body aches, and pain are also usually present. Acute (category I) and chronic (category II) bacterial prostatitis are the best understood, but least common of the prostatitis syndromes. CP/CPPS, with or without inflammation, is the third type of prostatitis syndrome. In CP/CPPS type IIIa (i.e., with inflammation), urine, semen, and other fluids from the prostate show no evidence of infection. In type IIIb, there is no evidence of inflammation. The type IIIb category of prostatitis is regarded as the most common but also least understood [22]. The fourth category of prostatitis is asymptomatic inflammatory prostatitis in which white blood cells are present in the semen but there are no symptoms.

CP/CPPS symptoms may vary without notable warning to the patient or physician [23]. The classic longstanding symptom of CP/CPPS is pain that can manifest itself in acute attacks or longstanding persistent pain or some combination of the two. Pain is located in several urogenital regions including the perineum, pelvic area, and/or genitalia [21, 24, 25]. As in other painful chronic conditions, CP/CPPS pain does not correspond strongly with medical findings [26, 27]. Although CP/CPPS may include patients with inflammatory findings in the prostate, no pathognomonic, histologic, or radiologic findings exist to provide a confirmatory diagnosis. Thus, CP/CPPS may be described as a symptom complex rather than specific disease [28, 29]. Currently, the National Institutes of Health (NIH) definition of CP/CPPS is pelvic pain for 3 of the previous 6 months, with or without voiding symptoms [30].

The North American prevalence of CP/CPPS-like symptoms is variable but estimated between 2% and 16% across community dwelling and other samples [31, 32]. A prostatitis diagnosis is common and accounts for as many as 8% of urology outpatient visits in the USA and almost 3% in Canada [33]. For many men, symptoms peak at 35–65 years [34] and symptoms range considerably by socioeconomic status, race, and age [21]. Recent research also suggests that male adolescent populations in Canada and in Africa present with significant CP-like symptoms suggesting that adolescence needs to be examined in greater detail [35, 36]. Unfortunately, symptoms experienced by men suffering from CP/CPPS do not routinely remit and in community-based research 66% of patients continue experiencing symptoms one year later [33]. Further, treatment successes in patients suffering CP/CPPS have been described as bleak, with strategies based on sequential monotherapies for patients with long histories of severe CP/CPPS called suboptimal [22]. CP/CPPS QoL is reported as terrible and ranks as comparable to those suffering severe congestive heart failure, diabetes, myocardial infarction, unstable angina, hemodialysis-dependent end-stage renal disease, or active Crohn's disease [20, 37].

## The Psychology of Urogenital Pain

It is general understanding that biomedical pain models focused purely on etiological and pathophysiological explanations for chronic pain are deficient. In the following sections, a brief literature review is offered on the catastrophizing and social support literature that applies to CP/CPPS outcomes such as QoL and pain. Models of social support will then be discussed in reference to implications for current treatment of CP/CPPS and other urogenital medical conditions like prostate cancer.

Previous reviews of the association of psychological factors within CP/CPPS QoL suggested that physical disease and psychiatric disorders coexist to a large degree [38]. Further, the high degree of comorbidity between symptom severity and psychosocial symptoms reported by patients with CP/CPPS (e.g., low mood, poor sleep, libido) has been noted as significant. Personality assessments of men suffering from CP/CPPS have shown that a heterogeneous personality type may be prevalent (e.g., psychosomatic, alexithymic, borderline, narcissistic), lending complexity to individual treatment prognosis. This early review has been followed by a series of papers showing that a biopsychosocial model is an appropriate fit to understanding patient symptoms in CP/CPPS pain and QoL and that psychological factors like catastrophizing are strongly associated with both outcomes [39, 40].

Pain-related "catastrophizing" is broadly considered as a set of negative, exaggerated cognitive schema engaged when a patient is undergoing pain or is anticipating pain [41]. Pain catastrophizing can be assessed using the reliable and valid

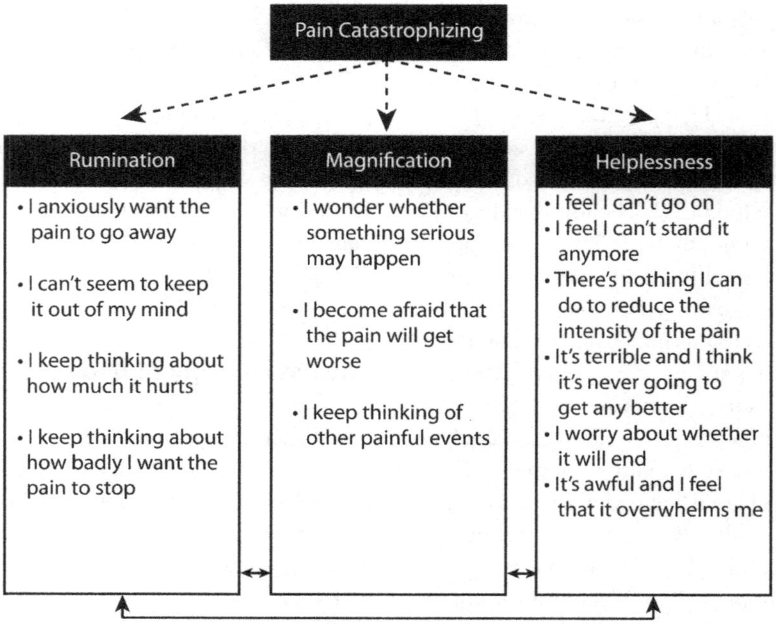


**Fig. 18.2** The pain catastrophizing scale items, subscales (*dotted lines*), and relations among subscales (*solid lines*)

Pain Catastrophizing Scale [41]. As a construct, catastrophizing captures three correlated factors consisting of three components of negative pain referenced thinking: *rumination*, *magnification*, and *helplessness* (see Fig. 18.2). As captured in the language of the components listed in the figure, rumination and magnification tend to be considered reactionary or proximal cognitive responses to pain experience, whereas helplessness may develop at a later time following ruminatory or magnifying thoughts about pain. Helplessness is associated with feelings of despair and may represent one's internal belief that they do not have appropriate resources to manage their pain and its impact.

Catastrophizing is one of the most robust predictors of pain across many clinical and nonclinical samples [19]. The first study examining pain catastrophizing in CP/CPPS found catastrophizing was associated with greater disability, depression, urinary symptoms, and pain [39]. Further, helplessness catastrophizing (e.g., "it's awful and I feel that it overwhelms me") was the strongest predictor of overall pain, even when the significant relations of urinary symptoms and depression were controlled [39]. Another recent study investigated QoL determinants in CP/CPPS showing that poorer mental health status was predicted by greater helplessness catastrophizing (e.g., "it's terrible and I think it is never going to get any better") and lower social support from friends and family, beyond the demographic, medical status, and other competing psychosocial variables in the analyses [40]. Helplessness catastrophizing is a predominant pain and QoL predictor in CP/CPPS and is expressed by patients reporting longer pain durations (e.g., 4–7 years) [42]. Therefore, the present relation between helplessness and pain may not be specific to UCPPS but perhaps can be a manifestation of suffering from long-term pain.

Of particular recent interest, a community-dwelling sample of Canadian adolescent males (16–19 years) not only reported a high prevalence of chronic prostatitis-like symptoms (8.3%), but also reported pain, urinary symptoms, depressive symptoms, and catastrophizing as all being associated with poorer QoL [35]. Catastrophizing magnification of pain (e.g., "I keep thinking of other painful events") was the lone predictor of poorer adolescent QoL when statistically controlling for pain and urinary status in this paper [35].

It is unfortunate that this study did not examine symptom and pain onset because these data may indicate that for the adolescent samples pain may be a relatively new experience. It is imperative that longitudinal research follow such young men to examine if helplessness follows magnification and if interventions designed to help these young men distract themselves or use other basic pain management strategies can be helpful in alleviating their catastrophizing.

The CP/CPPS catastrophizing findings have directed current efforts in the area of clinical assessment and management of psychosocial factors for improved patient adjustment. Using the clinically practical UPOINT phenotyping classification system for patients diagnosed with CP/CPPS [43], the psychosocial domain of UPOINT suggested that pain catastrophizing is a key target for clinical intervention. As noted, it is possible that stable negative symptoms (e.g., pain) combined with noncurative medical therapies could cause or assist in the development of helplessness in these men. Indeed, it has been suggested that helplessness is likely a product of feeling unempowered to make positive changes in one's ability to manage pain [41]. Interventions targeting catastrophizing and helplessness in particular may be valuable in programs for men with CP/CPPS. It has been suggested that such programs be developed from an empirically supported base [44] with a particular emphasis on de-catastrophizing.

A psychotherapy model has been proposed for the treatment of empirically supported UCPPS psychosocial risk factors (e.g., depressed mood, social support, catastrophizing) [45]. Examining research-validated factors associated with negative patient outcomes is as important to the promotion of empirically supported therapies in the area of mental health as it is in medicine. A recent study has examined the amenability of these specific risk factors to psychosocial intervention in men suffering from CP/CPPS [43]. The authors sought to determine the feasibility of a cognitive-behavioral symptom management program, for the acute improvement of psychosocial risk factors of diminished QoL in CP/CPPS. CP/CPPS symptoms and impact and psychosocial risk factors (i.e., catastrophizing, negative mood, and social support) and general pain were assessed at baseline and weekly throughout the 8 one-hour session weekly program. The eight sessions were designed in such a way as to teach the patient how to identify, dispute and replace pessimistic, catastrophic thinking about pain, relationships, and physical functioning with health-focused thinking and new coping behaviors.

Discussion of catastrophizing (or distorted cognitions) concerning pain and its "meaning" to our patients can be critical to improving patient management. The basic type of therapy model used by Tripp et al. [46] is amenable to the physician–patient relationship and can provide extremely valuable insights that can assist physicians. In particular, such patient interactions are keys in directing patients to examine their fears and worries about their treatment and disease management in a collaborative manner.

Figure 18.2 provides the subscales and the items of the Pain Catastrophizing Scale [41]. These items can be discussed or reviewed with the patient and physician to initiate or lead a discussion into the types of pain catastrophizing they can "acknowledge." Looking at Fig. 18.2 with a patient, a physician could lead a discussion as suggested below:

> Everyone experiences pain at some point in their lives. Such experiences may include headaches, tooth pain, joint or muscle pain. People also have pains that can be chronic or pains that repeat sporadically overtime and are experienced as chronic.
>
> I am interested in the types of thoughts and feelings that you have when you are in pain. Here are some statements describing different thoughts and feelings that may be associated with pain. Please tell me how often you believe you have these thoughts and feelings when you are experiencing pain. This may help us find a pattern that your pain creates. That is important because if we know when and how your pain makes you feel and think, we can start to look at possible solutions to battle these negative effects of your pain… that may include medical and self-management suggestions.

In the Tripp et al. [46] study, the mean baseline scores showed significant linear reductions for pain, disability, and catastrophizing. Also, changes were made in depressive symptoms and social support but these were modest and not significant for the group. The CP/CPPS symptom scores compared to follow-up scores were also significantly reduced, as was negative QoL impact. Further analyses showed that the change in scores from baseline to the 8-week termination mark for CP/CPPS symptoms and psychosocial risk factors was predicted by associated reductions in pain catastrophizing but were not significant likely due to the small sample size in this study.

The authors concluded that psychosocial management programs could target and significantly reduce several empirically supported psychosocial risk factors associated with poorer CP/CPPS outcomes. It would seem, from these initial data, that psychosocial management for risk factors of increased CP/CPPS symptoms is feasible, but it is cautioned that a randomized controlled trial with longitudinal follow-up is necessary to properly estimate the value of such an approach. Catastrophizing can be treated successfully in patients with CP/CPPS, and it is suggested that patients would benefit from interventions that discuss and help problem solve catastrophic thinking about pain and disability.

## Social Support and Chronic Pain

The literature on social support and health outcomes is enormous and for that reason is presented following the UCCPS catastrophizing data. For the sake of parsimony and connection to the main theme of this chapter, we provide a brief review of social support and then focus on an emerging research area in UCPPS support.

To put it lightly, chronic pain conditions are not only pervasive, but they also impair daily functioning, disable the sufferer, are associated with marital discord, and negatively impact both men and women at alarming rates in North America. Individuals who experience chronic pain are faced with a consistent health/life stressor that increases demand for support from one's social network and spouse in particular. The general chronic pain literature suggests that perceptions of low social support are associated with diminished QoL, depression, disability, pain severity, and pain behavior [47].

There have been three longstanding types of social support described by Barrera [48], including perceived, received, and social integration support. Perceived support is simply the patient's subjective evaluation that support providers will offer them effective help during stressful times. Received support is defined by specific supportive actions (e.g., behavioral or verbal) offered by providers. Finally, social integration refers to how connected inside of a social network is the patient. These supportive networks are flexible and can be Internet or communal networks for example, with family and friends also contributing. The research has shown that these types of social support may be quite different from each other in impact for patients and that each is associated with patient health or personality in various ways [49]. Perceived support is associated with less depression and anxiety whereas received support and social integration support are not significant [49]. In contrast, social integration support has been associated with better physical health such as heart disease [49]. Received support is surprisingly the least effective, or associated with positive outcomes for patients [48, 49]. Research suggests there are three main causes of perceived support [50]. Perceptions of support or recipient influences can be influenced by the personality traits of the patient, the influence that the support provider has with the patient (i.e., are they supportive or have been in the past), and the quality of the relations they share (or relational support). The recent meta-analysis by Lakey [50] examining the recipient, provider, and relational influences on social support showed that *relational influences* are robust, accounting for about 60% of perceived support. Recipient trait influences about 25% of perceived support and provider influences account for 5–10%. Thus, the personal tastes of support recipients may be a deciding factor in who perceives social support. In another recent paper reviewing the latest on relational regulation and social support impact, it was suggested that social support has roots in everyday contact and interactions and not just in coping with distress as discussed in previous models [51]. This statement suggests that social support occurs frequently in people who have relations that provide consistent contact opportunities, such as spouses.

## Spouses and Social Support

The chronic pain literature on supportive spousal coping behaviors has operationalized couples' interactions in the form of positive and negative responses to pain behavior by the significant other. There have been three categories of spousal responses including: *solicitous* (e.g., "tries to get me to rest"), *distracting* (e.g., "tries to get me involved in some activity") and *negative* or punishing (e.g., "gets angry with me"). As expected, negative responses to a partner's chronic pain by a spouse are associated with increased depression and anxiety [52], greater disability [53], higher pain [54], and greater endorsement of pain catastrophizing [55] by the patient. Solicitous spousal responses to chronic pain are also negatively associated with patient outcomes and are associated with greater pain severity [56], pain behavior [57], physical disability [58–60], depression [61, 62], and pain catastrophizing [55, 63]. Finally, distracting spousal responses to pain are associated with greater pain [54, 56, 60], physical disability [57, 60], pain behaviors [57], and psychological distress [64]. Overall, these results suggest that social responses by spouses to pain behavior are important predictors of a wide range of pain outcome variables.

Although spousal support has been initially examined in UCPPS samples [40, 65], much remains unknown beyond bivariate relationships between spousal support and, for example, QoL. Sufferers of CP/CPPS frequently report depressive symptoms [66], disability [40], and diminished QoL [67]. For instance, in one reported study, 13% of men with CP/CPPS compared to 4% of otherwise healthy men met criteria for a mental health diagnosis [68].

## Stress-Buffering Model of Social Support

Studying such differences in spousal support in chronic pain is of particular importance as social support is associated with greater physical health [69, 70], mental health [71, 72], and marital satisfaction [73–75]. The stress-buffering model of social support [71] suggests that social support benefits individuals by attenuating the negative effects of stress on well-being. This model suggests that social support enhances efficacy, esteem, and confidence, and thus the individual feels that they can cope with a particular stressor [76].

The stress-buffering model of social support has been studied most heavily in the depression literature, but the outcomes of studies have been mixed [77–81]. The degree of life threat and functional impairment may determine which types of support are beneficial. For example, individuals who are faced with a life-threatening disease may benefit most from emotional support as it may prevent depression, whereas as an individual who suffers from a condition which renders them physically unable to carry out daily functions may benefit most from instrumental support [82]. Individuals with CP/CPPS suffer from both emotional distress and functional disability. Thus, these patients may benefit from a number of different types of spousal support.

Whereas spousal support is purported to diminish the effects of pain on patient outcomes, other factors studied in the pain literature may amplify the effects of pain such as pain catastrophizing (i.e., magnification, helplessness, and rumination) [41]. As suggested earlier in this chapter, the appraisal process is dynamic and shifts as individuals evaluate continuing circumstances [83]. The Communal Coping Hypothesis [19, 84] posits that patients catastrophizing may actually have a function of eliciting support and intimacy from significant others, although it may not always been seen as interpersonal outreach. Indeed, it has been demonstrated that catastrophizing is associated with negative and solicitous spousal responses to pain [55].

## UCCPS Spousal Support

By investigating spousal support for pain behavior as buffering agents to poor patient outcomes such as pain or disability, recent research has provided some tangible insights in UCPPS and how social support from spouses may be an important target for future interventions. In a study examining

**Table 18.1** Factors and the items that can be used for conversations about spousal support between physicians and patients

| Distracting | Solicitous | Negative/punishing |
|---|---|---|
| Reads to me | Asks me what he/she can do to help | Ignores me |
| Talks to me about something else to take my mind off the pain | Takes over my jobs or duties | Expresses irritation at me |
| Tries to involve me in some activity | Tries to get me to rest | Expresses anger at me |
| Encourages me to work on a hobby | Gets me some pain medications | Expresses frustration at me |
| | Gets me something to eat or drink | |
| | Turns on the TV to take my mind off the pain | |

the perceived spousal support to patient pain behavior, solicitous spouse responses to patient pain was associated with poorer patient adjustment in CP/CPPS [85]. Specifically, the analyses examined changes in the association between pain and the outcome variables (i.e., patient QoL, depressive symptoms, and disability) at varying levels of spouse responses to patient pain behavior. Of all of the outcomes assessed, only mental QoL and disability were significantly predicted, and the association between pain and the outcome variables did not vary as a function of distracting and negative spousal responses [85]. Interestingly, at higher levels of spouse solicitousness (e.g., "tries to get me to rest"), pain was more highly associated with level of disability than at lower levels of spouse solicitousness. In fact, at lower levels of spouse solicitousness, pain was not significantly associated with disability. This can be interpreted as greater levels of solicitous responses from a spouse for a patient's pain behavior may increase the negative impact that pain can have on disability for men with CP/CPPS. Further, this could mean that spouses may respond solicitously as a reaction to the patient's pain and level of disability (i.e., patients are physically incapable of completing certain tasks, and thus, require the help of their spouse). Alternatively, solicitous responding may help create or maintain the patient's pain and disability by reinforcing pain behavior.

Surprisingly, the Ginting et al. study also found that distracting and negative spouse responses did not impact the association between pain and mental QoL [85]. This result supports the notion that spouse responses to pain behavior may be differentially associated with patient adjustment in men and women with chronic pain [86] and may be impacted by a series of inter and intrapersonal variables as suggested by Lakey et al. [50, 51]. Indeed, identification of the potential role that catastrophizing plays in social support has been one area of little investigation to date in UCCPS.

The Ginting et al. data set has also produced a novel finding yet to be published. A recent analysis examining the moderating potential of catastrophizing on patient outcomes (i.e., patient QoL, depressive symptoms, and disability) was performed. Here, the association between pain and mental QoL was stronger at higher levels of catastrophizing than it was at moderate and lower levels of pain catastrophizing in the patient. Therefore, catastrophizing appears to be increasing the negative impact of pain on mental QoL. Catastrophic appraisals of pain are likely to lead to the experience of distress, and thus, creating a strong association between pain and poorer mental QoL.

Given the cross-sectional nature of the Ginting et al. study, no conclusions on the direction of the relationships can be offered and both are equally plausible. Regardless, discussion of such social interactions is important because they can assist physicians in directing patient and spouse relations to support their disease management. Table 18.1 provides the items that patients have responded to in regard to spousal support. These items could be discussed or reviewed by the patient and physician to initiate or lead a discussion into the types and benefit of spousal support. Looking at Table 18.1 with a patient, a physician could lead a discussion as suggested below:

> I am interested in knowing how your significant other responds to you when they know you are in pain. In this table is a list of possible responses

from spouses. After reading these, let's discuss them for a minute and then you tell me how often your significant other responds to you in that particular way when you are in pain.

Another recent and related study sought to repeat these spousal support analyses in women suffering from Interstitial Cystitis/Painful Bladder Syndrome (IC/PBS), a urogenital pelvic pain condition suggested as similar in symptom profile to CP/CPPS [87]. The primary aim of the study was to examine patient adjustment in light of various types of negative, solicitous, and distracting responses from the spouses of patients suffering pain as in the CP/CPPS study. In particular, spousal responses to patient pain would alter the association between pain and patient QoL, depression, and disability. Using a sample of 96 women with IC/PBS (*mean* age=50.6 (13.8)), the authors examined the changes in association between pain and adjustment variables at high, moderate, and low levels of negative, solicitous, and distracting spousal responses. They found that for women, the association between pain and all outcome variables did not vary as a function of levels of solicitous and negative spousal responses. However, the association between pain and mental QoL was stronger at lower levels of distracting responses than it was at moderate and higher levels of distracting responses from spouses (e.g., "tries to get me involved in some activity"). This means that greater levels of distracting responses for pain from a spouse acts to decrease the negative impact that pain can have on the mental QoL for IC/PBS patients. These findings are in contrast to the spousal support findings from the male CP/CPPS study where this effect was not found. It seems likely that distracting spousal responses may act to "buffer" the deleterious effects of pain on mental QoL for women suffering from IC/PBS, but this type of support does not function similarly in men with CP/CPPS.

In sum, this novel UCPPS social support research provides insights into patient management that hopefully starts new academic and clinical discussions about gender differences in spousal support. Such findings have important clinical implications for couples suffering from UCPPS where adjunctive psychosocial interventions should be considered. Previous research has already shown that brief psychoeducational interventions for spousal responses to expressions of patient pain have benefits for couples suffering with arthritis [88]. It is our suggestion that such programs could be modified and delivered by an attending nurse or from within a support group setting within primary care or tertiary care centers.

The take home messages are straightforward. It is suggested that solicitous responses from a spouse were to be avoided, suggesting that men need to be more active in their lives to counter the high association between pain and disability [85]. These suggestions can be followed up by conversations with men about how pain influences "how they live their life" probing for the types of social support they perceive and receive from their spouses and others. Encouraging men to stay as active as possible in their lives despite their pain and symptoms is likely an important component to preventing disability. Recent work would support such claims showing that exercise programs for CP/CPPS showed significant reductions in total CP/CPPS symptoms, pain measures, and symptom quality life impact [89].

## Prostate Cancer and Social Support

It is documented that individuals with more social support experience less cancer pain, take less pain medication, report less labor pain and are less likely to use epidural anesthesia during childbirth or suffer from chest pain after coronary artery bypass surgery [90]. The workup and diagnosis of cancer and of course its following treatment is a hugely stressful event for patients associated with fear, uncertainty, pain, and depressed moods. Estimates are that between 10% and 50% of cancer patients experience high levels of psychosocial distress [91–93].

Recent research has argued that men and women are very different when it comes to the expressed desire for social support when diagnosed with cancer [94]. In particular, assessing cancer patients' needs and desire for psychological support and contrasting it with demographic and psychosocial information, 26% of women desired psychological support compared to 11% of the men surveyed. Interestingly, patients' desire for psychological support found more in younger patients that also endorsed a tendency for support-seeking coping. What was also interesting in this study was that the level of psychological distress in the women or men was not associated with their desire for such support. This study adds to the discussion of support needs in cancer patients and suggests that women are more amenable to outwardly desiring support. As previous research suggests, this gender difference is not a novel suggestion as women tend to be more socially accepting of seeking help for distress [95, 96] and that men are generally unenthusiastic to do so [97, 98]. The focus of this chapter is on men and urogenital pain, thus the larger literature on cancer and support may be bridged to in this discussion but cannot be reviewed here. Thus, prostate cancer was selected for review in common.

Research suggests that other than skin cancer, prostate cancer is the most common cancer in US males and is a significant risk for cancer-associated mortality [99]. Many of the men who receive curative therapies (i.e., radiation or radical prostatectomy) report troublesome adverse events following treatment, like urinary and sexual dysfunction [100, 101]. For years it has been suggested that for many men, the novel and taxing nature of these difficulties negatively impact patients' self-confidence that they can manage creating deficits in self-efficacy [102]. When considered together, diminished physical function and low beliefs in one's ability to manage is likely the fuel needed to create depressive symptoms [103, 104]. It is plausible that supportive therapies may act to reduce such feelings of low self-management ability. Researchers have been examining social support as a buffer to poor outcomes in prostate cancer survivors for several years now with interesting and positive findings [105–107].

In one prostate cancer therapy pilot study, patients were matched with male therapy providers who were survivors of prostate cancer for more than 3 years themselves [107]. These dyadic support partners (i.e., therapy that was one-to-one) in this study were selected in an attempt to avoid the male tendency to not engage in therapeutic relationships. It has been suggested previously that men typically do not take advantage of support group opportunities perhaps based on their disinclination to talk about issues surrounding urinary and sexual dysfunction that may be discomforting to discuss in the group setting typically offered at tertiary care centers [108]. It is also understood that the average man tends to deny or diminish problems for the simple reason of avoiding the burden such claims may have on others, avoid being perceived as vulnerable or helpless, avoid negative affect, or to maintain a damaged positive self [109, 110]. The results of this study showed that dyadic intervention might be effective at reducing depression between controls and patients receiving the dyadic intervention at 4 weeks, and at increasing self-efficacy at 8 weeks in men who have undergone radical prostatectomy. This study is also important because it suggested that men may be more accepting of this type of treatment versus a group setting, primarily substantiated by its low attrition rate of 6%.

Other research has suggested that the male tendency to avoid expression of distress and associated feelings might be useful short-term strategies allowing a patient to seem in control with the appearance of sufficient QoL. But, these types of cognitive, affective, or behavioral strategies may also lead to unexpressed sadness and anger, which may show itself in terms of social isolation. Given that support is of benefit to prostate cancer patients, the efficacy of a cognitive-behavioral intervention designed to improve QoL was examined. This program was designed to educate the prostate cancer patients on stress-management skills training using a 10-week, group-based program. In comparison with a half-day seminar in improving QoL, the intervention group reported improved QoL following the 10 weeks, even when ethnicity, patient income, and baseline QoL were accounted for in the analyses. This study showed that men can benefit from a group setting and that treatment was useful in improving the QoL in men treated for prostate cancer. The teaching of stress-management skills is to be promoted in prostate cancer survivors.

In a more recent follow-up to their original effort, Penedo et al. also examined the efficacy of their group-based psychosocial intervention with the Hispanic ethnic minority to test the impact of cultural factors on group processes [106]. They found that the 10-week group-based cognitive-behavioral stress management intervention was successfully adapted for Hispanic monolinguals treated for prostate cancer. As in their previous study, after controlling for covariates, the intervention condition reported significantly greater physical well-being, emotional well-being, sexual functioning, and total well-being. This is promising because one cannot expect that one intervention created for a particular general ethnicity (i.e., white male) is adaptable to other cultures.

Further research into the anxiety and depression experienced by prostate cancer patients has been advanced recently. It has been proposed that anxiety and depression in these men may weaken relationships and potentials support with partners and family members. In an attempt to define some mechanisms that may underlie the development of negative affect, Sharpley et al. examined the coping strategies reported by prostate cancer patients in regard to the stressors and standard of living changes that patient experienced from their cancer [111]. Interestingly, they found that the most common patient coping strategies were acceptance, the use of exercise, the use of medication, keeping a positive attitude, or seeking out support from their wives or families. It is important to note that this study suggested a wide range of coping strategies were being reported across patients with many reporting that they used their significant others for support on issues associated with "feeling worse," "feeling disorganized," "feeling sad or disappointed," "feeling angry," or "social issues." The primary coping was reported as using "Acceptance," that the authors described as "just getting on with life" or "biting my lip and putting up with it." These data may lead to future investigations that focus on mechanisms of such coping.

Other researchers have suggested that depression and anxiety may be associated with patient reactivity and exposure to the novel aversive intra and interpersonal changes and events associated with prostate cancer [112]. These authors reported that negative gains reported by the patients (i.e., the acknowledgement of onset of previously absent negative events) play a substantial role in the development of depression and anxiety in prostate cancer. Issues such as pain, fatigue, depression, and having lessened tolerance of others were associated with anxiety, whereas general feelings of sadness, loss of social relations, and anger were more associated with depressed affect. It was suggested that these aversive responses due to disease-based events might stem from poor or diminished coping and the belief that events are to a certain degree uncontrollable. This type of helpless orientation has been reflected in the urogenital research in this chapter again and again. Further investigation of the possible mechanisms or causes for adverse patient responses to daily life-events could aid in treating these exacerbated patient responses.

### Couples and Prostate Cancer

The relationship between cancer and patient/spouse adjustment cannot be described as a direct one but can nevertheless be described in models that discuss various methods of influence like mediation or moderation [113, 114]. In these earlier studies, the cognitive responses displayed by the caregivers of cancer patients' acted to mediate (i.e., or explain) the psychological reactions of patient caregivers' to the disease-related burdens they were recognizing in patients [113].

Also, it had been reported that relationship factors were argued to be either present or not changed the association between cognitive patterns and distress in married cancer patients. The study by Manne et al. examined whether perceived spouse criticism and avoidance impacted cognitive processing in cancer patients [114]. The results showed that a moderating effect for spouse criticism existed between the association of early negative thought patterns and later patient distress. This means that high levels of spousal criticism are likely to promote the chance the depression will occur in patients with cancer.

These earlier couple relations' studies in cancer have promoted two specific variables of interest in the psychosocial oncology: coping processes and dyadic adjustment. The work of Banthia et al. examined dyadic adjustment and coping styles and their association with psychological distress following prostate cancer diagnoses in couples [115]. This study sought to test the strength of the association between coping and distress when accounting for the strength of the couples dyadic functioning was considered. Dyadic function was defined as the ability of the relationship to offer useful social support, love, and functional assistance to spouses. The moderational model was supported for patients, showing that when the dyadic strength was high the effects of avoidant coping and intrusive thinking on mood disturbance were lower. These findings are interesting because they suggest that even though patients reported maladaptive coping (i.e., avoidant coping), patients who were members of stronger dyads reported less distress than those in more dysfunctional relationships. In sum, the relationship between coping and distress depends on the quality of dyadic functioning and better quality is protective from distress for patients. These results, as those of Ginting et al. [85] suggest that interventions that strengthen communication and overall couple support are likely to have wide ranging benefits to couples with urogenital pain conditions or cancers. Indeed, regardless of the target of intervention, increased support resources and instructional therapies are suggested for cancer patients and spouses to facilitate each member of the couple to help each other.

Following on the general concepts examined in the Banthia paper, Kershaw et al. [116] examined a theory-based longitudinal analysis of factors associated with the QoL of prostate cancer patients and spouses. This paper is important because it provides information on the processes of patient and spouse adjustment over time. Their results showed that the patient's personal, social, and illness-related variables had the most significant effects on their own negative appraisal at 4 months, and ultimately on their own QoL. Patient's self-efficacy (i.e., belief they can manage) was also noted as a strong predictor of positive outcomes for patients. Indeed, less self-efficacy at baseline led to more negative appraisals of illness/caregiving, more hopelessness, and greater uncertainty for both patients and spouses at the 4-month follow-up and diminished QoL outcomes at the 8-month follow-up. Of the mediators examined, patient's cognitive appraisals such as hopelessness served as an important mediator of these associations for patient's QoL.

## Concluding Comments

By their very nature, urogenital illnesses that are associated with pain are more than a physical phenomenon but rather a complex physical, emotional, and interpersonal fusion associated with negative patient outcomes. The research reviewed in this chapter suggests the roles that psychosocial risk factors play in patients' responses to symptoms like pain are significant. This chapter also highlights the salient role of social and spousal support and pain catastrophizing as concerns for men suffering from CP/CPPS and prostate cancer. The narrative from these studies compels the primary care physician and the urologist to consider the influences of an individual's prior history with pain, their cognitive pain appraisals (i.e., catastrophizing) and the social milieu in which the pain occurs [43].

It is generally understood that male patients often have difficulty identifying, expressing or reporting the details of distressing experiences. To alleviate such social pressures, patients have been treated in one-to-one settings [46, 107], but group treatments have also been shown as successful even across ethnicities [105, 106]. Together, these findings are seen as hopeful for better management of urogenital pain syndromes in men and are strongly suggested as clinical treatment options for these men.

The basic mechanism of change across all studies reviewed here seems to be one of patient *activation*, or in other words, having the patients identify, discuss, and problem solve the mental and physical hurdles their disease has place in front of them. The particular reduction of catastrophizing in men is a significant target for future intervention, especially because it is considered to be inflammatory to greater pain perception, perceptions of disability, social isolation, and difficulties in dyadic relationships. As suggested in this chapter, a simple dialog can be used to start addressing this type of catastrophic thinking pattern or spousal support problems in patients. The dialog here is not meant to be a standalone intervention but can provide patients with a greater sense of being understood and cared for by their attending physician. This quality alone, if it has been lacking in the provider relationship, can be associated with positive change in patients' outlook and hope, which can be a catalyst to patients trying new things in regard to self-management. Indeed, analyzing difficult doctor–patient relationships, it was suggested that a physician's interpersonal stance can be a benefit to cooperative relationships or inflammatory to conflicts or difficulties with treating patients [117]. Physician factors such as workload, communication skills, personality, level of experience, and practice setting, should also be considered. When patients are suffering from comorbid depression or serious mental health issues immediate referral is recommended. Note that this referral should not alter the suggested patient–physician discussions on catastrophizing or spousal support. Approached with sensitivity, these basic conversations can provide unique insight into disease management and patient QoL for all patients.

Brief psychoeducational interventions for spouses are strongly recommended. This type of support is being shown repeatedly to be of value in QoL, pain, negative affect or disability. Nurses in support group settings can economically offer spousal support therapy to patient dyads but some settings may not have the personnel or resources to offer such a service. Couple therapy works for patients in pain [88] and adaptations of such work to urogenital illness is exciting. Physicians can open dialogs on the types of coping support patients' are receiving from their significant others as a starting point to understanding the environmental supports of their patients. Based on the emerging literature, some strategies are suggested to be better than others. For example, men with CP/CPPS may benefit from a reduction in solicitous spousal responses [85] and perhaps an increase distracting responses to decrease the impact of pain on disability.

It is our hope and expectation that the following years of research will expand upon the literature reviewed in this chapter. Treatments that are informed by this new research may provide further emphasis on therapies that occur outside of a strict biomedical model. This in no way is a slight to the potential medical advances in curing urogenital diseases that we hope flourish in the near future, but rather is a strong recommendation for psychosocial support of our patients. The urogenital patient care maps of tomorrow must use all avenues to combat the multidimensional nature of such conditions [43].

## References


1. Bonica JJ. The need of a taxonomy. Pain. 1979; 6(3):247–8.
2. Turk DC, Dworkin RH. What should be the core outcomes in chronic pain clinical trials? Arthritis Res Ther. 2004;6(4):151–4.
3. Cordell WH, Keene KK, Giles BK, Jones JB, Jones JH, Brizendine EJ. The high prevalence of pain in emergency medical care. Am J Emerg Med. 2002; 20(3):165–9.
4. Hasselstrom J, Liu-Palmgren J, Rasjo-Wraak G. Prevalence of pain in general practice. Eur J Pain. 2002;6(5):375–85.
5. Breivik H, Borchgrevink PC, Allen SM, et al. Assessment of pain. Br J Anaesth. 2008;101(1): 17–24.
6. Turk DC, Okifuji A. Pain terms and taxonomies of pain. In: Bonica JJ, Loeser JD, Chapman CR, Turk DC, Butler SH, editors. Bonica's management of pain. Hagerstown: Lippincott Williams & Wilkins; 2001. p. 17–25.
7. Spanswick CC, Main CJ. Pain management: an interdisciplinary approach. Edinburgh: Churchill Livingstone; 2000.
8. Thienhaus O, Cole BE. Classification of pain. In: Weiner R, editor. Pain management: a practical guide for clinicians. Boca Raton: CRC; 2002. p. 28.
9. Rey R. History of pain. Paris: La Decouverte; 1993.
10. Descartes R. L'Homme. Paris: C. Angot; 1664.
11. Goldscheider A. Die spezifische Energie der Gefuhlsnerven der Haut. Prakt Derm. 1884;3:283.
12. Hill HE, Kornetsky CH, Flanary HG, Wikler A. Effects of anxiety and morphine on discrimination of

intensities of painful stimuli. J Clin Invest. 1952;31(5):473–80.
13. Beecher HK. Relationship of significance of wound to pain experienced. J Am Med Assoc. 1956;161(17):1609–13.
14. Melzack R, Wall PD. Pain mechanisms: a new theory. Science. 1965;150(699):971–9.
15. Melzack R, Wall PD, Ty TC. Acute pain in an emergency clinic: latency of onset and descriptor patterns related to different injuries. Pain. 1982;14(1):33–43.
16. Melzack R. From the gate to the neuromatrix. Pain. 1999;(Suppl 6):S121–6.
17. Turk DC. A diathesis-stress model of chronic pain and disability following traumatic injury. Pain Res Manag. 2002;7(1):9–19.
18. Loeser JD, Butler SD, Chapman CR, Turk DC. Bonica's management of pain. Philadelphia: Lippincott Williams & Wilkins; 2001.
19. Sullivan MJ, Thorn B, Haythornthwaite JA, et al. Theoretical perspectives on the relation between catastrophizing and pain. Clin J Pain. 2001;17(1):52–64.
20. McNaughton Collins M, Pontari MA, O'Leary MP, et al. Quality of life is impaired in men with chronic prostatitis: the Chronic Prostatitis Collaborative Research Network. J Gen Intern Med. 2001;16(10):656–62.
21. Schaeffer AJ, Datta NS, Fowler Jr JE, et al. Overview summary statement. Diagnosis and management of chronic prostatitis/chronic pelvic pain syndrome (CP/CPPS). Urology. 2002;60 Suppl 6:1–4.
22. Nickel JC, Downey J, Ardern D, Clark J, Nickel K. Failure of a monotherapy strategy for difficult chronic prostatitis/chronic pelvic pain syndrome. J Urol. 2004;172(2):551–4.
23. Nickel JC. Prostatitis/chronic pelvic pain syndrome. Rev Urol. 2002;4(2):95–6.
24. Krieger JN, Nyberg Jr L, Nickel JC. NIH consensus definition and classification of prostatitis. JAMA. 1999;282(3):236–7.
25. Litwin MS, McNaughton-Collins M, Fowler Jr FJ, et al. The National Institutes of Health chronic prostatitis symptom index: development and validation of a new outcome measure. Chronic Prostatitis Collaborative Research Network. J Urol. 1999;162(2):369–75.
26. Deyo RA, Weinstein JN. Low back pain. N Engl J Med. 2001;344(5):363–70.
27. Egan KJ, Krieger JL. Chronic abacterial prostatitis—a urological chronic pain syndrome? Pain. 1997;69(3):213–8.
28. Nickel JC. Words of wisdom. Re: Clinical phenotyping in chronic prostatitis/chronic pelvic pain syndrome and interstitial cystitis: a management strategy for urologic chronic pelvic pain syndromes. Eur Urol. 2009;56(5):881.
29. Nickel JC. Chronic prostatitis/chronic pelvic pain: the syndrome. J Urol. 2009;182(1):18–9.
30. Nickel JC. Prostatitis and related conditions. In: Walsh PC, Retik AB, Vaughan ED, et al., (eds.) Campbell's urology. Philadelphia: WB Saunders; 2002. p. 603–30.
31. Nickel JC, Downey J, Hunter D, Clark J. Prevalence of prostatitis-like symptoms in a population based study using the National Institutes of Health chronic prostatitis symptom index. J Urol. 2001;165(3):842–5.
32. Nickel JC, Teichman JM, Gregoire M, Clark J, Downey J. Prevalence, diagnosis, characterization, and treatment of prostatitis, interstitial cystitis, and epididymitis in outpatient urological practice: the Canadian PIE Study. Urology. 2005;66(5):935–40.
33. Nickel JC, Downey JA, Nickel KR, Clark JM. Prostatitis-like symptoms: one year later. BJU Int. 2002;90(7):678–81.
34. Collins MM, Stafford RS, O'Leary MP, Barry MJ. Distinguishing chronic prostatitis and benign prostatic hyperplasia symptoms: results of a national survey of physician visits. Urology. 1999;53(5):921–5.
35. Tripp DA, Nickel JC, Ross S, Mullins C, Stechyson N. Prevalence, symptom impact and predictors of chronic prostatitis-like symptoms in Canadian males aged 16–19 years. BJU Int. 2009;103(8):1080–4.
36. Tripp DA, Nickel JC, Pikard JL, Katz L. Chronic prostatitis-like symptoms in African males aged 16–19 years. Can J Urol. 2012;19(1):6081–7.
37. Wenninger K, Heiman JR, Rothman I, Berghuis JP, Berger RE. Sickness impact of chronic nonbacterial prostatitis and its correlates. J Urol. 1996;155(3):965–8.
38. Ku JH, Kim SW, Paick JS. Quality of life and psychological factors in chronic prostatitis/chronic pelvic pain syndrome. Urology. 2005;66(4):693–701.
39. Tripp DA, Nickel JC, Wang Y, et al. Catastrophizing and pain-contingent rest predict patient adjustment in men with chronic prostatitis/chronic pelvic pain syndrome. J Pain. 2006;7(10):697–708.
40. Nickel JC, Tripp DA, Chuai S, et al. Psychosocial variables affect the quality of life of men diagnosed with chronic prostatitis/chronic pelvic pain syndrome. BJU Int. 2008;101(1):59–64.
41. Sullivan MJL, Bishop SR, Pivik J. The Pain Catastrophizing Scale: development and validation. Psychol Assess. 1995;7(4):524–32.
42. Sullivan MJ, Stanish W, Sullivan ME, Tripp D. Differential predictors of pain and disability in patients with whiplash injuries. Pain Res Manag. 2002;7(2):68–74.
43. Shoskes DA, Nickel JC, Dolinga R, Prots D. Clinical phenotyping of patients with chronic prostatitis/chronic pelvic pain syndrome and correlation with symptom severity. Urology. 2009;73(3):538–42. discussion 542–3.
44. Nickel JC, Mullins C, Tripp DA. Development of an evidence-based cognitive behavioral treatment program for men with chronic prostatitis/chronic pelvic pain syndrome. World J Urol. 2008;26(2):167–72.
45. Shoskes DA, Nickel JC, Rackley RR, Pontari MA. Clinical phenotyping in chronic prostatitis/chronic

pelvic pain syndrome and interstitial cystitis: a management strategy for urologic chronic pelvic pain syndromes. Prostate Cancer Prostatic Dis. 2009; 12(2):177–83.

46. Tripp DA, Nickel JC, Katz L. A feasibility trial of a cognitive behavioral symptom management program for chronic pelvic pain for men with refractory chronic prostatitis/chronic pelvic pain syndrome. Can Urol Assoc J. 2011;5(5):328–32.
47. Leonard MT, Cano A, Johansen AB. Chronic pain in a couples context: a review and integration of theoretical models and empirical evidence. J Pain. 2006; 7(6):377–90.
48. Barrera M. Distinctions between social support concepts, measures, and models. Am J Community Psychol. 1986;14:413–45.
49. Uchino BN. Understanding the links between social support and physical health: a life-span perspective with emphasis on the separability of perceived and received support. Perspect Psychol Sci. 2009;4:236–55.
50. Lakey B. Social support: basic research and new strategies for intervention. In: Maddux JE, Tangney JP, editors. Social psychological foundations of clinical psychology. New York: Guilford; 2010. p. 177–94.
51. Lakey B, Orehek E. Relational regulation theory: a new approach to explain the link between perceived social support and mental health. Psychol Rev. 2011;118(3):482–95.
52. Cano A, Gillis M, Heinz W, Geisser M, Foran H. Marital functioning, chronic pain, and psychological distress. Pain. 2004;107(1–2):99–106.
53. Cano A, Johansen AB, Franz A. Multilevel analysis of couple congruence on pain, interference, and disability. Pain. 2005;118(3):369–79.
54. Cano A, Weisberg JN, Gallagher RM. Marital satisfaction and pain severity mediate the association between negative spouse responses to pain and depressive symptoms in a chronic pain patient sample. Pain Med. 2000;1(1):35–43.
55. Buenaver LF, Edwards RR, Haythornthwaite JA. Pain-related catastrophizing and perceived social responses: inter-relationships in the context of chronic pain. Pain. 2007;127(3):234–42.
56. Flor H, Turk DC, Rudy TE. Relationship of pain impact and significant other reinforcement of pain behaviors: the mediating role of gender, marital status and marital satisfaction. Pain. 1989;38(1):45–50.
57. Turk DC, Kerns RD, Rosenberg R. Effects of marital interaction on chronic pain and disability: examining the down side of social support. Rehabil Psychol. 1992;37(4):16.
58. Clark LA, Watson D. Tripartite model of anxiety and depression: psychometric evidence and taxonomic implications. J Abnorm Psychol. 1991;100(3):316–36.
59. Romano JM, Turner JA, Jensen MP. The family environment in chronic pain patients: comparison to controls and relationship to patient functioning. J Clin Psychol Med Settings. 1997;4(4):383–95.
60. Williamson D, Robinson ME, Melamed B. Pain behavior, spouse responsiveness, and marital satisfaction in patients with rheumatoid arthritis. Behav Modif. 1997;21(1):97–118.
61. Burns JW, Johnson BJ, Mahoney N, Devine J, Pawl R. Anger management style, hostility and spouse responses: gender differences in predictors of adjustment among chronic pain patients. Pain. 1996;64(3): 445–53.
62. Flor H, Kerns RD, Turk DC. The role of spouse reinforcement, perceived pain, and activity levels of chronic pain patients. J Psychosom Res. 1987;31(2):251–9.
63. Giardino ND, Jensen MP, Turner JA, Ehde DM, Cardenas DD. Social environment moderates the association between catastrophizing and pain among persons with a spinal cord injury. Pain. 2003;106(1–2):19–25.
64. Kerns RD, Haythornthwaite J, Southwick S, Giller Jr EL. The role of marital interaction in chronic pain and depressive symptom severity. J Psychosom Res. 1990;34(4):472–503.
65. Warwick R, Joseph S, Cordle C, Ashworth P. Social support for women with chronic pelvic pain: what is helpful from whom? Psychol Health. 2004;19:28.
66. Pontari MA. Chronic prostatitis/chronic pelvic pain syndrome and interstitial cystitis: are they related? Curr Urol Rep. 2006;7(4):329–34.
67. Tripp DA, Curtis Nickel J, Landis JR, Wang YL, Knauss JS. Predictors of quality of life and pain in chronic prostatitis/chronic pelvic pain syndrome: findings from the National Institutes of Health Chronic Prostatitis Cohort Study. BJU Int. 2004;94(9): 1279–82.
68. Clemens JQ, Brown SO, Kozloff L, Calhoun EA. Predictors of symptom severity in patients with chronic prostatitis and interstitial cystitis. J Urol. 2006;175(3 Pt 1):963–6. discussion 967.
69. Cunningham MR, Barbee AP. Social support. In: Hendrick C, Hendrick SS, editors. Close relationships: a sourcebook. Thousand Oaks: Sage; 2000. p. 272–85.
70. Sarason BR, Sarason IG, Gurung RAR. Close personal relationships and health outcomes: a key to the role of social support. In: Duck S, editor. Handbook of personal relationships. 2nd ed. Chichester: Wiley; 1997. p. 547–73.
71. Cohen S, Wills TA. Stress, social support, and the buffering hypothesis. Psychol Bull. 1985;98(2):310–57.
72. Schwarzer R, Leppin A. The possible impact of social ties and support on morbidity and mortality. In: Veiel H, Baumann U, editors. The meaning and measurement of social support. Washington: Hemisphere; 1992. p. 65–83.
73. Conger RD, Rueter MA, Elder Jr GH. Couple resilience to economic pressure. J Pers Soc Psychol. 1999;76(1):54–71.
74. Pasch LA, Bradbury TN. Social support, conflict, and the development of marital dysfunction. J Consult Clin Psychol. 1998;66:219–30.
75. Saitzyk AR, Floyd FJ, Kroll AB. Sequential analysis of autonomy-interdependence and affiliation-disaffiliation in couples' social support interactions. Pers Relat. 1997;4:341–60.

76. Bova C. Adjustment to chronic illness among HIV-infected women. J Nurs Scholarsh. 2001;33: 217–24.
77. Burton E, Stice E, Seeley JR. A prospective test of the stress-buffering model of depression in adolescent girls: no support once again. J Consult Clin Psychol. 2004;72:689–97.
78. Zimmerman MA, Ramirez-Valles J, Zapert KM, Maton KI. A longitudinal study of stress-buffering effects for urban African-American male adolescent problem behaviors and mental health. J Community Psychol. 2000;28:17–33.
79. Carlsson AH, Bjorvatn C, Engebretsen LF, Berglund G, Natvig GK. Psychosocial factors associated with quality of life among individuals attending genetic counseling for hereditary cancer. J Genet Couns. 2004;13(5):425–45.
80. Lee TC, Yang YK, Chen PS, et al. Different dimensions of social support for the caregivers of patients with schizophrenia: main effect and stress-buffering models. Psychiatry Clin Neurosci. 2006;60(5): 546–50.
81. O'Donovan A, Hughes B. Social support and loneliness in college students: effects on pulse pressure reactivity to acute stress. Int J Adolesc Med Health. 2007;19(4):523–8.
82. Penninx BW, van Tilburg T, Boeke AJ, Deeg DJ, Kriegsman DM, van Eijk JT. Effects of social support and personal coping resources on depressive symptoms: different for various chronic diseases? Health Psychol. 1998;17(6):551–8.
83. Cervone D. The architecture of personality. Psychol Rev. 2004;111(1):183–204.
84. Sullivan MJL, Tripp DA, Santor D. Gender differences in pain and pain behaviour: the role of catastrophizing. Cogn Ther Res. 2000;24:121–34.
85. Ginting JV, Tripp DA, Nickel JC. Self-reported spousal support modifies the negative impact of pain on disability in men with chronic prostatitis/chronic pelvic pain syndrome. Urology. 2011;78(5):1136–41.
86. Fillingim RB, Doleys DM, Edwards RR, Lowery D. Spousal responses are differentially associated with clinical variables in women and men with chronic pain. Clin J Pain. 2003;19(4):217–24.
87. Ginting JV, Tripp DA, Nickel JC, Fitzgerald MP, Mayer R. Spousal support decreases the negative impact of pain on mental quality of life in women with interstitial cystitis/painful bladder syndrome. BJU Int. 2011;108(5):713–7.
88. Keefe FJ, Caldwell DS, Baucom D, et al. Spouse-assisted coping skills training in the management of osteoarthritic knee pain. Arthritis Care Res. 1996; 9(4):279–91.
89. Giubilei G, Mondaini N, Minervini A, et al. Physical activity of men with chronic prostatitis/chronic pelvic pain syndrome not satisfied with conventional treatments–could it represent a valid option? The physical activity and male pelvic pain trial: a double-blind, randomized study. J Urol. 2007;177(1):159–65.
90. Eisenberger NI, Lieberman MD. Why it hurts to be left out: the neurocognitive overlap between physical and social pain. In: Williams KD, Forgas JP, von Hippel W, editors. The social outcast: ostracism, social exclusion, rejection, and bullying. New York: Cambridge University Press; 2005. p. 109–27.
91. Zabora J, BrintzenhofeSzoc K, Curbow B, Hooker C, Piantadosi S. The prevalence of psychological distress by cancer site. Psychooncology. 2001; 10(1):19–28.
92. Derogatis LR, Morrow GR, Fetting J, et al. The prevalence of psychiatric disorders among cancer patients. JAMA. 1983;249(6):751–7.
93. Chochinov HM, Wilson KG, Enns M, Lander S. Prevalence of depression in the terminally ill: effects of diagnostic criteria and symptom threshold judgments. Am J Psychiatry. 1994;151(4):537–40.
94. Merckaert I, Libert Y, Messin S, Milani M, Slachmuylder JL, Razavi D. Cancer patients' desire for psychological support: prevalence and implications for screening patients' psychological needs. Psychooncology. 2010;19(2):141–9.
95. Neal MB, Ingersoll-Dayton B, Starrels ME. Gender and relationship differences in caregiving patterns and consequences among employed caregivers. Gerontologist. 1997;37(6):804–16.
96. Fiorentine R, Anglin MD, Gil-Rivas V, Taylor E. Drug treatment: explaining the gender paradox. Subst Use Misuse. 1997;32(6):653–78.
97. Galdas PM, Cheater F, Marshall P. Men and health help-seeking behaviour: literature review. J Adv Nurs. 2005;49(6):616–23.
98. Addis ME, Mahalik JR. Men, masculinity, and the contexts of help seeking. Am Psychol. 2003; 58(1):5–14.
99. Society AC. What are the key statistics about prostate cancer? 2011. http://www.cancer.org/Cancer/ProstateCancer/DetailedGuide/prostate-cancer-key-statistics. Accessed 5 Aug 2011.
100. Fowler Jr FJ, Barry MJ, Lu-Yao G, Wasson J, Roman A, Wennberg J. Effect of radical prostatectomy for prostate cancer on patient quality of life: results from a Medicare survey. Urology. 1995;45(6):1007–13. discussion 1013–5.
101. Stanford JL, Feng Z, Hamilton AS, et al. Urinary and sexual function after radical prostatectomy for clinically localized prostate cancer: the Prostate Cancer Outcomes Study. JAMA. 2000;283(3):354–60.
102. Beckham JC, Burker EJ, Lytle BL, Feldman ME, Costakis MJ. Self-efficacy and adjustment in cancer patients: a preliminary report. Behav Med. 1997; 23(3):138–42.
103. Massie MJ, Gagnon P, Holland JC. Depression and suicide in patients with cancer. J Pain Symptom Manage. 1994;9(5):325–40.
104. McDaniel JS, Musselman DL, Porter MR, Reed DA, Nemeroff CB. Depression in patients with cancer. Diagnosis, biology, and treatment. Arch Gen Psychiatry. 1995;52(2):89–99.

105. Penedo FJ, Dahn JR, Molton I, et al. Cognitive-behavioral stress management improves stress-management skills and quality of life in men recovering from treatment of prostate carcinoma. Cancer. 2004;100(1):192–200.
106. Penedo FJ, Traeger L, Dahn J, et al. Cognitive behavioral stress management intervention improves quality of life in Spanish monolingual hispanic men treated for localized prostate cancer: results of a randomized controlled trial. Int J Behav Med. 2007;14(3):164–72.
107. Weber BA, Roberts BL, Resnick M, et al. The effect of dyadic intervention on self-efficacy, social support, and depression for men with prostate cancer. Psychooncology. 2004;13(1):47–60.
108. Deans G, Bennett-Emslie GB, Weir J, Smith DC, Kaye SB. Cancer support groups—who joins and why? Br J Cancer. 1988;58(5):670–4.
109. Boehmer U, Clark JA. Communication about prostate cancer between men and their wives. J Fam Pract. 2001;50(3):226–31.
110. Hess U, Senecal S, Kirouac G, Herrera P, Philipot P, Kleck RE. Emotional expressivity in men and women: stereotypes and self-perceptions. Cogn Emot. 2000;14:609–42.
111. Sharpley CF, Bitsika V, Christie DRH. How prostate cancer patients cope with the effects of diagnosis and treatment: development of the Effects of Prostate Cancer Coping Strategies Scale. J Men's Health. 2011;8(1):56–65.
112. Bitsika V, Sharpley CF, Christie DRH. Positive (but not negative) punishment predicts anxiety and depression among prostate cancer patients: an exploration of the behaviour analytic model of depression. Behav Change. 2009;26(4):235–44.
113. Kurtz ME, Kurtz JC, Given CW, Given B. Relationship of caregiver reactions and depression to cancer patients' symptoms, functional states and depression—a longitudinal view. Soc Sci Med. 1995;40(6):837–46.
114. Manne SL. Intrusive thoughts and psychological distress among cancer patients: the role of spouse avoidance and criticism. J Consult Clin Psychol. 1999;67(4):539–46.
115. Banthia R, Malcarne VL, Varni JW, Ko CM, Sadler GR, Greenbergs HL. The effects of dyadic strength and coping styles on psychological distress in couples faced with prostate cancer. J Behav Med. 2003;26(1):31–52.
116. Kershaw TS, Mood DW, Newth G, et al. Longitudinal analysis of a model to predict quality of life in prostate cancer patients and their spouses. Ann Behav Med. 2008;36(2):117–28.
117. Vegni E, Visioli S, Moja EA. When talking to the patient is difficult: the physician's perspective. Commun Med. 2005;2(1):69–76.

# Index


**A**
Abdominal aortic aneurysm (AAA), 6
Abrams, P., 60
ADAM. *See* Androgen decline in aging male (ADAM)
Age-appropriate PHE. *See* Preventive health evaluation (PHE)
Albertsen, P.C., 141
Alexander, R.B., 30–32
Alfuzosin
  CPPS, 31
  LUTS, 58
Alpha-blockers
  CPPS, 29–33
  nonselective, LUTS
    doxazosin, 57–58
    prazosin, 56
    terazosin, 57–58
  selective (*see* Selective alpha blockers, LUTS)
5-Alpha reductase inhibitors (5ARIs), 59
American Cancer Society (ACS), 7–8
AMS Ambicor penile prosthesis®, 122, 123
AMS 700 CX inflatable penile prosthesis®, 122, 124
Anastomotic urethroplasty, 158
Anderson, R.U., 34
Androgen decline in aging male (ADAM)
  clinical presentation and diagnosis, 90–91
  epidemiology, 89–90
  TRT
    clinical benefits of, 93
    monitoring of patients, 92–93
    and prostate cancer, 93–94
    in USA, 91, 92
Angermeier, K.W., 163
Antibiotics, CPPS, 31, 33
Anti-inflammatories, CPPS, 31, 33
Antimuscarinics, 60
Antisperm antibodies, 174–175
5ARIs. *See* 5-Alpha reductase inhibitors (5ARIs)
Arousal/erection, 112
ART. *See* Assisted reproductive techniques (ART)
Arterial revascularization, 121
Artificial urinary sphincter (AUS)
  components, 135
  outcomes, 136–137
  surgical technique, 135–136
  surgical variations, 136
Aspirin, 5
Assisted reproductive techniques (ART), 177–178
Athanasopoulos, A., 62
AUS. *See* Artificial urinary sphincter (AUS)
Aversa, A., 19

**B**
Banthia, R., 202
Barrera, M., 196
Bates, S.M., 31
BCR. *See* Biochemical recurrence (BCR)
Beecher, H.K., 190
  Benign prostatic hyperplasia (BPH). *See also* Lower urinary tract symtoms (LUTS)
  AUA guidelines, 56, 57
  beta-sitosterol supplements, 77–79
  combination therapy, 61–63
  medications for, 56
  surgical treatment
    intraprostatic stents, 74
    laser therapy (*see* Laser therapy, BPH)
    open simple prostatectomy, 67–68
    TUIP, 73–74
    TUMT, 70–71
    TUNA, 69–70
    TURP, 68–69
Berglund, R.K, 163
Biochemical recurrence (BCR), 142, 143
Biopsychosocial relation diagram, 192
Bladder neck contracture (BNC), 132
Bladder outlet obstruction, 41
Blood pressure, 2
Botox, 133
Brachial artery FMD, 15, 17
Bruskewitz, R., 69, 70


D.A. Shoskes (ed.), *Urological Men's Health: A Guide for Urologists and Primary Care Physicians*, Current Clinical Urology, DOI 10.1007/978-1-61779-900-6,
© Springer Science+Business Media New York 2012

Buccal mucosal graft onlay urethroplasty
- complications, 160
- indication, 158–159
- postoperative care, 160
- surgical technique, 159–160

**C**

Campo, B., 69
Cancer of Prostate Risk Assessment (CAPRA), 143–144
Carotid artery stenosis (CAS), 8
Catheters, 43
Celecoxib, 31, 33
Cernilton, 32, 34
Chapple, C., 56
Cheah, P.Y., 30, 31
Chen, Y., 31
Cholesterol
- PHE, 2, 4
- reduction mechanisms, 77–79

Chronic pain
- description, 189, 191
- and social support
  - spouses, 197
  - stress-buffering model, 197
  - types, 196
  - UCCPS, 197–199
- VZV, 9

Chronic pelvic pain syndrome (CPPS)
- complementary medicine, 79–80
- monotherapies for
  - antibiotics, 33
  - anti-inflammatories, 33
  - α-blockers, 29–33
  - hormonal agents, 33
  - neuroleptic, 34
  - nonpharmacological therapy, 34
  - phytotherapy, 33–34
- multifactorial etiology of, 29, 30
- NIH classification of, 29, 30
- UPOINT, 34–36

Chronic prostatitis (CP). *See* Chronic pelvic pain syndrome (CPPS)
Chronic scrotal content pain
- algorithm for, 185
- diagnosis, 182–183
- epidemiology and etiology, 181–182
- pathophysiology, 181–182
- surgical management, 185–187
- treatment, 183–186

Chung, D.E., 63
Ciprofloxacin, 31, 32
Coloplast Titan inflatable penile prosthesis®, 122, 124
Colorectal cancer, 6
Complementary interventions
- bladder/kidney/prostate cancers, 80–81
- BPH/LUTS, 77–79
- chronic nonbacterial prostatitis, 79–80
- infertility, 81–82
- sexual dysfunction, 82–83
- stones and urinary tract infections, 83

Complicated urethroplasty
- long bulbar and panurethral strictures, 163–164
- PFUDDs, 164–165
- prostate cancer therapy, 166–167
- restenosis after urethral stent placement, 165–166
- urethral strictures after hypospadias repair, 162–163

Cooperberg, M.R., 164
Coronary heart disease (CHD) risk levels, 5
Couples and prostate cancer, 201–202
CPPS. *See* Chronic pelvic pain syndrome (CPPS)
Cutaway diagram, EndoPAT device sensor, 16

**D**

Dalpiaz, O., 164
D'Amico, A.V., 145
D'Amico classification, 143, 145
De Rose, A.F., 31
Descartes' biomedical pain model, 190
Detumescence, 14
Diabetes, 4
Digital plethysmography, vascular function, 15–18
Dmochowski, R., 63
Double graft technique, long bulbar urethral stricture, 163
Doxazosin
- CPPS, 31, 32
- LUTS, 57–58

Duloxetine, 132
Dutasteride, 60

**E**

EBRT. *See* External-beam radiotherapy (EBRT)
Eisenberg, M.L., 157, 165
Eisenberg, R.A., 157
Elist, J., 32
Elliot, S.P., 166
Endocrine causes, male infertility, 173–174
Endo-PAT 2000 machine, 17
Epididymectomy, 185
Epididymitis
- definition, 181
- diagnosis, 182–183
- epidemiology and etiology, 181–182
- pathophysiology, 181–182

Erectile dysfunction (ED)
- complementary interventions, 82–83
- consultation, 116–117
- CVD risk, 113
- design improvements, 126
- educational and psychosocial interventions, 113–114
- endothelial function
  - assessment of, 15–18
  - biomarkers, 18
  - and cardiovascular risk, 19–20
  - measurement of, 15

physiologic considerations, 13–14
practical considerations, 15
testing, 20
ultrasound-based measurement, FMD, 15
follow-up, 116
lifestyle and medication changes, 114
management, 110–111
next step after identification, 110
partner satisfaction, 126–127
patients and partners
sexual disorders, 109
sexual matter discussion, 108
PDEIs, 115–116
pharmacologic treatment, 114–115
primary care evaluation
arousal/erection, 112
initial, 111
inquiry and management, 106–107
medications, 112
orgasm/ejaculation, 112
sex counseling, 110
sexual health, 105–106
surgical treatment, 114–115
device coatings, 126
penile prosthesis implantation, 122
penile vascular surgery, 121–122
Esposito, K., 19
European Randomized Study of Screening or Prostate Cancer (ERSPC), 23–26
Evidence-based PHE. *See* Preventive health evaluation (PHE)
External-beam radiotherapy (EBRT), 148–149

**F**
Finasteride
BPH, 59–60
CPPS, 31, 32
FitzGerald, M.P., 32
Flouro-urodynamic image, overactive bladder, 132, 133
Flow-mediated dilatation (FMD), measurement of, 15
Follicle-stimuating hormone (FSH), 173

**G**
Gate control theory of pain, 190
Gelman, J., 166
Ginting, J.V., 198
Goldmeier, D., 31
Goldscheider, A., 190
Grade A and B recommendations, PHE, 7–8
Green light laser, 73
Gul, O., 31

**H**
Hanley, J.A., 24
Harvested and defatted buccal graft, 159
Holmium:YAG laser, 72–73
Hormonal agents, CPPS, 31, 33
Hourglass-deformity, 99
HPV vaccine. *See* Human papilloma virus (HPV) vaccine
Human immunodeficiency virus (HIV) screening, 6–7
Human papilloma virus (HPV) vaccine, 9
Hyperprolactinemia, 174
Hypogonadotropic hypogonadism (HH), 173–174

**I**
Ignarro, L.J., 13
Immunizations, recommended adult
HPV vaccine, 9
influenza vaccine, 9
pneumococcal vaccine, 10
Td and Tdap vaccines, 9
VZV vaccine, 9–10
Infertility
algorithm, for treatment, 172
ART, 177–178
complementary interventions, 81–82
definition, 169
medical treatment
antisperm antibodies, 174
endocrine causes, 173–174
retrograde ejaculation, 175
presentation, 169–170
surgical treatment
sperm delivery, 176–177
sperm production, 177
sperm retrieval, 175–176
workup
indications, 171
male infertility, causes of, 171–172
Inflatable penile prostheses, 122–124
Influenza vaccine, 9
Intensive counseling, obese adults, 4
Interstitial cystitis (IC), 79–80
Intracytoplasmic sperm injection (ICSI), 177, 178
Intraprostatic stents, 74
Intrauterine insemination (IUI), 177, 178
In-vitro fertilization (IVF), 177, 178
IUI. *See* Intrauterine insemination (IUI)

**J**
Jeong, C.W., 32
Jeong, Y.B., 61
Johanson urethroplasty
complications, 162
indication, 161
postoperative care, 162
surgical technique, 161

**K**
Kamischke, A., 175
Kaplan, S.A., 62

Kawabe, K., 58
Kershaw, T.S., 202
Kirby, R.S., 56
Klotz, L., 147

L
Lakey, B., 196, 198
Laser therapy, BPH
  green light laser, 73
  holmium:YAG laser, 72–73
  Nd:YAG laser, 72
Laumann, E., 111
La Vignera, S., 19
Lepor, H., 57, 58
Leskinen, M., 31
Leukocyte esterase, 40
Levofloxacin
  acute epididymitis, 184
  CPPS, 31, 32
LGX cylinders, 123, 125
Localized prostate cancer
  history, 142–143
  risk stratification
    CAPRA, 143–144
    nomograms, 144
    progression-free probability, 145
  transperineal permanent interstitial brachytherapy, 149
  treatment guidelines
    active surveillance, 147
    ADT, 146
    EBRT, 148–149
    NCCN, 145
    primary androgen deprivation therapy, 150
    radical prostatectomy, 148
Lower urinary tract symptoms (LUTS)
  alpha blockers, 56
  assessment of, 55–56
  beta-sitosterol supplements, 77–79
  bladder outlet obstruction
    evaluation, 42
    management, 42
    signs and symptoms, 41–42
  catheters, 43
  combination therapy, 61–63
  groups, 129
  nonselective alpha blockers
    doxazosin, 57–58
    prazosin, 56
    terazosin, 57–58
  phytotherapy, 56
  prevalence of, 129
  prophylaxis, 43–44
  selective alpha blockers
    alfuzosin, 58
    antimuscarinics, 60
    5ARIs, 59
    dutasteride, 60
    finasteride, 59–60
    naftopidil, 59
    PDE-5 inhibitors, 60–61
    silodosin, 58–59
    tamsulosin, 58
LUTS. *See* Lower urinary tract symptoms (LUTS)

M
Malleable/rod penile prostheses, 122, 123
Mangera, A., 163
Manne, S.L, 201
Marks, L.S., 58
Massachusetts Male Aging Study, 89
Mathur, R.K., 164
MDSC. *See* Microdenervation of spermatic cord (MDSC)
Meeks, J.J., 162
Mehik, A., 31
Mehrotra, A., 1
Melzack, R., 191
Meparticin, 31
Microdenervation of spermatic cord (MDSC), 186
Microsurgical (PESA) approach, 176
Millard, R.J., 69
Mulhall, J.P., 61

N
Naftopidil, 59
Narayan, P., 58
National Comprehensive Cancer Center Network (NCCN), 145
Nd:YAG laser, 72
Neurogenic hypothesis, 130
Neuromatrix pain model, 191
Nickel, J.C., 31
Nitrite positivity, 40
Nonpharmacological therapy, CPPS, 34
Nonselective alpha blockers, LUTS
  doxazosin, 57–58
  prazosin, 56
  terazosin, 57–58

O
OAB. *See* Overactive bladder (OAB)
Obesity, 4–5
Open simple prostatectomy, 67–68
Orandi, A., 73, 74
Orgasm/ejaculation, 112
Overactive bladder (OAB)
  behavioral therapies, 131
  definition, 129
  diagnosis and initial treatment
    behavioral therapies, 131
    medications, 131–132
  epidemiology, 129
  medications, 131–132
  pathophysiology, 130
  surgical treatment, 132–134

## P


Pain
  and biomedical model, 189–192
  description, 189
  gating, 190, 191
  urogenital
    description, 192–193
    psychology of, 193–196
Pain catastrophizing scale items, 194
Palminteri, E., 163
PCA3, 27
PCSM. *See* Prostate cancer-specific mortality (PCSM)
PDEIs. *See* Phosphodiesterase type 5 inhibitors (PDEIs)
Pelvic fracture urethral distraction defects (PFUDDs), 164–165
Penedo, F.J., 201
Penile incontinence clamp, 132
Penile prosthesis implantation
  description, 122
  informed consent for, 124–126
Penile vascular surgery, 121–122
Pentosan polysulfate, 31, 33
Perceived support, 196
Percutaneous (PESA) approach, 176
Perineal slings, 134–135
Pertussis. *See* Whooping cough
Peyronie's disease
  anatomy of, 97, 98
  diagnostic evaluation, 98–100
  goals of therapy, 100
  management algorithm, 102
  treatment, 100–102
PFUDDs. *See* Pelvic fracture urethral distraction defects (PFUDDs)
PHE. *See* Preventive health evaluation (PHE)
Phosphodiesterase type 5 (PDE-5) inhibitors
  erectile dysfunction, 115–116
  LUTS, 60–61
Phytotherapy
  CPPS, 32–34
  LUTS, 56
Pneumococcal vaccine, 10
Pollen extract, 32–34
Pontari, M.A., 32
Porst, H., 61
Post hoc analysis, PLCO trial, 24
Post-vasectomy pain syndrome, 181–182
Post-void dribbling, 131
Prazosin, 56
Prednisolone, 31, 33
Pregabalin, 32, 34
Preventive health evaluation (PHE)
  abdominal aortic aneurysm, 6
  aspirin, to prevent CVD, 5
  blood pressure, 2
  cholesterol, 2, 4
  colorectal cancer, 6
  diabetes, 4
  grade A, B and D recommendations, 7–8
  human immunodeficiency virus screening, 6–7
  immunizations
    HPV vaccine, 9
    influenza vaccine, 9
    pneumococcal vaccine, 10
    Td and Tdap vaccines, 9
    varicella zoster virus vaccine, 9–10
  obesity and health diet counseling, 4–5
  purpose of, 1
  USPSTF A and B recommendations, 2, 3
Primary androgen deprivation therapy (ADT), 150
Prophylaxis, 43–44
Prostate cancer. *See* Localized prostate cancer
Prostate cancer prevention trial (PCPT), 24–26
Prostate cancer-specific mortality (PCSM), 141–143
Prostate specific antigen (PSA) screening
  controversies
    overdiagnosis, of harmless cancers, 25
    prostate biopsy, 24
    randomized controlled trials, 23–24
  opportunities
    biomarkers, 27
    diagnostic accuracy, 26
    risk calculator, 25–26
    testing, 26–27
Prostatitis
  classification
    management, 49
    signs and symptoms, 47–48
    workup, 48–49
  description, 47
Psychosocial factors, in urogenital conditions, 189. *See also* Pain; Social support
Pyuria, 40


## Q


Quercetin, 32–36


## R


Radical prostatectomy, 148
Ramon, J., 69
Reactive hyperemia PAT (RH-PAT), 15–17, 19–20
Received support, 196
Referred pain, 181
Retrograde ejaculation, 175
Retropubic approach, 67
Rodriguez Jr, E., 166
Roehrborn, C.G., 58, 62, 69
Rofecoxib, 31, 33
Rosario, D.J., 69


## S


Sacral neuromodulation (SNM), 133, 134
Sairam, K., 61
Santucci, R.A., 157
Saw palmetto, 56, 79
Scandinavian prostate cancer, 142
Schellhammer, P.F., 186

Schulman, C.C., 69
Sclerosing lymphangitis, 99
Selective alpha blockers, LUTS
  alfuzosin, 58
  antimuscarinics, 60
  5ARIs, 59
  dutasteride, 60
  finasteride, 59–60
  naftopidil, 59
  PDE-5 inhibitors, 60–61
  silodosin, 58–59
  tamsulosin, 58
Sex hormone binding globulin (SHBG), 90
Sexually transmitted infections (STIs), 7
Sharlip, I.D., 121
Sharma, A., 164
Sharpley, C.F., 201
Shenfeld, O.Z., 164
Shores, M.M., 90
Shoskes, D.A., 32
Silodosin, 58–59
Sinclair, A.M., 184
Sleep, D.J., 69
SNM. *See* Sacral neuromodulation (SNM)
Social integration, 196
Social support
  and chronic pain
    spouses and social support, 197
    stress-buffering model, 197
    types, social support, 196
    UCCPS social support, 197–199
  and prostate cancer, 199–201
Steele, G.S., 69
Steenkamp, J.W., 156
Stief, C.G., 62
Stoner, E., 59
Stress-buffering model, social support, 197
Stress UI
  medications, 132
  surgical treatment, 134
Suprapubic prostatectomy, 67

**T**
Tamsulosin
  CPPS, 31, 32
  LUTS, 58
Td and Tdap vaccine, 9
Terazosin
  CPPS, 31
  LUTS, 57–58
Testosterone replacement therapy (TRT)
  clinical benefits of, 93
  monitoring of patients, 92–93
  and prostate cancer, 93–94
  in USA, 91, 92
Tetracycline hydrochloride, 31
Tewari, A., 58
Three-piece inflatable prostheses, with girth- and length-expanding cylinders, 123–124
Transperineal permanent interstitial brachytherapy, 149
Transurethral bulking agents, 134
Transurethral incision of prostate (TUIP), 73–74
Transurethral microwave therapy (TUMT), 70–71
Transurethral needle ablation (TUNA), 69–70
Transurethral resection of prostate (TURP), 68–69
Transvesical prostatectomy, 67
Tripp, D.A., 195
TRT. *See* Testosterone replacement therapy (TRT)
Tugcu, V., 30–32
TUIP. *See* Transurethral incision of prostate (TUIP)
TUMT. *See* Transurethral microwave therapy (TUMT)
TUNA. *See* Transurethral needle ablation (TUNA)
Tuncel, A., 63
TURP. *See* Transurethral resection of prostate (TURP)

**U**
UCCPS spousal support, 197–199
UI. *See* Urinary incontinence (UI)
Ultrex cylinders, 123, 125
UPOINT
  description, 34
  diagnostic criteria, 36
  domains and associated therapies, 34, 35
Upper urinary tract
  anatomic abnormalities, 46
  foreign objects, 46–47
  imaging, 45
  management, 45–46
  signs and symptoms, 44
Ureterovesical reflux, 46
Urethral strictures
  after hypospadias repair, 162–163
  anastomotic urethroplasty, 158
  anatomy, 155
  buccal mucosal graft onlay urethroplasty
    complications, 160
    indication, 158–159
    postoperative care, 160
    surgical technique, 159–160
  diagnosis and evaluation, 156
  etiology, 155–156
  johanson urethroplasty
    complications, 162
    indication, 161
    postoperative care, 162
    surgical technique, 161
  long bulbar and panurethral strictures, 163–164
  open reconstruction, 157
  PFUDDs, 164–165
  prostate cancer therapy, 166–167
  restenosis, 165–166
  treatment, 156
  urethral dilation and internal urethrotomy, 156–157
  urethral stents, 157
Urethritis, 49–50
Urethroplasty
  anastomotic, 158
  buccal mucosal graft onlay, 160

complications, 160
indication, 158–159
surgical technique, 159–160
johanson (*see* Johanson urethroplasty)
Urinary incontinence (UI)
adjunctive measures, 132
behavioral therapies, 131
diagnosis and initial treatment
adjunctive measures, 132
behavioral therapies, 131
medications, 131–132
epidemiology, 129–130
medications, 132
pathophysiology, 130
surgical treatment
AUS (*see* Artificial urinary sphincter (AUS))
patient selection, 137
perineal slings, 134–135
transurethral bulking agents, 134
Urinary stasis, 41–43
Urinary tract infections (UTIs)
antibiotic therapy, 41
complementary interventions, 83
definition, 40
diagnosis of, 40
lower (*see* Lower urinary tract)
prevalence, 39
symptoms, 40
upper (*see* Upper urinary tract)
urinalysis, elements of, 40
Urodynamic testing, 132, 133
Urologic chronic pelvic pain syndromes (UCPPS), 192
Urolume stent, 166
Urotheliogenic mechanism, 130
US penile prostheses, 122, 123

**V**
Varicella zoster virus (VZV) vaccine, 9–10
Varicocele grading system, 177
Veno-occlusive ED, surgery for, 121–122
Ventral urethrotomy and ventral buccal graft placement, 160
Vickers, A.J., 26

**W**
Wagenlehner, F.M., 32
Wang, P., 164
Welch, H.G., 141
Whooping cough, 9

**X**
Xu, Y.M., 164

**Y**
Yamanishi, T., 58
Ye, Z.Q., 32

**Z**
Zafirlukast, 31, 33
Zhao, T., 31
Zhou, Z., 31

Made in the USA
Las Vegas, NV
26 June 2026

49922320R00129